Hand
Ambu

Handbook of Ambulatory Cardiology

Victor F. Froelicher, M.D.
Professor of Medicine, Division of Cardiovascular
Medicine, Stanford University School of Medicine,
Stanford; Director, ECG and Exercise Laboratory, Veterans
Affairs Palo Alto Health Care System, Palo Alto, California

Susan Quaglietti, R.N.P., M.S.
Assistant Clinical Professor, School of Nursing, University
of California, San Francisco; Adult Nurse Practitioner,
Cardiology Division, Veterans Affairs Palo Alto Health
Care System, Palo Alto, California

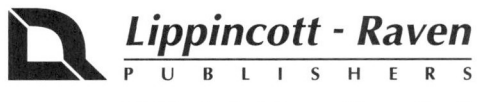

Lippincott - Raven
P U B L I S H E R S

Philadelphia • New York

Acquisitions Editor: Ruth Weinberg
Developmental Editor: Renee Gagliardi
Manufacturing Manager: Dennis Teston
Production Manager: Maxine Langweil
Cover Designer: Jeane Norton
Indexer: Alexandra Nickerson
Compositor: Focus Graphics
Printer: R. R. Donnelley and Sons

Printed in the United States of America

9 8 7 6 5 4 3 2 1

Library of Congress Cataloging-in-Publication Data

Froelicher, Victor F.
    Handbook of ambulatory cardiology / Victor F. Froelicher, Susan Quaglietti.
      p. cm.
    Includes bibliographical references and index.
    ISBN 0-316-29447-0
    1. Heart—Diseases—Handbooks, manuals, etc. 2. Ambulatory medical
care—Handbooks, manuals, etc. I. Quaglietti, Susan. II. Title.
    [DNLM: 1. Cardiovascular Diseases—diagnosis—handbooks.
2. Cardiovascular System—physiopathology—handbooks. 3. Ambulatory
Care—handbooks.   WG 39 F926ha 1997]
    RC681.F84   1997
    616.1—DC21
    DNLM/DLC
    for Library of Congress   96-39468
                                                    CIP

To Susie . . . thanks for your patience,
carefulness, the charts, and
the ADVIsE.

V.F.F.

I dedicate this book
to the one I love . . .
with whom I discuss
all matters of the heart.

S.Q.

Contents

Preface

One of the goals of this handbook is to address and help the practitioner meet the needs of the current trends in health care. These trends include the following:

1. *A shift to ambulatory care from hospital care.* Disease-related groupings (DRGs) have resulted in shortened hospital stays (for instance, the length of hospitalization for an uncomplicated myocardial infarction has dropped from 2 weeks to 3 days), outpatient surgery has replaced in-hospital surgery for many procedures, hospices are often chosen for terminal care, and advanced directives let patients choose less-intensive care at the end of their lives. *This handbook is designed for the practitioner delivering ambulatory care.*

2. *A transition to capitation from fee-for-service, to contain costs.* The system of medical services reimbursement according to fee-for-service was like letting the hangman or housewrecker be paid per unit [1]. Another approach to controlling medical costs, yet maintaining fee-for-service, involves resource value units (RVUs) developed so that there would be equal pay for cognitive services and technical procedures. *This handbook takes a cost-effective approach to patient evaluation and treatment.*

3. *More generalists and less subspecialists, to contain costs.* In a study conducted by the American College of Physicians, subspecialists were found to be the most expensive clinicians, often introducing expensive technology before adequate evaluation. The study also discovered that the number of procedures performed in a population was not related to the prevalence of disease but to the number of specialists [2]. The response has been to curtail the number of subspecialists. *This handbook is designed for the nonspecialist.*

Thus, for better or worse, health care is being redirected both from subspecialists to generalists and from inpatient care to outpatient care. Subspecialization has led to technological advances that require a high level of training in order to initiate and maintain them. Medications and devices that have been developed, while sometimes lifesaving or life enhancing, can have uncomfortable and even dangerous side effects. The thought of applying and following these therapies can appear to be an impossible task for practitioners without specialized knowledge. The problem is intensified in the outpatient setting, where consultation and technical support are not as available as in the hospital setting.

Our aim with this book is to provide a simplified approach to the ambulatory patient presenting in the clinic with cardiac complaints. The approach, using the acronym ADVIsE, has been empirically developed and tested in our practice and has been applied in an expert system and database. It can empower the general practitioner with a paradigm for dealing with the complexities of cardiovascular pathophysiology. Using the ADVIsE spreadsheet box-by-box approach simplifies patient management, helping the clinician decide which tests are needed, what the results mean, which therapies may be administered, and when referral to a cardiologist is necessary.

This book concentrates on *common conditions* rather than rare diseases or unusual presentations of common diseases. The basic methods of patient evaluation are stressed. This book primarily applies to patients with *stable disease.* Treatment for acute presentations of cardiac disease are left for emergency-oriented textbooks. Hopefully, this handbook will help the clinician decide when patients should be referred to the hospital for possible admission.

The wide range of potential pharmacologic therapies for cardiac disease are extensively discussed in this book because they are better accessed using a local, current formulary. However, ***must-use*** medications that are known to improve outcome are highlighted; there is even a special section in Appendix B dedicated to these ***must-use medications.***

Another goal is to present a book that can be read cover to cover like the two editions of Arthur Seltzer's *Cardiology*. There are a number of excellent cardiology reference texts, but nothing like Arthur's books is currently available. In fact, we hope that the reader at least quickly reads the first three chapters and then references the fourth and fifth chapters and the appendixes when confronted with specific problems, tests, and symptoms. When reading the book, please keep in mind that the repetition is intentional—consider it like a travel guide that repeats areas of interest when focusing on various cross-referenced points such as shopping, museums, or dining. The concepts in the first three chapters have been "field tested" as part of our training program for the past 10 years. We use the ADVIsE approach spreadsheet on every patient we see!

Health care is going back to the basics of medicine (the history and physical examination plus the standard ECG and treadmill test are used for "gatekeeping") and that is the direction of this handbook. The first chapter introduces the ADVIsE approach used throughout the handbook. Following the stepwise approach, Chapter 2 covers the medical history and physical examination, Chapter 3 outlines the ECG and the chest x-ray, and Chapter 4 covers other specialized tests. Chapter 5 presents the diagnosis and management of specific disorders grouped under the five key features. The appendixes include extensive charts on differential diagnoses of basic symptom presentations associated with the key features.

REFERENCES

1. Shaw GB. *The Doctor's Dilemma.* London: Penguin, 1946.
2. American College of Physicians. The role of the future general internist defined. *Ann Intern Med* 1994;121: 616–622.

Acknowledgments

There are a lot of people to thank and give credit. Bob Eastlack worked with us while he was a Stanford undergraduate student. Bob developed many of the graphics using Corel Draw and helped gather the ECGs from our Marquette ECG Management System. Bob is now in medical school at San Antonio, Texas. Dat Do has been our technical right hand for several years and does anything we need requiring computer wizardry, from scanning to graphics. He worked on the parallel expert system that uses the ADVIsE rules, and drew the logo. Dat is our most recent "graduate" to medical school. Julie Johnson did the first editing and organization of the figures and tables for the book. Karen and Christine finalized the charts. Frank Yanowitz provided the most constructive criticisms. Eddie Atwood continues to inspire us as the consummate clinician and teacher. Jon Myers approved the exercise portions of the book. John Giacommini does the administration so we have time to write. Anthony Umann has networked us, scanned some of the artwork, and put us on the Worldwide Web—he is the first person we call when we have problems downloading a reference from The National Library of Medicine.

The book would not be if it were not for Nancy Megley, who put us under contract. Thanks also to Jo-Ann Strangis, who has visited us in person and given us suggestions and guidance. The patience and competence of Richard Wilcox and Kevin Sullivan have made the final steps of the book easy.

Thanks must also go to our patients and students.

Please let us know about any shortcomings of the book, particularly those that can be improved in a second edition. Comments that help us generate the energy to do a second edition will also be appreciated, through conventional mail, via the internet (vicmd@aol.com), or on our web page (www.cardiology.org). We hope this book helps you be successful in this era of difficult transitions.

The ADVIsE Approach to Ambulatory Care Cardiology

The ADVIsE approach to cardiology requires that the clinician consider whether a patient has any of the five key *prognostic features of heart disease* shown in Figure 1-1 rather than focus on the major syndromes of heart disease. The grouping of the key features is empirical, having evolved from clinical experience in ambulatory care cardiology and from clinical research. Traditionally, the approach to the work-up of the cardiac patient was targeted to explaining the symptoms by searching for associations with specific disease processes. Unfortunately, the end result with this approach was that cardiac patients were often directed to cardiac tests and prescribed cardiac medications, rather than to the tests and the medications specific for their condition. The ADVIsE approach incorporates symptoms and syndromes; however, it emphasizes common presentations, the basics of evaluation, and prognostic stratification. ADVIsE deemphasizes rare presentations and provides a systematic approach to rule out "confounders," diagnoses that have similar presentations but are not due to the key features. ADVIsE was developed to provide the general practitioner with a new paradigm for managing outpatients. This handbook indicates specific situations when referral to a subspecialist is indicated. Emphasis is on the basic methods of evaluation for stable patients and discussions of acute treatments are left to textbooks dealing with emergency and acute care.

ADVIsE is an acronym for the five key features represented by an *A* for arrhythmias (and conduction abnormalities), *D* for myocardial dysfunction or damage, *V* for valvular dysfunction, *Is* for ischemia, and *E* for exercise capacity or intolerance. Exercise capacity is included because of its powerful and independent association with prognosis.

As discussed later, these key features are the appropriate focal points because they help the practitioner:

1. Explain symptoms.
2. Make the diagnosis.
3. Determine which tests are needed.

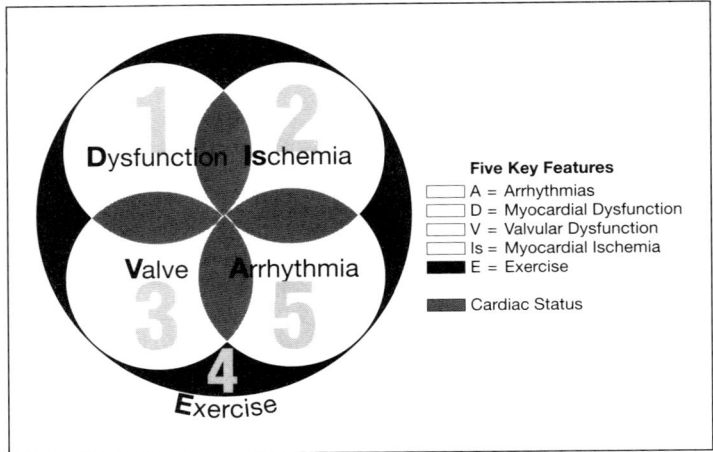

Five Key Features

☐ A = Arrhythmias
☐ D = Myocardial Dysfunction
☐ V = Valvular Dysfunction
☐ Is = Myocardial Ischemia
■ E = Exercise

▨ Cardiac Status

Fig. 1-1.   Flow diagram illustrating how a patient enters the ADVIsE approach to evaluating cardiac condition.

4. Direct therapy and indicate the need for interventions.
5. Independently predict prognosis.

KEY FEATURE ORDER
While the ADVIsE acronym helps one to remember the five features, the order of the importance of the features differs from their appearance in the acronym. By order of *prevalence* in the outpatient setting and *prognostic impact,* myocardial dysfunction is first, myocardial ischemia second, valvular dysfunction third, exercise capacity fourth, and arrhythmias last. This order by importance is followed throughout the book.

1. Myocardial dysfunction
2. Myocardial ischemia
3. Valvular dysfunction
4. Exercise capacity
5. Arrhythmias

Considering the five key features in the ADVIsE approach provides a *logic* that will continue to apply as advances in knowledge occur. Consider how the concepts of coronary thrombosis, the exercise programs for patients who have had a myocardial infarction (MI), and the hemodynamic versus neurohumoral basis for congestive heart failure (CHF) have changed over time and how the indications for nitroglycerin (NTG) have expanded from angina to MI and CHF. Understanding the *pathophysiology* of the five key features of heart disease facilitates adjustment to such changes in clinical practice.

THE PATHOPHYSIOLOGIC BASIS OF THE KEY FEATURES

The following explains the basis of the ADVIsE key features:

1. Myocardial *D*ysfunction or damage incorporates the pathophysiologic etiologies of the most common causes of heart muscle disease. The main determinant of prognosis is the amount of myocardium damaged or lost by the disease process, while symptoms are mainly dependent on the amount of myocardial dysfunction present.
2. Myocardial *I*schemia is the pathophysiologic basis of coronary artery disease.
3. *V*alvular dysfunction is mainly either insufficiency (causing regurgitation) or stenosis (causing obstruction). The main lesions of concern are aortic stenosis (which causes myocardial damage and ischemia) and mitral insufficiency (which can lead to myocardial damage).
4. *E*xercise capacity is the amount of exercise that can be performed. Poor exercise capacity, or exercise intolerance, is associated with symptoms of dyspnea and fatigue with exercise that can be due to inactivity (deconditioning) and many disease processes. It is included as a key feature because of its independent and consistent impact on prognosis.
5. *A*rrhythmias and conduction disturbances are associated with multiple mechanisms, symptoms, and syndromes. The mechanisms include atrial and ventricular origins, bradycardia, tachycardia, and heart block. The symptoms include palpitations, syncope, dyspnea, and fatigue. The syndromes include paroxysmal supraventricular tachycardia (PSVT), atrial fibrillation, complete heart block, and sudden death.

THE IMPORTANCE OF THE KEY EMPIRICAL FEATURES

Expanding on the importance of the five key empirical prognostic groupings or characteristics, they are the basis for the following:

1. Explaining symptoms: Shortness of breath and chest pain have many causes, but the mechanism should be

sought. Are they due to myocardial dysfunction or ischemia?

2. Making the diagnosis: For instance, a middle-aged man with exertional substernal chest pain has a 90% probability of having coronary artery disease.

3. Deciding which tests are needed: As an example, screening asymptomatic individuals with an exercise test is inappropriate because of the false-positive rate, whereas other patients are appropriately tested.

   Which tests are appropriate for ischemia? (stress tests or coronary angiography)

   Which tests are appropriate for damage? (echocardiography, nuclear multigated acquisition [MUGA] for left ventricular [LV] function, LV angiography)

   Which tests are appropriate for valvular dysfunction? (echocardiography, cardiac catheterization)

   Which tests are appropriate for arrhythmias? (ECG, Holter monitoring)

   Which tests are appropriate for exercise intolerance? (treadmill or ergometer test)

4. Directing therapy and indicating the need for interventions: Ischemic chest pain should be treated to alleviate pain, but many patients are treated for noncardiac pain with antianginal medications. If the symptoms associated with the key features cannot be tolerated or treated medically, the physician and patient must consider surgery or other interventions.

5. Determining prognosis independently: These features, except for arrhythmias, have independent predictive power for determining risk of cardiac death. The prognostic capabilities of the features are critical to estimating the major outcomes of disease for a patient.

PROGNOSIS AND THE KEY FEATURES

The prognoses for different types of conditions associated with the key features are listed in Table 1-1. Prognostic indicators within each grouping determine outcomes including angina, MI, and death. The identified variables in each feature help direct risk stratification. The key features use presenting symptoms (the usual presenting symptoms being chest pain, dyspnea, syncope, and fatigue) and test results to initiate stratification as well as prognostic scores when applicable. Myocardial dysfunction is associated with a high mortality (10–20% annual) and prognosis is objectively determined by ejection

Table 1-1.   The Etiologies and Prognoses for Different Types of Conditions Associated With the Five Key Features of Heart Disease

Key Features	Type	Etiology	Prognosis
Myocardial dysfunction	Systolic (dilated cardiomyopathy)	Viral, alcohol, MI, HBP (damage from)	10 to 25% annual mortality
	Diastolic (hypertrophic)	HBP, congenital, IHSS (due to stiffness of LV)	Depends on cause; lower mortality than dilated cardiomyopathy
Myocardial ischemia	Angina	Atherosclerosis, aortic stenosis	2 to 4% annual mortality
	Post MI	Atherosclerosis, thrombus	2 to 30% mortality in the first year
	Variant angina	Spasm	Uncertain mortality; low prevalence
Valvular disorders	Original	Rheumatic, congenital, degenerative	Poor when valvular or myocardial dysfunction occurs
	Prosthetic	Tissue or mechanical	Depends on type
Exercise intolerance	Cardiac cause	Peripheral changes, decreased cardiac output	Prognostic equation scores include METs
	Noncardiac cause	Pulmonary, anemia, etc.	Underlying disease determines the prognosis
Arrhythmias	Atrial fibrillation	"Lone" or cardiac/metabolic	Expected mortality doubles; 5% annual risk for cerebrovascular accident
	Complete heart block	Degenerative, ischemic	If syncope occurs, mortality increases
	Ventricular tachycardia	Ischemic, re-entry	Depends on associated conditions

MI = myocardial infarction; HBP = high blood pressure; IHSS = idiopathic hypertrophic subaortic stenosis; LV = left ventricle.

fraction (EF) and exercise capacity. Variables indicating severity of dysfunction would be presence of symptoms such as dyspnea on exertion and fatigue, exercise capacity measured in multiples of basal ventilatory oxygen consumption (METs), and inability of systolic BP to rise with exercise. Prognostic scores for patients with myocardial ischemia include variables such as systolic BP during exercise, angina, ST-segment changes, and MET level, to help estimate severity of coronary artery disease. Exercise capacity is closely associated with prognosis, particularly in patients with myocardial dysfunction, myocardial ischemia, and valvular disease. Exercise intolerance, whether due to cardiac disease such as ischemia or dysfunction or illnesses such as lung disease or cancer, is associated with a poor prognosis. The diagnosis of valvular disease is also associated with a high mortality secondary to progressive LV damage. Surgery can greatly alter this prognosis, but the timing recommendations for valve replacement or repair require follow-up by a subspecialist. In general, whenever a patient with valvular disease has a change in symptoms suggesting progression of disease, he or she should be referred to a subspecialist. The prognostic indicators associated with arrhythmias are less clear, in part due to the difficulty of documenting the event and their poor reproducibility. However, in general, the prognosis in patients with arrhythmias is determined by the underlying cardiac disease, with myocardial damage being the most important predictor.

APPLYING THE KEY EMPIRICAL FEATURES
Evaluation of each patient should begin with the history and physical examination for the five empirical features and for the degree of severity of the features. As shown in Figure 1-2, the patient's entry into the ADVIsE approach is usually via the patient's chief complaint. Previous test results are also used to determine which of the key features are present, because the patient's chief complaint may be a new problem or an exacerbation of a previously stable complaint. The chief complaints associated with cardiac disease are chest pain, dyspnea, syncope, and fatigue so we address them relative to the key features.

The ADVIsE approach using the five key features is a logical and efficient way to evaluate all patients who present with cardiac symptoms and signs. The five key empirical prognostic groupings of heart disease, representing the basic pathophysiologic mechanisms of the symptoms

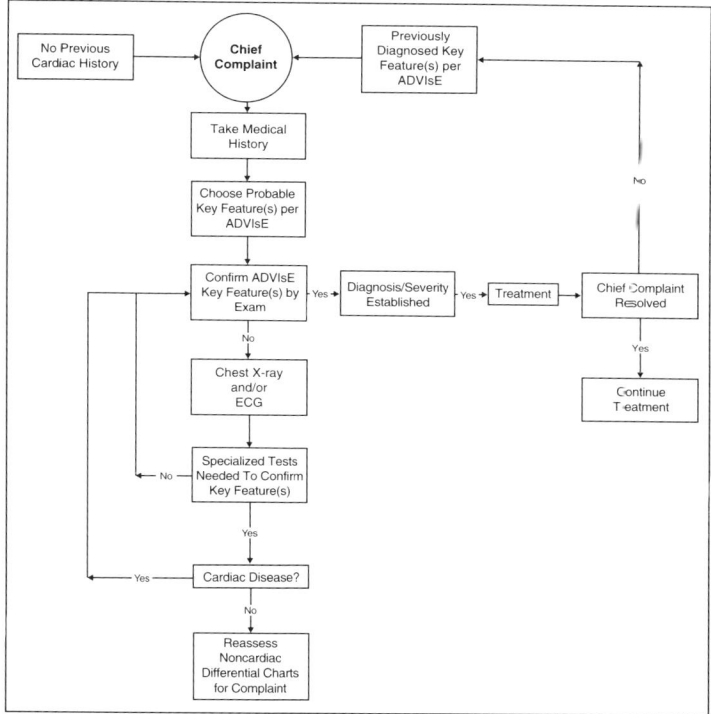

Fig. 1-2.   The ADVIsE approach diagram. CV = cardiovascular.

and signs that are treated, provide an organizational structure (see Fig. 1-1). This structure directs the practitioner in a most logical fashion to the most cost-effective way to "work up" the patient with possible heart disease.

THE ADVIsE SPREADSHEET
The ADVIsE approach is facilitated by considering the ADVIsE spreadsheet for every patient, entering the available data, looking for inconsistencies, considering confounders, obtaining missing information, and ordering the appropriate tests. Table 1-2 illustrates the ADVIsE spreadsheet evaluation of historical information and of results obtained from ECGs, echocardiograms, nuclear medicine studies, Holter monitoring, exercise and nonexercise stress testing, and angiograms. At first it is easiest to actually fill out the spreadsheet on paper, but later this can be done mentally. Do not be confused by the interaction between the key features: Myocardial ischemia or a

Table 1-2.   Key Features and Evaluation Methods for the ADVIsE Approach

Key Features	History and Physical Examination	ECG and Chest X-Ray Films	Echo-cardio-gram	Nuclear Medicine Tests	Ambulatory ECG Monitoring	Stress Tests (Exercise and Nonexercise)	Cardiac Catheterization/ Angiography
1: Myocardial damage							
2: Myocardial ischemia							
3: Valvular status							
4: Exercise capacity							
5: Arrhythmias							

dysfunctioning valve can cause myocardial damage, and exercise intolerance and arrhythmias are multifactorial and due to many conditions. When these overlaps occur, one should focus on the more common occurrences and the primary key feature.

As the spreadsheet indicates, the ADVIsE approach begins with the medical history and physical examination. From the history and physical examination the practitioner can establish the pretest probability for the abnormality causing the feature to be present and determine what further tests are indicated. The basic tests are the ECG and chest x-ray study, and most patients being evaluated for a cardiac problem need these two tests. Beyond the basics, the usual tests include echocardiography (for valve status and LV function), stress tests (for ischemia and exercise capacity), nuclear medicine tests, and Holter monitoring (for arrhythmias and syncope). There has been concern that referral for these tests by cardiologists who are reimbursed for performing these tests leads to excessive utilization. The key feature approach considering the history and physical examination prioritizes additional tests as to their indication for each of the key features. Specialized tests other than cardiac catheterization include cardiac tomography, positron emission tomography, and magnetic resonance imaging. In general, these are only needed for unusual conditions and their performance characteristics have yet to be demonstrated.

Not all the tests need to be performed on every patient, so all of the ADVIsE spreadsheet boxes *do not* need to be filled with data to evaluate a patient! Many studies have proved the importance of the history and physical examination. For instance, the major symptom and syndrome of ischemia, angina pectoris, is associated with a 90% probability for obstructive coronary artery disease in a middle-aged man; the other major syndrome, CHF (with the symptoms of shortness of breath on exertion and fluid retention), is associated with a 25% annual mortality. Remember that all of the testing procedures, even imaging techniques, have limitations for diagnosis (sensitivity and specificity) and prognostication. The tests are not definitive and clinical judgment is required to interpret and apply the results.

STUDIES ESTABLISHING THE PERFORMANCE CHARACTERISTICS OF TESTS

Clinical studies have been performed to demonstrate how well a test separates those with disease from those without a disease. In order to accept findings of these studies, they must not break Guyatt's rules [1] for believing an evaluation of a diagnostic test:

1. Identification of comparison groups, with one group free of disease
2. Consecutive or randomly selected patients for whom the diagnosis is in doubt (this rule avoids the major evaluation errors of work-up bias and limited challenge)
3. Separate analysis of patients likely to have the disease (e.g., post-MI patients are likely to have coronary disease)
4. Blind comparison of the test with a reliable standard (such as coronary or LV angiography)

If these believability criteria are met, and the study fulfilling these criteria proves the test can differentiate disease from nondisease, the test can be put into practice. Although most tests have not been evaluated by studies that fulfill these criteria, many of the tests are in clinical use. The physician should be skeptical of new procedures and wait for validation by studies that have fulfilled these criteria! Following the ADVIsE approach will help one to decide which tests are needed; the various tests are ranked as to their value in Chapter 4. However, test performance varies according to location and to the technical capabilities of the laboratory performing the test. Clinicians may choose one test over another based on their experience or quality assurance data from the laboratory available in their area.

THE SPREADSHEET—BOX BY BOX
As shown in Figure 1-1, the patient enters the ADVIsE approach with his or her chief complaints and test results from previous evaluations. The complaints could be new, exacerbated, recurrent, or chronic. The first step is to take a detailed, structured history, review any available test results from previous evaluations and then perform a physical examination. The following sections provide an overview of the basis of the features and gives a spreadsheet box-by-box description of how each of the features of heart disease can be assessed by the history, physical examination, and the tests currently available for evaluating patients (see Table 1-2). Myocardial dysfunction is the first row and the approach involves stepping across each of the procedures used for evaluating it. The first spread-

sheet box explains how the cardiac history applies to the assessment of myocardial dysfunction.

Myocardial Dysfunction or Damage (Row 1)

Pathophysiology

Myocardial damage is the pathophysiologic basis of heart muscle disease, resulting in myocardial dysfunction. Myocardial dysfunction can be divided into systolic and diastolic dysfunction. Systolic function relates to the emptying characteristics of the LV, and diastolic function relates to its filling properties. Systolic dysfunction due to myocardial damage is most common and usually leads to LV dilation. The ventricle dilates to take advantage of the Frank-Starling relationship (i.e., increased contractility with stretching of the sarcomeres). Anything that causes ventricular damage or scarring (e.g., muscle loss) leads to systolic dysfunction.

Approximately 80% of patients with CHF have systolic dysfunction, while the remainder have diastolic dysfunction. In patients with the latter, systolic function and EF can be normal but filling pressure is elevated due to a stiff, noncompliant ventricle. Usually, diastolic dysfunction is secondary to hypertension, pathologic hypertrophy, infiltrative diseases of the myocardium, and at times, ischemia. All patients with systolic dysfunction have diastolic dysfunction and when systolic dysfunction is compensated, diastolic dysfunction remains. Currently, the treatment for acute CHF in both conditions is the same. This is fortunate because they can be difficult to distinguish clinically. For chronic CHF, digoxin should be avoided in the setting of isolated diastolic dysfunction, and contrary to what was first thought, calcium antagonists are not specific treatment for diastolic dysfunction.

Definition of Congestive Heart Failure

CHF can be defined as a syndrome consisting of signs and symptoms of intravascular and interstitial volume overload, including shortness of breath, rales, and edema; and manifestations of inadequate tissue perfusion, such as fatigue and poor exercise tolerance.

Key Points

1. CHF is the major manifestation of LV damage. It is associated with systolic dysfunction and dilated cardiomyopathy. Patients with systolic dysfunction always have diastolic dysfunction and the latter often

remains after the systolic component is compensated. Left-sided failure can lead to right-sided failure.

2. Diastolic dysfunction can exist independently and cause CHF due to a stiff, hypertrophied (but normal-size) ventricle caused by chronically high BP or congenital abnormalities.

3. Abnormalities in the periphery (anemia, beriberi heart disease, arteriovenous fistulas, thyrotoxicosis) can cause CHF associated with a high cardiac output.

4. Pneumonia, chronic obstructive pulmonary disease (COPD), restrictive heart disease, and cardiac tamponade are confounders often mistaken for CHF due to systolic dysfunction.

Symptoms and Physical Examination
for Myocardial Damage
The symptoms and physical findings of the major syndrome due to myocardial damage (CHF) include the historical features (and symptoms) and physical findings of left-sided failure and right-sided failure.

LEFT-SIDED FAILURE. Patients report symptoms of fatigue, dyspnea on exertion, and paroxysmal nocturnal dyspnea. They usually have a history of MI, alcoholism, myocarditis, or hypertension. The following are precipitators for episodes of CHF in patients with systolic dysfunction: atrial fibrillation, excessive salt intake, illness, MI, and noncompliance.

Physical findings include an S_3 gallop, cardiomegaly, and rales.

RIGHT-SIDED FAILURE. Patients report weight gain and swelling. The most common cause of right-sided failure is left-sided failure.

Physical findings include edema, hepatomegaly, neck vein distention, and ascites (when tricuspid regurgitation results from dilation and increased pressure, hepatic and jugular vein pulsations are more obvious).

Evaluation Options
The options for evaluating myocardial dysfunction or damage include:

Physical examination (cardiac size, apical impulse, gallops)
Chest x-ray study and ECG
Echocardiography: Mitral regurgitation can be seen with Doppler echocardiography, while it is not seen using other noninvasive modalities. This factor makes echo-

cardiography the preferred modality for evaluation of myocardial function and mitral regurgitation.

Radionuclide ventriculography: This is based on radiation counts in an area, so no geometric assumptions are required.

LV angiography: The equations are based on a proloid ellipse; therefore, Simpson's rule is more appropriately used. Biplane views are more accurate. Regardless of any limitations, this remains the "gold standard."

Ejection Fraction

EF is the best and most practical index of myocardial function. This is the percentage of end-diastolic volume (EDV) expelled with each cardiac contraction and is calculated using the following equations:

SV (stroke volume) = EDV − ESV (end-systolic volume)

$$EF = \frac{SV}{EDV}$$

EF can be estimated using any of the above-mentioned techniques (normal, 55–70%). Although it can be affected by heart rate, afterload, and preload, EF is inversely related to the severity and complications of MI or valvular disease. In coronary artery disease, it has an independent impact on mortality. Even patients with left main coronary artery disease have a better prognosis if their EF is normal, and patients with single-vessel disease have a worse prognosis if their EF is low. Patients with EFs of 30 to 50% seem to benefit the most in terms of longevity from bypass surgery, while those with EFs less than 30% have a higher surgical mortality. EF can be misleading in patients with mitral regurgitation because of the unloading effect of the regurgitation. These patients may have a relatively good EF that actually worsens after valve surgery, or they may have a surprisingly difficult time coming off of cardiopulmonary bypass because of poor LV function. This is in contrast to patients with aortic stenosis, whose EF will often improve after valve surgery because the afterload is removed.

Prognosis and Congestive Heart Failure

CHF (when due to dilated cardiomyopathy) is associated with a 10 to 25% annual cardiac mortality; survival is improved by angiotensin-converting enzyme (ACE) inhibitors [2] and organized follow-up [3]; symptoms are treated by diuretics, digoxin. Analysis of 34 years of follow-up of Framingham Study data provided clinically relevant insights into the prevalence, incidence, secular trends, prognosis, and modifiable risk factors for the occurrence of heart failure in a general population sample [4]. Heart failure was found in about 1% of persons in their 50s and 10% of persons in their 80s. The annual incidence also increased with age, from about 0.2% in persons 45 to 54 years old to 4.0% in men 85 to 94 years old, with the incidence approximately doubling with each decade of age. Women had a lower incidence at all ages. Male predominance was due to coronary heart disease, which conferred a fourfold increased risk of heart failure. Once heart failure was present, one-third of men and women died within 2 years of the diagnosis. The 6-year mortality rate was 82% for men and 67% for women, which corresponded to a death rate fourfold to eightfold greater than that of the general population of the same age. Sudden death was common, accounting for 28% of the cardiovascular deaths in men with heart failure and for 14% in women with heart failure. Hypertension and coronary disease were the predominant causes for heart failure and accounted for more than 80% of all clinical events. Factors reflecting deteriorating cardiac function were associated with a substantial increase in risk of overt heart failure. These included low vital capacity, sinus tachycardia, and LV hypertrophy on the ECG.

Myocardial Ischemia (Row 2)
Myocardial ischemia is important to document because it forms the pathophysiologic basis of angina pectoris and indicates underlying coronary artery disease or coronary artery spasm. The manifestations of myocardial ischemia are angina pectoris and exercise-induced ST-segment depression, regional (wall motion abnormalities) and global myocardial dysfunction, and thallium-detected postexercise defects ("cold spots" that fill in later after exercise or are not present on resting scans). Not all of these features are always present in a given ischemic patient (i.e., silent ischemia). Unfortunately, they have surprisingly poor correlation with one another. Muscle in jeopardy by ischemia (i.e., myocardium to be lost if the ischemic area becomes infarcted) can be roughly estimated by the degree of test abnormalities.

Pathophysiology of Ischemic Syndromes
Ischemic syndromes involve an inadequate supply of and an increased demand for oxygen. Primary causes (due to coronary artery disease) are fixed atherosclerotic lesions or change in tone (spasm around fixed lesions), thrombosis,

and silent ischemia, a low-prevalence phenomenon with less risk than angina. Secondary causes are aortic stenosis, hypertrophy, and anemia. Confounders are esophageal reflux, costochondritis, pulmonary artery hypertension, aortic stenosis, pericarditis, aortic dissection, and variant angina (coronary spasm in normal vessels).

Symptoms and Physical Examination of Angina Pectoris
The major presentation of myocardial ischemia is typical angina pectoris, the characteristics of which include a dull pressure or squeezing sensation and usually a dull pain, never a sharp pain. The sensation is substernal and radiates down the left arm and to the neck. Angina pectoris is precipitated by exercise or anger in a consistent manner. It can occur during and up to 6 minutes after exercise and lasts for 2 to 15 minutes. Angina pectoris is relieved by rest and sublingual NTG.

Any prior cardiac or atherosclerotic event or procedure is a historical feature that makes ischemia more likely to be the explanation of chest pain. Confounders are multiple types of pain, stoicism or fear to identify a sensation as pain, concern over normal sharp pains, and referral of pain over old injuries.

The physical findings that can be associated with angina include tendon xanthoma, earlobe creases, arcus senilis, and peripheral arterial bruits, but these are rarely present in ischemic patients.

Symptoms and Physical Examination
of Myocardial Infarction
MI (due to prolonged ischemia that results in damage to the LV) is characterized by

- Prolonged anginal pain (longer than 15 minutes but less than several hours); constant pain lasting for hours is usually not ischemic, though infarction or unstable angina pain may be intermittent and last for days
- Increases in myocardial enzyme levels
- ECG changes

The physical findings can include gallops, rub, murmur, and a precordial bulge, but these are often neither present nor appreciated. Neck vein distention can be due to CHF or right ventricular infarction. They are differentiated by the presence or absence of rales, which suggests CHF or right ventricular infarct, respectively. Their identity is important because CHF is treated by diuresis while a right ventricular infarct is treated by increasing fluids.

Whereas a small or uncomplicated MI can be a marker for ischemia, a large or complicated MI is a marker for myocardial damage.

Evaluation Options
Exercise ECG with treadmill, the *first choice* for cost-effective evaluation of the patient with nonacute chest pain: If the clinical impression is that the treadmill result is false positive or false negative, then the next best test available should be performed. This could be coronary angiography but a nuclear perfusion test would be acceptable to diagnose ischemia.
Exercise add-ons: These include echocardiography and nuclear perfusion for increased sensitivity and localization, and are also indicated if ECG shows left bundle-branch block or Wolff-Parkinson-White syndrome.
Holter (ambulatory monitoring) ECG during everyday activities
Pharmacologic stressors (if the patient cannot exercise or gives an inadequate response or effort to an exercise test)
    Dipyridamole (Persantine) or adenosine with imaging using thallium or isonitriles (sesti-MIBI)
    Dobutamine or arbutamine echocardiography

Prognosis and the Ischemic Syndromes
MYOCARDIAL INFARCTION.   Ten percent of patients die prior to admission (this could be decreased by patient education and bystander CPR), 10% die in a hospital (aspirin, thrombolysis, and beta-blockers have decreased this by 25%), and 10% die in the first year after hospital discharge (beta-blockers given during this period lower mortality by 25%). An MI can be classified as complicated when shock, CHF, or ischemia occurs versus uncomplicated when these do not occur. Mortality is concentrated in those with complicated MIs and those resulting in an abnormally low EF.

ANGINA PECTORIS.   Stable angina pectoris has a 2% annual cardiac mortality and unstable angina pectoris has a 4% rate. Coronary artery bypass surgery (CABG) can decrease mortality only in high-risk subsets determined by clinical and angiographic patterns (left main coronary artery or three-vessel disease with EF < 50%). Prognosis can be determined easily using clinical scores for individual patients with angina.

Valvular Function (Row 3)
Valvular dysfunction manifests itself as insufficiency (causing regurgitation) or stenosis (causing obstruction).

Echocardiography is the first choice for cost-effective evaluation of the patient with possible valvular disease. The main lesions of concern are aortic stenosis (which causes myocardial damage and ischemia) and mitral insufficiency (which can cause damage). Mitral stenosis is very rare in developed countries and thus need not be considered here. Aortic insufficiency is well tolerated because it is associated with flow work rather than pressure work; therefore, the only concerns in ambulatory care are antibiotic prophylaxis to prevent subacute bacterial endocarditis (SBE) and sudden worsening of the valve's dysfunction. When caused by cystic medial necrosis and Marfan's syndrome, aortic insufficiency is more alarming because it can result in aortic root enlargement and dissection. Prognosis for the various lesions is discussed in the treatment section.

Exercise Capacity (Row 4)
Exercise intolerance is associated with symptoms of dyspnea and fatigue with exercise that can be due to inactivity as well as many other disease processes [5]. The exercise capacity of a patient has an independent effect on the prognosis of heart disease [6]. The amount of exercise that a patient can do is determined by both central cardiac, pulmonary, and peripheral features. Because of this, EF does not imply a certain exercise capacity; to identify exercise intolerance even in patients with a low EF, exercise capacity should be measured. The peripheral determinants of exercise capacity are independent of cardiac function and imply a good prognosis if they are operative, even in a patient with severe heart disease. Maximal ventilatory oxygen uptake (VO_2 max) is the greatest amount of oxygen that a person can extract from inspired air while performing dynamic exercise involving a large part of the total-body muscle mass. As VO_2 max is equal to the product of cardiac output and arterial-venous oxygen (a-VO_2) difference, it is a measure of the functional limits of the cardiovascular system. Maximal a-VO_2 difference is physiologically limited to roughly 15 to 17 vol%. Thus, maximal a-VO_2 difference behaves more or less as a constant, making maximal oxygen uptake an indirect estimate of maximal cardiac output. Myocardial oxygen demand is actually complicated to measure or estimate because of the various factors involved, but it can be estimated clinically by the product of heart rate and systolic BP (or double product); angina and ST-segment depression usually occur at the

same double product. The factors involved in the hemodynamic responses to exercise are illustrated in the flow chart in Figure 1-3.

In clinical practice, exercise capacity can be either estimated from treadmill speed and grade or measured by expired gas analysis [7]. Measuring expired gases is more accurate than estimating because it avoids the problems of hanging on (the patient hangs onto the side rails), serial testing (which leads to increased efficiency), and oxygen cost differential between running and walking (running is less efficient than walking).

Types of Exercise
Three types of exercise performed by the body can be used to stress the cardiovascular system: isometric, dynamic, and a combination of the two. Isometric exercise, defined as constant muscular contraction without movement (e.g., handgrip), imposes a disproportionate pressure load on the LV relative to the body's ability to supply oxygen. Dynamic exercise is defined as rhythmic muscular activity resulting in movement, and it initiates a more appropriate increase in cardiac output and oxygen exchange. As a delivered workload can be calibrated accurately and the physiologic response measured easily, dynamic exercise is preferred for clinical testing. By imposing progressive workloads of dynamic exercise, the examiner can protect patients with coronary artery disease from rapidly increasing myocardial oxygen demand. Although bicycling is a dynamic exercise, most individuals perform more work on a treadmill because greater muscle mass is involved and most subjects are more familiar with walking than with cycling.

Dynamic exercise is preferred to isometric exercise for testing because it can be graduated and controlled, and also because it puts a volume rather than a pressure stress on the heart. However, most activities usually combine both types of exercise to varying degrees. Dynamic exercise can be classified according to intensity and duration. Endurance or resistance to fatigue is characterized by the amount of time the exercise is performed (measured by calories), whereas multiples of basal total-body oxygen consumption (METs) relate to the intensity of exercise.

METs
For convenience, ventilatory oxygen consumption is expressed in multiples of a basal ventilatory oxygen

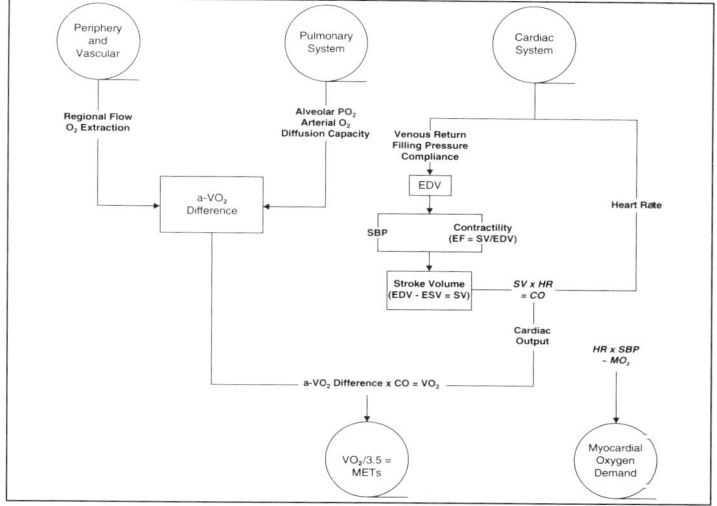

Fig. 1-3. The factors involved in the hemodynamic responses to exercise. EDV = end-diastolic volume; SBP = systolic BP; EF = ejection fraction; SV = stroke volume; HR = heart rate; CO = cardiac output; MO_2 = myocardial oxygen consumption; VO_2 = volume of oxygen.

requirement (METs). One MET is equal to a unit of basal oxygen consumption measuring approximately 3.5 ml O_2/kg/min. This value is the average oxygen requirement from inspired air to maintain life in the resting state. The maximal MET capacity depends on many factors, including natural physical endowment, activity status, age, and gender, but it is the best index of exercise capacity and maximal cardiovascular function. As a rough reference, the maximal oxygen uptake of the normal sedentary middle-aged adult is approximately 30 ml O_2/kg/min (8.5 METs), and the minimal level for physical fitness is 40 ml O_2/kg/min (11 METs). Aerobic training can increase maximal oxygen uptake by up to 25% and bed rest, the converse. This increase depends on the initial level of fitness and age as well as the intensity, frequency, and length of training sessions. Individuals performing aerobic training such as distance running can have maximal oxygen uptakes as high as 60 to 90 ml O_2/kg/min.

A review of previous studies [8] of VO_2 max and its variation with age and activity yielded the following regression equation:

Predicted METs = $16.2 - (0.11 \times \text{Age})$

Nomograms that present METs in a percentage as expected for age are the best way to represent exercise capacity (see Chapter 4).

Questionnaires
The functional status of patients with heart disease is frequently classified by symptoms during daily activities. The New York Heart Association, Canadian, and Weber classifications are common examples (see Appendix C). These have been replaced by specific activity questionnaires (Duke, V.A. Medical Center) that record usual activities and their associated exercise energy expenditures.

**Ventricular Arrhythmias
and Atrial Fibrillation (Row 5)**
Arrhythmias and conduction abnormalities have multiple mechanisms, symptoms, and syndromes:

Premature ventricular contractions (PVCs), which can cause palpitations but their risk depends on associated diseases

Premature atrial contractions (PACs), which are totally benign

Supraventricular tachycardia, which can cause palpitations, angina, CHF, and rarely syncope

Ventricular tachycardia, which can cause syncope and sudden death

Atrial fibrillation, which can occur in patients free of heart disease ("lone") or in patients with cardiac disease (it can precipitate CHF in patients with cardiac dysfunction but its major risk is cerebral embolic stroke)

Heart block which can cause low cardiac output, fatigue, and syncope

Ventricular arrhythmias should be classified as to frequency, form, and timing relative to the T wave. Ventricular tachycardia should be classified as to the number of beats in succession and to its form relative to whether the R waves are always in one direction or whether they point on either side of the isoelectric line (torsades de pointes). Torsades needs to be distinguished because it does not respond to lidocaine or quinidine, but should be treated with isoproterenol, overdrive pacing, and at least a trial of intravenous magnesium. Torsades can be caused by antidysrhythmic agents such as quinidine or disopyramide (Norpace) by prolonging the QT interval. QT prolongation can also be caused by nonsedating anti-histamines, such as terfenadine (Seldane), combined with antifungal agents and antibiotics [9]. In general, the malignancy or prognostic implications of ventricular arrhythmias and atrial fibrillation relate to "the company they keep." In other words, frequent PVCs, atrial fibrillation, and even ventricular tachycardia can occur in healthy individuals and not indicate high risk, while in the patient with a cardiomyopathy, valvular disease, or acute MI, they may be problematic and dependent risk markers. However, referral to arrhythmia specialists is only indicated for patients with serious, symptomatic arrhythmias [10].

Atrial fibrillation results from a circus dispersion of conduction through the atria with suppression of sinus node activity. Figure 1-4 is an ECG showing atrial fibrillation. Loss of the atrial kick and rapid conduction through the atrioventricular (AV) node can result in symptoms of fatigue and shortness of breath. The latter can be controlled by slowing conduction through the AV node with digoxin or calcium antagonists. Agents like quinidine that can speed conduction can be used to convert to sinus rhythm but must be avoided until AV conduction is blocked [11]. Patients must receive anticoagulation therapy to avoid cerebral emboli, the major danger of atrial fibrillation. *The appearance of atrial fibrillation is associated with a doubling of the annual mortality* [12]. Most supraventricular rhythms are benign and their danger is really due to associated conditions; for example, tachycardia can precipitate ischemia in a patient with coronary disease or can precipitate CHF in a patient with valvular disease or LV dysfunction.

Heart block can be due to structural disease (degenerative or acute), ischemia or infarction, high vagal tone, medications, and electrolyte abnormalities. Third-degree heart block usually requires pacemaker insertion.

Confounders and Rare Confounders

As the focus of the ADVIsE approach is on the most common and usual presentations, only a brief mention is made of the confounders that simulate the five key prognostic groupings and of the rare confounders that can be confused with the key feature groupings.

1. Myocardial dysfunction or damage: Its most common presentation is CHF. Confounders are anxiety, diastolic dysfunction, athletic heart, thromboembolism and pul-

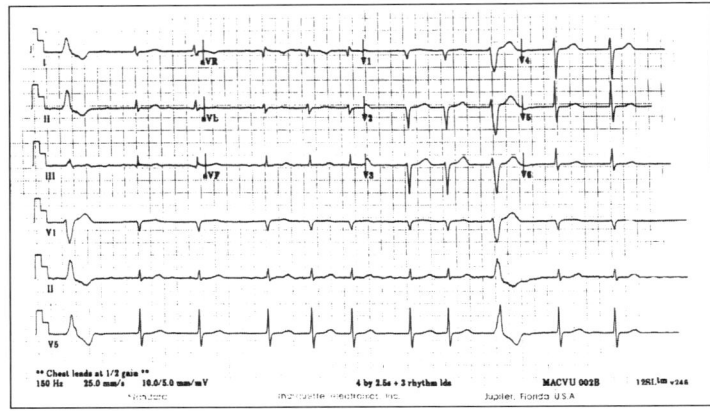

Fig. 1-4.   Atrial fibrillation with premature ventricular or aberrantly conducted complexes. Notice the absence of P waves. The ECG format is four 2.5-second groupings of three leads plus 10 seconds of three leads; the precordial leads are at one-half standard.

monary disease including pulmonary embolism and cardiac tamponade. Rare confounders that simulate CHF due to myocardial damage are high-output failure, radiation heart disease, and right ventricular infarction.

2. Myocardial ischemia: Its most common presentation is angina pectoris. Confounders are esophageal reflux, pulmonary embolism or pulmonary hypertension, aortic stenosis, pericarditis, and costochondritis. Rare confounders are aortic dissection and coronary spasm.

3. Valvular status: Its most common presentations are CHF and angina. Confounders are functional murmurs, asymmetric septal hypertrophy (idiopathic hypertrophic subaortic stenosis), bacterial endocarditis, and Marfan's syndrome.

4. Exercise capacity: Its main presentation is exercise intolerance. Confounders are deconditioning, pulmonary disease, obesity, and good endurance but decreased aerobic capacity (e.g., the patient who claims to be able to walk miles but takes all day to do so).

5. Arrhythmias and conduction abnormalities: Their main symptomatic presentations are palpitations, syncope, fatigue, and sudden death. Confounders are anxiety and vasomotor syncope. Rare confounders are long QT syndrome and right ventricular dysplasia.

While the confounders can confuse the diagnosis, the rare confounders are interesting but unusual. However, the practitioner should not miss either of them. When the tests do not confirm the clinician's impression based on the ADVIsE key feature classification and there are major incongruities, one of these confounders may be present and referral to a cardiologist is appropriate.

EXAMPLES OF THE ADVIsE APPROACH*

Myocardial Ischemia Spreadsheet Box Row

A 50-year-old white female physician who was chief of staff at a large medical center presented with new-onset chest pain. She had had no previous medical problems but was under considerable job stress and had a physician husband who was recovering from an MI. She described the pain as substernal, coming on with confrontations at work and with hurrying at airports. It did not occur at rest nor was it cyclic. (This history puts her in the myocardial ischemia spreadsheet box row.) Her cholesterol level was in the low 200s, her BP normal, and she did not smoke. The pain went away with rest but she had not tried NTG. The pain began on a recent trip and there was no other pertinent history. Findings on physical examination were normal. She showed no tendon xanthoma, xanthelasma, murmurs, or bruits. A recent chest x-ray film appeared normal and a current ECG showed nonspecific ST-segment depression but was otherwise normal. This is consistent with normal ventricular function and a good prognosis. (These additional data negate any need for evaluation of the other key features at this time.)

Given the patient's inability to remove herself from her important job, the possibility of false-positive results on stress tests, and the new onset of angina pectoris (unstable angina), she was sent for cardiac catheterization the next day. Her coronary arteries were totally normal and there was no evidence for spasm. (This removes her from the ADVIsE approach spreadsheet box since she does not have cardiac disease.) In retrospect, she described GI complaints of some duration and taking antacids, which she forgot to mention. She was reassured and provided with a reference of the excellent prognosis of persons with normal coronary arteries [13]. She did well and never returned with chest pain.

---

*These examples involve actual patients.

Key Feature	History/Physical Examination	ECG/Chest X-Ray	Exercise Test	Catheterization
Myocardial damage	None	Normal		Normal
Ischemia	Angina pectoris		Too unstable	Normal
Valves	No murmur			
Exercise capacity	Normal			
Arrhythmias	None			
There was no need for nuclear, Holter, or echocardiography studies nor had they ever been performed.				

Myocardial Damage Spreadsheet Box Row

A 55-year-old hairdresser developed cardiogenic shock and ventricular tachycardia after CABG. He had myocardial damage and the EF was 20%. He recovered after a difficult hospital course. He was treated with digoxin, ACE inhibitors, amiodarone, and diuretics. He had a mild cough with the ACE therapy but was convinced to tolerate it because of the survival benefits. He did well working every day, never complained of chest pain or specifically of angina, and in fact did hiking and other activities. He understood the importance of fluid intake, diuretics, and his weight, but occasionally was admitted for weight gain and dyspnea. He responded nicely to intravenous diuretics and returned to work. Any time cardiac transplantation was proposed, he said he was doing too well. (Based on the ADVIsE approach, the data gathered and placed in the spreadsheet box confirm that he has myocardial dysfunction. There is nothing to suggest residual ischemia, the valves are normal, his exercise capacity satisfies him and sounds good, and his arrhythmias are secondary to myocardial damage but are stable.)

At an appointment he was tachycardic and dyspneic, without any weight gain. His physical examination revealed increased cardiomegaly, S_3 gallop, rales, and neck vein pulsations, still visible with him sitting. His ECG was unchanged except for a new left atrial abnormality, and he denied having chest pain or palpitations. Anxiety and a tremor seemed appropriate for his acute distress. He was admitted to the hospital based on concern regarding some other precipitator for his CHF since his weight had not increased; a murmur was not appreciated but did he have torn chordae or become ischemic? (Was the new CHF due to valvular dysfunction, ischemia, or arrhythmias?) Elevated triiodothyronine levels confirmed the possibility of hyperthyroidism due to amiodarone. Since he had had no recurrence of ventricular tachycardia with the amiodarone therapy [14], despite the recent data showing no improved survival in cardiomyopathy patients [15], his physicians were reluctant to stop it. He responded to propylthiouracil, later received radiation thyroic ablation, and did well.

Key Feature	History/ Physical Examination	ECG/ Chest X-Ray	Holter	Echocardiography	Catheterization
Myocardial damage	+ +	+ +		+ +	+ By history
Ischemia	CABG				
Valves	− −			No abnormalities	− −
Exercise capacity	− By history				
Arrhythmias	Ventricular tachycardia	− −	No recurrence		
Exercise testing and nuclear tests were not indicated and were not previously performed. Diagnostic value: + + = very helpful; + = helpful; − = moderately helpful; − − = not helpful.					

Spreadsheet Boxes Filled but Noncardiac Cause

A 50-year-old white obese Vietnam veteran (underwent surgery for war wounds) was transferred to our care after his health insurance coverage was exceeded at a local hospital. He had presented there with flash pulmonary edema, BP of 270/140 mm Hg, and a normal creatine phosphokinase; stabilized quickly; and was told that cardiac catheterization and percutaneous transluminal coronary angioplasty (PTCA) or CABG would "fix him." He denied having any previous health problems except for obesity (5 feet, 9 inches tall and 320 lb), which led to stomach stapling 15 years ago and weight loss to 160 lb, but he was back to 200 lb). He admitted to light smoking and occasional heavy drinking in the past but currently had a regular job and a family. He denied having chest pain, exercise limitations, syncope, or other symptoms. He denied snoring or having a sleeping disorder. His physical examination was unremarkable except for carotid bruits; there were no murmurs, gallops, or cardiomegaly. ECG showed LV hypertrophy with strain; chest x-ray study was normal. An exercise test was negative for ischemia but revealed a poor exercise capacity (40% for age) due to dyspnea. An echocardiogram showed normal ventricular and valvular function but there was dyskinesia (bulging outward) of the posterior wall. Pulmonary function showed restrictive abnormalities and decreased diffusion capacity. Because of recurrent dyspnea and the uncertainty of his diagnosis, he underwent cardiac catheterization. It revealed a normal left anterior descending coronary artery and total occlusion of the left circumflex and right coronary arteries, which would have supplied an aneurysmal posterior wall. There was no residual ischemia shown by perfusion testing or any hemodynamic abnormalities due to the posterior wall infarct. (By the ADVIsE approach, he was removed from the myocardial dysfunction and ischemia spreadsheet boxes for treatment but was directed to pulmonary for probable hypersensitivity lung disease.) The acute event may have been either a hypertensive crisis causing papillary muscle dysfunction in an area of previous damage or all totally due to his lung condition. His only complaint 1 year later was orthopnea without any findings of LV dysfunction. He had no ascites to explain this but there was evidence for diaphragmatic nerve dysfunction. A follow-up exercise test was unremarkable.

Key Feature	History/ Physical Exami- nation	ECG/ Chest X-Ray	Exercise Test	Echocar- diography	Cathe- teriza- tion
Myocardial damage	+	+ +		Normal	Post WMA
Ischemia	− −	−	Too unstable	Post WMA	Two-vessel disease
Valves	No murmurs			Normal	− −
Exercise capacity	Poor				
Arrhythmias	None				

Holter and nuclear tests were not indicated and not performed previously. Post WMA = posterior wall motion abnormality.
Diagnostic value: + + = very helpful; + = helpful; − = moderately helpful; − − = not helpful.

Dilated Cardiomyopathy

A 40-year-old female physician presented with dyspnea and fatigue. She related a problem with anorexia nervosa and depression but denied having chest pain, drinking, or smoking. She was seen a year before when she requested a treadmill test to enter the US Air Force Reserves. The test was remarkable for a superb level of fitness (150% of expected for age) and was totally normal. Her family history was negative; results of ECGs and laboratory studies had always been normal. A physical examination revealed cardiomegaly, a systolic murmur, and an S_3 gallop. There were no murmurs or bruits. The ECG revealed LV hypertrophy with strain and a left atrial abnormality; the chest x-ray film showed cardiomegaly. An echocardiogram revealed dilated cardiomegaly and no valvular abnormalities. A careful dietary history was consistent with thiamine deficiency (beriberi heart disease) and her abnormalities and symptoms responded over the following year, along with her anorexia nervosa, to psychotherapy.

Key Feature	History/ Physical Examination	ECG/ Chest X-Ray	Exercise Test	Echocardi- ography
Myocardial damage	None	Cardio- megaly		Dilated CM
Ischemia	None		None previously	
Valves	No murmurs			Normal
Exercise capacity	OK		Excellent previously	
Arrhythmias	None			
Nuclear studies, catheterization, and Holter monitoring were unnecessary and not previously performed.				

Myocardial Ischemia

A 50-year-old male smoker presented with chest fullness and dyspnea on exertion. He was relatively sedentary and had had an elevated cholesterol level. His family history was incomplete but he did not have diabetes or high BP or an alcohol problem. He also described a sharp chest pain that seemed to worry him more. On physical examination there were no cardiac abnormalities or signs of COPD—forced expiration with his mouth open was quick. An ECG and chest x-ray study were normal. The treadmill test had the following results: His chief complaint was reproduced and accompanied by 1.5-mm horizontal ST-segment depression at a heart rate of 135 bpm, systolic BP of 200 mm Hg, and 6 METs. Cholesterol measurements revealed a total of 275 mg/dl and a high-density-lipoprotein (HDL) level of 30 mg/dl. He received 50 mg of atenolol, which he tolerated nicely. On a repeat treadmill test he reached 8 METs (normal for his age) without symptoms, but still had ST-segment depression. After he started lovastatin (20 mg qd), his lipid levels were much improved.

Key Feature	History/Physical Examination	ECG/ Chest X-Ray	Exercise Test
Myocardial damage	Dyspnea	Normal	
Ischemia	Atypical angina pectoris		Compatible with ischemia
Valves	No murmurs	Normal	
Exercise capacity	OK		Good after treatment
Arrhythmias	None		

Nuclear studies, echocardiography, catheterization, and Holter monitoring were unnecessary and not previously performed.

PROBLEM-BASED LEARNING FOR CARDIOLOGY*

Case 1   Ischemia Due to Coronary Atherosclerosis

Chest Pain Charlie

A 55-year-old white man presents with chest pain. He has no other complaints though he does admit to vague leg pain that makes him stop walking (if this turns out to be claudication, it increases the chance of him having coronary artery disease). He is a smoker and inactive, has no family history of coronary artery disease except for a grandfather who died at age 80 of a heart ailment. He denies drinking much but does admit to consuming a couple glasses of red wine each week. BP is 120/80 mm Hg and he denies any history of high BP. His physical examination is unremarkable; specifically there are no tendon xanthoma, xanthelasma, bruits, murmurs, gallops, or other cardiac findings (this is typical of coronary artery disease patient). On questioning, he tells you he is most worried about an indigestion type of pain that is relieved by eating and a sharp stabbing left-sided chest pain that comes on with stress at work. (This is noncardiac chest pain!!)

*These two examples are fictitious cases designed for teaching.

You order some tests and counsel him to stop smoking cigarettes and to walk briskly for 30 minutes at least five times a week and have him return in 3 months. You also give him information regarding the American Heart Association (AHA) low-fat diet.

1. What tests should you order?
    Lipid profile with low-density-lipoprotein (total cholesterol)/HDL cholesterol ratio (265 mg/dl total, 28 mg/dl for HDL, ratio 8.2) and a resting ECG (normal ECG) are all the cost-effective physician needs, but some might add a chest x-ray study, CBC count, and blood chemistries.
2. What is atherosclerosis and what are the origins of the word?
    Athero means gruel and *sclero*, hard, for the hard gruel-like substance that the Greek anatomists found when cutting diseased arteries. These are lipid deposits that occlude the lumen as well as generate a plaque that is "dirty," gathering platelets and thrombus.
3. What are the four major risk factors for atherosclerosis?
    Serum cholesterol (total cholesterol/HDL ratio), high BP, cigarette smoking, and physical inactivity are the four risk factors. Physical inactivity was just raised to the status of the fourth risk factor by the Centers for Disease Control and Prevention (CDC) and AHA [16, 17].
4. Is red wine or alcohol protective?
    Maybe.
    Is it a good public health policy to recommend drinking?
    No. Consider all those drunk drivers!
5. Is family history a risk factor?
    No, it is not a factor. The term *factor* implies more than an association and something that can be corrected. Perhaps family history is a risk marker only in those who have family members with events occurring before the age of 65 years.
6. Describe angina pectoris.
    Angina pectoris is a dull, squeezing substernal chest pain, pressure, or sensation brought on by exertion or anger.
7. How do you calculate his probability of developing coronary artery disease from the AHA-Framingham score [18] (see Appendix D)?
    The points add up to predicting a 19% chance of MI,

angina, or sudden death. The accuracy of this prediction approaches 85%, particularly when HDL cholesterol is included.

He returns in 3 months with the test results and some further history. After your reassurance regarding the chest pains that he presented with, these pains became less of a concern so he was able to focus on the squeezing, dull, constricting substernal chest sensation that comes on with exercise and when arguing with his teenage son. He describes this sensation while making a fist with his left hand (Levine's sign). It disappears within minutes of stopping exercise or the interaction with his son. He has not stopped smoking nor has he increased his exercise program. With this new historical data you decide to order another test and repeat a previous test.

8. What tests would you order?
   Standard treadmill test and repeat lipid profile are ordered.
9. What medication do you give him to try and why?
   Sublingual NTG is given for therapeutic and diagnostic reasons.
10. Is his symptom complex now classic angina pectoris?
    Yes.

When you get back the treadmill test and laboratory results, you add another three medications. The treadmill test shows abnormal ST-segment depression and predicts a high probability of coronary artery disease. The cholesterol level is 263 mg/dl.

11. What should the first two drugs be?
    Beta-blocker and acetylsalicylic acid (ASA, 81 mg per day).
12. What are the side effects of these drugs.
    Depression, impotence, and gastritis are side effects but they are rare.
13. Before the third drug can be added, you should order certain laboratory studies. What tests and what is the class of drugs?
    A statin lipid lowering drug should be added after baseline liver function tests have been ordered.

You again stress his risk factors and their effect on the atherosclerotic process that he most likely has. You schedule him for repeat laboratory studies and a follow-up appointment in 3 months.

The laboratory results are normal, so you call him to start lovastatin.

In the interim, he stopped the ASA because of indigestion pains and the beta-blocker because of a possible decrement in his sexual function and fatigue. He continues to take lovastatin and to smoke but has increased his exercise level in spite of the chest pain.

Before he returns for his third visit, he presents to the emergency room with chest pain. There, his ECG shows ST-segment elevation in the inferior leads compatible with transmural ischemia and evolving inferior MI.

14. When his pain, which began less than 2 hours ago, does not respond to NTG, he is given what medications?

    Streptokinase and ASA are given. A tissue plasminogen activator (tPA) is a possibility but it is most important to give a thrombolytic agent soon. Emergent PTCA is another option.

15. A laboratory test was ordered as well. What is it?

    Measurement of CPK level, perhaps other enzyme levels as well, was ordered.

He does well and a follow-up ECG shows no Q waves but some minor T-wave changes and the laboratory test showed the reported value.

The patient has a CPK level of 1200 and MB of 15%. This CPK level is compatible with reperfusion rather than large MI since serial CPKs returned to normal quickly and the ECG exhibits no Q waves but does have ST-segment depression.

16. Did the patient have an MI and if so, what type of infarction did he have?

    Yes, he had a non-Q-wave or subendocardial MI, which has a lower associated mortality and damage but more residual ischemia and angina than a completed Q-wave MI.

17. What is the appropriate medication during and after hospitalization?

    Beta-blocker.

18. Is there any controversy regarding the choice of medication?

    Previously some clinicians favored calcium antagonists but the majority of studies showed that beta-

Problem-Based Learning Case One
Chest Pain Charlie

Key Feature	History/Physical Examination	ECG/Chest X-Ray	Exercise Test	Echocardiography	Nuclear Tests	Holter	Catheterization
Myocardial damage	None	None	No help		Post		None
Ischemia	Yes	Yes*	Yes				Two-vessel disease
Valves	No						
Exercise capacity	Poor						
Arrhythmias	No						

*Dynamic ECG changes.

blockers reduce mortality in the first year after MI by 25% for all types of MIs.

You counsel him again regarding the importance of stopping cigarette smoking and altering his risk factors . . . never give up!!!

A test is ordered prior to his discharge 4 days later. A treadmill test showed no ST-segment depression compatible with ischemia and reasonable exercise capacity. He "passes" this test and goes home.

At home, he stops cigarette smoking and returns to work. He has chest pain before returning to see you and is taken to another hospital. There cardiac catheterization reveals 50% stenosis of the mid left anterior descending coronary artery, 95% stenosis of the right coronary artery, no other occlusions, and an EF of 55%.

This patient had no ECG changes with the chest pain and had no further episodes of chest pain.

You decide to manage him conservatively with ASA, a statin drug, and a beta-blocker.

Case 2   Ischemic Cardiomyopathy

Dyspneic Dave

A 65-year-old white man presents to your clinic complaining of shortness of breath, dyspnea on exertion, and pedal edema. He gives a history similar to a patient you just treated for coronary artery disease but his ischemic symptoms began 15 years before this presentation. He developed a Q-wave infarction 12 years ago but did not receive streptokinase because the thrombolysis trials had not been performed and the current belief was that coronary thrombosis was a misnomer (pathologists taught that a thrombus was not the primary event at that time . . . there was confusion from the postmortem studies). His ECG several years later shows tiny R waves that grew back over large anterior Q waves.

1. Is this consistent with myocardial damage?
   Yes.
2. How much damage?
   A lot. A normal ECG is associated with normal LV function but an ECG with large anterior Q waves is associated with an EF of 30 to 40%.

He is lost to follow-up but is seen by other physicians and is known to have hypertension and to drink alcohol excessively rather frequently (so his dilated cardiomyopathy could be due to a combination of alcohol, hypertension, and ischemic damage/infarction).

On physical examination he is noted to have neck vein distention at 45 degrees including a large V wave, rales, cardiomegaly, and 2+ pitting edema. Auscultation reveals an S_3 and an S_4 plus a soft systolic murmur. His weight is up 15 lb from his last clinic visit.

3. What do these physical findings represent?
   These findings represent right- and left-sided CHF. Check the Framingham criteria for CHF below.
4. Why do these physical findings occur?
   There is increased fluid retention to compensate for poor LV function. Via the Frank-Starling mechanism, the heart dilates to maintain stroke volume but that causes a vicious cycle.
5. What laboratory tests would you order?
   BUN, creatinine, and electrolyte levels should be determined.
6. What cardiac tests would you order?
   ECG, chest x-ray, and echocardiography should be ordered.

The Framingham Criteria for Congestive Heart Failure
The subjectivity of the clinical diagnosis of CHF can be lessened by using standardized criteria. The Framingham criteria for CHF consist of a listing of historical and physical findings; a definitive diagnosis of CHF relies on the concurrent presence of two major or one major and two minor criteria.

• The major criteria include paradoxical nocturnal dyspnea or orthopnea, neck vein distention, rales, cardiomegaly, acute pulmonary edema, S_3, and hepatojugular reflux.

• The minor criteria include ankle edema, night cough, dyspnea on exertion, hepatomegaly, pleural effusion, and tachycardia greater than 120 bpm.

His ECG shows left branch-bundle block; the chest x-ray film shows cardiomegaly; and echocardiogram shows dilated LV with poor contraction.

7. Given these test results, what is the likely diagnosis?
   The likely diagnosis is dilated cardiomyopathy.

Problem-Based Learning Case 2
Dyspneic Dave

Key Feature	History/Physical Examination	ECG/ Chest X-Ray	Exercise Test	Echocardiography	Nuclear Tests	Holter	Catheterization
Myocardial damage	Yes	Yes	No help	Abnormal			EF42%
Ischemia	Yes	Yes	Yes				Three-vessel disease
Valves	No						
Exercise capacity	Poor						
Arrhythmias	No						

8. What is its likely cause(s)?
   The likely cause is systolic dysfunction due to ischemia-infarction and alcohol.
9. What medications should be started?
   ACE inhibitors, diuretics, and digoxin should be started.

He does better and turns out to be compliant with your advice. He stops smoking cigarettes and drinking. However, he cannot continue one of his medications (ACE inhibitor) because of an irritating cough and so has to switch to two others.

10. What were the replacement drugs?
    The patient was given long-acting nitrates and hydralazine (Apresoline).

He increases his exercise level only to develop recurrent substernal chest pain.

11. What test do you order?
    The standard treadmill test is ordered. Remember that the ST segments cannot be used to determine ischemia when left branch-bundle block is present; however, useful information is still obtained in a cost-effective way. Most worrisome are his exercise-limiting angina, exertional hypotension, and poor exercise capacity.

Given the exercise test results and his clinical improvement regarding CHF over the 4 months, you decide to order another test.

12. What is that test?
    Cardiac catheterization is ordered.

This reveals triple-vessel coronary artery disease with an EF of 42%. Based on these results you present his case to the cardiothoracic surgeons.

13. Do you argue for or against CABG and why?
    You argue for surgery because he fits in the group whose survival benefits from CABG. Consider the mortality estimates associated with CABG based on

clinical variables (range of 3 to 6% chance of dying during or after the operation).

CONCLUSION
As exemplified by these examples, the ADVIsE approach provides a simple way of organizing the complex data derived from evaluation of the patient with cardiac disease. When test results do not agree, this becomes very apparent, allowing decisions to be made regarding what is correct or erroneous. Rather than prescribing all cardiac medications or ordering all cardiac tests for the cardiac patient, following the ADVIsE approach helps the practitioner to manage cardiac patients in a logical and efficient manner.

REFERENCES
1. Guyatt GH. Readers' guide for articles evaluating diagnostic tests: what ACP Journal Club does for you and what you must do yourself. *ACP J Club* 1991; 115:A-16.
2. Yusuf S, Garg R, McConachie D. Effect of angiotensin-converting enzyme inhibitors in left ventricular dysfunction: results of the studies of left ventricular dysfunction in the context of other similar trials. *J Cardiovasc Pharmacol* 1993;22(suppl 9):S28–S35.
3. Stevenson WG, et al. Improving survival for patients with advanced heart failure: a study of 737 consecutive patients. *J Am Coll Cardiol* 1995;26:1417–1423.
4. Kannel WB, Belanger AJ. Epidemiology of heart failure. *Am Heart J* 1991;121:951–957.
5. Fletcher GF, et al. Exercise standards. A statement for healthcare professionals from the American Heart Association Writing Group. *Circulation* 1995; 91:580–615.
6. Mark DB, et al. Exercise treadmill score for predicting prognosis in coronary artery disease. *Ann Intern Med* 1987;106:793–800.
7. Myers J. *Cardiac Evaluation Using Expired Gas Analysis.* Champaign, Illinois: Human Kinetics Press, 1996. P. 7.
8. Dehn MM, Bruce RA. Longitudinal variations in maximal oxygen intake with age and activity. *J Appl Physiol* 1972;33:805–807.
9. Rosen M. Of oocytes and runny noses. *Circulation* 1996;94:607–609.

10.   Stevenson WG, Ridker P. Should survivors of myocardial infarction with low ejection fraction be routinely referred to arrhythmia specialists? *JAMA* 1996;276:481–485.

11.   Golzari H, Cebul RD, Bahler RC. Atrial fibrillation: restoration and maintenance of sinus rhythm and indications for anticoagulation therapy. *Ann Intern Med* 1996;125:311-323.

12.   Prystowsky E, et al. Management of patients with atrial fibrillation. A statement by the AHA subcommittee on ECG and electrophysiology. *Circulation* 1996;93:1262–1277.

13.   Kemp HG, Kronmal RA, Vlietstra RE, Frye RL. Seven year survival of patients with normal or near normal coronary arteriograms: a CASS registry study. *J Am Coll Cardiol* 1986;7:479–483.

14.   Podrid PJ. Amiodarone: reevaluation of an old drug. *Ann Intern Med* 1995;122:689–697.

15.   Singh SN, et al. Amiodarone in patients with congestive heart failure and asymptomatic ventricular arrhythmia. Survival Trial of Antiarrhythmic Therapy in Congestive Heart Failure. *N Engl J Med* 1995; 333:77–78.

16.   Morris CK, Froelicher VF. Cardiovascular benefits of improved exercise capacity. *Sports Med* 1993;16: 225–236.

17.   Fletcher GF, et al. Statement on exercise: benefits and recommendations for physical activity programs for all Americans. A statement from the American Heart Association. *Circulation* 1996;94:857–862.

18.   Anderson KM, Wilson PW, Odell PM, Kannel WB. An updated coronary risk profile. A statement of health professionals. *Circulation* 1991;83:356–362.

Basic Methods of Evaluation: The History and Physical Examination

HISTORY

The history initiates the medical evaluation. A complete composite of the patient including the medical issues and social context needs to be developed and reviewed. Accurate questioning requires identification of the chief complaint and associated symptoms. Remember always to capture the chief complaint in the patient's own words and put it in quotation marks. Symptoms should be evaluated for onset, pattern, and changes including frequency and severity. Immediate consideration should be given to whether a disease state is stable or unstable. Various circumstances ranging from medical to social to environmental should be investigated for explaining changes in symptoms. Eventual treatment is greatly altered by precipitating factors. All changes noted in the history and examination must be compared to previous results. These basic techniques will enable a very accurate initial diagnosis.

It is always important to consider the mental status of the patient; if the clinician has any concern, he or she should question the patient specifically as to person, place, and time. Patients who confabulate can provide fascinating but meaningless histories. The patient's significant other is often helpful but beware of the rare "folio duo" or couple who share delusions.

Calling or writing previous health care providers, reviewing old records that the patient has obtained, and mastering any computerized data bases with information are part of the "detective work" of piecing together a complete medical history. Perhaps someday medical records will be on the Internet, but problems regarding confidentiality will delay that. Some patients already update us on their progress or ask questions via the Internet or fax. Progressive health care organizations are already providing patients with health maintenance and access to health care information via the World Wide Web.

Disease Temporal Pattern

The first consideration is whether or not the patient's disease is stable (chronic) or unstable (acute). This seems rather simple, but a careful history is the most important assessment tool. The changes in symptoms, rather than caused by the disease, may be due to psychosocial (family, financial stresses) or environmental circumstances (temperature, weather). In that case, the physician should react to the instability by means other than medication adjustment or hospitalization. It is always recommended that the patient's test results be compared, to look for changes. Even physicians unaccustomed to interpreting ECGs can compare them and see if there are serial changes, even if they do not understand the significance of the discrepancies. However, when serial changes are noted and suggest instability of the disease, one must remember that there are reproducibility limitations to all procedures.

General Concepts

Figure 2-1 illustrates the importance of the history. The history should be structured in an outline compulsively followed when interviewing a patient. The patient's chief complaint(s) should always be recorded in his or her own words. The following list should be helpful:

1. History of current illness: chest pain or sensation pattern, dyspnea on exertion (DOE), paroxysmal nocturnal dyspnea (PND), change in weight, claudication, orthopnea, syncope, palpitations, cough, exercise status
2. Past medical history: usual activities, hospitalizations, illnesses and injuries, cigarettes and alcohol, medications used, results of prior tests, myocardial infarctions (MIs), cerebrovascular accidents, previous surgeries, results of prior cardiovascular and pulmonary tests, recent laboratory results, specific cardiovascular events, risk factors
3. Review of systems: head-eyes-ears-nose-throat, thyroid, pulmonary, cardiovascular, GI, genitourinary (venereal disease), renal, hematologic, neurologic
4. Family history: the usual plus coronary heart disease in those less than 65 years old, sudden death or hyperlipidemia, questions regarding the occurrence of diabetes, hypertension
5. Habits: tobacco, alcohol, and drug use
6. Social: employment status, living situation, social support system
7. Diet: fat, sodium, caloric, and fluid intake
8. Activity status: weekly activity pattern and activity-

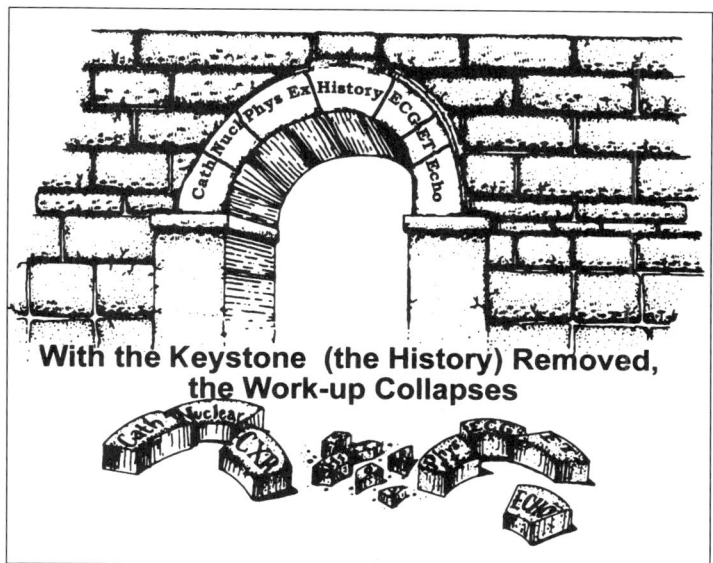

With the Keystone (the History) Removed, the Work-up Collapses

Fig. 2-1. The "arch" of the tools of evaluation symbolizes the importance of careful recording of cardiovascular history in the evaluation of every patient with a cardiovascular problem. CXR = chest x-ray; Nucl = nuclear medicine tests; Phys Ex = physical examination; ET = exercise test; Cath = cardiac catheterization; Echo = echocardiography.

limiting symptoms; use questionnaires to estimate daily MET level

A recent study of 100 consecutive patients seen in a general medicine clinic reported that 80% of the diagnoses were made by the history taking, an additional 10% by the physical examination, and the remainder by further laboratory tests [1]. The box-by-box spreadsheet approach of ADVIsE supports a rigorous and organized approach to the history and physical examination.

The Key Symptoms of Cardiac Disease
The four major symptoms of heart disease are fatigue, dyspnea, chest pain, and syncope. Because of their importance they are charted extensively in Appendix F.

Fatigue
Fatigue as a symptom is often frustrating to the health care provider because it is so pervasive as a complaint and so nonspecific. However, it is very rewarding when treatment or advice alleviates this problem. Though a diagno-

sis of exclusion, depression often explains the complaint of fatigue. It is often good to discuss this with the patient while beginning the work-up so he or she is prepared for this possibility. Deconditioning can either be due to an illness or be the primary cause of fatigue (i.e., sedentary lifestyle). In either situation, maintenance of a daily walking program can combat the fatigue due to deconditioning. This is even the case for claudication; in fact, walking can improve the peripheral circulation, decreasing atrophic changes and pain. The adage "Don't use it, lose it" is something patients seem to grasp.

CARDIAC CAUSES.   A decreased cardiac output due to cardiac damage or dysfunction, limited heart rate response to stress, arrhythmias, or valvular heart disease can be a cause of fatigue. Tachyarrhythmia or bradyarrhythmia can affect cardiac output as can loss of the atrial kick with atrial fibrillation. Rate control or a pacemaker can correct these problems and lessen fatigue. Treatment of the other symptoms and signs of congestive heart failure (CHF) or valvular disease can lessen fatigue. All of these conditions are discussed elsewhere. It is very unusual for these conditions to present only as fatigue since other signs and symptoms usually predominate. Cardiac cachexia due to a chronically lowered cardiac output is always accompanied by fatigue.

OTHER CAUSES.   Hypothyroidism should always be considered in the differential diagnosis of fatigue. Many types of lung disease including asthma, sleep apnea, and chronic obstructive pulmonary disease (COPD) can cause fatigue. It is easy to rule out major dysfunction of the kidneys or liver as well as anemia or infection, but diagnosing AIDS or chronic fatigue syndrome can be more challenging. Malingering often has obvious motivations associated with it. The following list is not all inclusive but we have found it helpful:

Cardiac: myocardial dysfunction, tachyarrhythmias or bradyarrhythmias, valvular disease
Pulmonary: COPD, asthma, sleep apnea
Other organ systems: renal, liver, hemopoietic, peripheral vascular disease, endocrine (particularly thyroid)
Systemic illness: collagen vascular disease, cancer, infection, obesity, chronic fatigue syndrome
Psychogenic: depression, malingering

Dyspnea
Dyspnea is a common symptom that is difficult to define and can result from a wide variety of causes. By one defini-

tion, dyspnea is an uncomfortable awareness of breathing occurring at times other than during exhaustive exertion. It is frequently the first complaint of the patient with myocardial dysfunction. This complex sensation that arises from multiple stimuli involves both subjective perceptions and objective reactions. In the assessment of patients with dyspnea, use of a systematic approach to determine the precipitating factors and the degree of breathlessness is important [2].

Although many diseases can produce dyspnea, in two-thirds of patients it results from a pulmonary or cardiac disorder. Neuromuscular, metabolic, and psychogenic causes should also be considered. Dyspnea can occur at rest or with exertion; however, as the disease process progresses, rest dyspnea is usually eventual. Patients who have dyspnea at rest that goes away with exertion usually have a psychogenic etiology for their symptoms. A comprehensive history, physical examination, and basic laboratory tests are important in the initial assessment; however, the diagnosis may depend on specialized testing, the results of which may differ from the initial clinical impression. If the history reveals a history of cigarette abuse or exposure to lung irritants and the physical examination reveals hyperinflated lungs, wheezing, or other signs of lung disease, certainly a pulmonary work-up is indicated. Initial testing should include ECG, chest x-ray study, hemoglobin determination, thyroid function tests, and spirometry with use of a bronchodilator and diffusion capacity. More specialized evaluation includes detailed pulmonary function testing and echocardiography. Accurate diagnostic data are critical for choosing appropriate treatment.

CARDIAC CAUSES.   As previously mentioned, dyspnea is frequently associated with cardiac disease. While there are other causes, the most common differential is cardiac versus pulmonary. Some patients may have a component of both; however, either a cardiac or pulmonary cause should be prominent. Dyspnea can be associated with valvular disease, left ventricular (LV) failure due to a cardiomyopathy (systolic or diastolic dysfunction), coronary artery disease, arrhythmias, and pericardial disease. Orthopnea and paroxysmal nocturnal dyspnea (PND) are associated with LV failure. Orthopnea is relief of dyspnea due to pulmonary congestion by propping up the head and thorax, thus lowering filling pressure; however, it can be due to pressure on the diaphragm due to ascites. PND occurs when patients are supine for several hours and awaken with dyspnea due to increased venous volume. Table F-29 in Appendix F reviews associated symptoms, precipitating factors, and clinical findings. Dyspnea can also be an anginal equivalent due to a stiff ventricle from ischemia, but this presentation is uncommon. In addition, dyspnea can be caused by CHF due to high-output states such as pregnancy, thyroid disease, anemia, or infection.

Chest Pain

Chest pain is a common cardiac symptom expressed by patients. It is fundamentally important to obtain a specific history regarding the characteristics of the chest pain in order to diagnose its etiology. Not all chest pain should be called angina and rigorous questioning is necessary to conclude if angina is present. Patients can experience myocardial ischemia or angina from aortic stenosis and not have coronary artery disease. Other chest pains such as that due to pericarditis have a cardiac source but are not angina nor are they due to ischemia. As shown in Tables F-17 to F-28 in Appendix F, chest pain can be caused by cardiac, pulmonary, GI, neuromuscular, and psychogenic problems. Sharp pain can be associated with pulmonary disease, and lingering pain lasting days is not angina. Occasionally, dyspnea or GI disturbance can be an "anginal equivalent" and be indicative of coronary artery disease. Care should always be taken to distinguish angina pectoris, which is a specific chest pain or sensation pattern, from other forms of chest pain. More information concerning angina is provided later.

ANGINA PECTORIS.   The history of classic angina pectoris has a high probability for underlying significant coronary artery disease. Angina pectoris is usually described as a pain, though some patients will deny having pain and instead only admit to a pressure, squeezing, strange sensation or discomfort in their chest. It is usually brought on by exercise, but variations are walk-through angina which lessens after an initial warm-up phase, and pain that occurs within 3 to 4 minutes after exercise. It also can be brought on by anger or emotional upset. It is usually worse after meals, in the morning, and in the cold. Prolonged angina (lasting constantly from 10 to 15 minutes up to several hours), particularly when accompanied by diaphoresis, nausea, and radiation, usually indicates an MI is occurring. Such pain should always be treated with nitroglycerin (NTG) and an aspirin and thrombolysis given if ST-segment elevation is noted on the ECG.

UNSTABLE ANGINA AND VARIANT ANGINA. True anginal pain at rest implies unstable angina or variant angina. Unstable angina has been described as angina occurring at rest, angina increasing without any change in medications or stress, or new onset of angina. Unstable angina can be intermittent and last for days. Variant angina is a relatively rare syndrome related to coronary artery spasm. The chest pains usually occur at rest. They are often cyclic, occurring at the same time of day. The angina is also frequently marked by ST-segment elevation (or depression) and dysrhythmias, including heart block and even ventricular tachycardia. The spasm can occur in normal coronary vessels or in proximity to fixed lesions. Unstable angina and variant angina are two forms of myocardial ischemia that have a higher risk associated with them than does stable, chronic angina.

Syncope
Syncope is a brief sudden loss of consciousness and muscle tone secondary to cerebral ischemia or inadequate oxygen or glucose delivery to the brain. Syncopal episodes are relatively common [3]. The causes of syncope may be benign and require very little in the way of evaluation or treatment. Micturition syncope and a vasovagal syncope after the sight of blood are common in healthy young individuals. However, syncope may be the harbinger of sudden death, and extensive evaluation and monitoring may be appropriate. The history including use of medications such as vasodilators and antidepressants is the most important clue when attempting to identify which patient with syncope is at risk for sudden death. Cardiogenic syncope is usually not associated with the aura and postictal phases of neurogenic syncope and has both a sudden onset and offset. A careful cardiac and neurologic examination should be performed in any patient presenting with syncope including measurement of orthostatic BP. Selective use of laboratory testing and cardiac monitoring may assist the practitioner in making the diagnosis. Most often patients with syncope will have a benign cause such as vasovagal events, hyperventilation, or orthostatic hypotension. The cause is frequently problematic if the diagnosis is not made quickly after the initial clinical and laboratory evaluation. The periodic and unpredictable frequency of events with days to years separating spells and a high remission rate are obstacles to diagnosis.

Patients with a cardiac condition causing their syncope are at increased risk for sudden death [4]. The ominous, cardiac-related causes of syncope in the younger population include hypertrophic cardiomyopathy, aberrant coronary arteries, and aortic dissection secondary to Marfan's syndrome or cystic medial necrosis. In the older population, coronary or cerebral atherosclerosis and aortic stenosis may present as syncope. Dysrhythmias ranging from heart block to ventricular tachycardia may be the cause of syncope in both populations.

PHYSICAL EXAMINATION IN GENERAL
The physical examination is used to support symptoms and confirm the diagnosis. Accurate examinations require a thorough understanding of cardiovascular examination techniques. Findings are crucial to making a correct diagnosis. A complete history and a pertinent cardiovascular examination are basic critical tools for establishing accurate initial diagnoses. A basic review of examination techniques is presented.

1. General: Assess skin turgor and emotional state.
2. Vital signs: Measurements of heart rate, BP, respiration, and temperature give a general overview of the patient's status. Heart rate should be assessed for rate (normal, tachycardic, or bradycardic) and for rhythm (regular, irregular, or irregular-irregular). If the heart rate is irregular, a 1-minute reading should be calculated, considering that an apical count will be more accurate than using a peripheral pulse. Respiration can be assessed for rate, depth, and pattern. BP measurement should be manual, using the correct-size cuff for the individual patient [5]. Automatic cuff readings are inaccurate. An *auscultatory gap* is a phenomenon where systolic sounds appear and disappear between a higher and lower value, allowing one to think the true pressure is lower than it is. This can be detected by going to a relatively high systolic pressure or by palpating the peripheral pulse and noting where it disappears. An auscultatory gap has been associated with carotid atherosclerosis and with increased arterial stiffness in high BP patients, independent of age [6]. In the patient with suspected peripheral vascular disease (PVD), discrepancies between arm-to-arm and arm-to-leg measurements are important. Index measurements comparing arm-to-leg readings by the Doppler study can identify high-risk atherosclerotic patients. However, this practice

has not been recommended for routine screening for PVD. Since pulse pressure (the absolute difference between systolic and diastolic pressure) is affected by stroke volume, both wide and narrow readings should be recorded. Wide pulse pressure is associated with aortic regurgitation, and narrow pulse pressure is associated with valvular aortic stenosis. Other pulse variations such as pulsus paradoxus (which is a drop in systolic BP during inspiration greater than the normal decrease of 10 mm Hg or less) occurs with pericardial effusion, cardiac tamponade, COPD, and constrictive pericarditis. Pulsus alternans (which is differing intensities of Korotkoff's sounds or strength of the pulses) is present with rhythm disturbances such as ventricular ectopic contractions, bigeminal rhythm, or poor cardiac output associated with cardiogenic shock or CHF.

3. Lungs: Abnormal lung sounds including rales, rhonchi, wheezes, and rubs should be identified during auscultation. If any abnormal breath sounds are noted, these signs can distinguish between airway disease and heart failure. Pleural effusions can be noted by percussing the lung fields.

4. Abdomen: The abdomen should be palpated for hepatic or splenic enlargement, the former being associated with right-sided heart failure. Abdominal pain, especially in the upper right quadrant, can indicate right-sided heart failure. An enlarged abdomen from ascites and presacral edema is also a sign of venous congestion. A pulsatile liver occurs from hepatic congestion due to right-sided heart failure. A periumbilical bruit or a pulsatile fusiform shape can be indicative of an aortic aneurysm. Femoral bruits can be associated with PVD.

5. Extremities: Assessment of arterial and venous perfusion should be done. Clubbing and cyanosis are signs of diminished oxygen saturation. Rubor and slow capillary refill are signs of arterial insufficiency. Peripheral edema can be associated with chronic heart failure, venous valve insufficiency, or medication use. Venous dilatation and chronic brown discoloration can confirm a diagnosis of venous insufficiency.

6. Arterial pulses: The arterial pulse is influenced by stroke volume and ejection velocity, heart rate, distance from the heart, and the compliance and capacity of the arterial system. The contour (shape) is composed of several waves: the early systolic component of the arterial pulse, called the percussion wave (upstroke), and the later systolic peak, labeled as the tidal wave. The upstroke

wave is normally brisk and if it is delayed as in aortic stenosis, an anacrotic notch will be present. The dicrotic notch is formed during diastole and is the negative (down-stroke) portion of the pulse wave. Usually, either the percussion or the tidal wave is dominant during percussion, and the anacrotic and dicrotic notches are not easily palpated. The following characteristics should be noted when examining the arterial pulse: cardiac rhythm, volume or amplitude, contour or shape, speed or rate of ejection, and stiffness of the vessel wall.

Carotid pulses should be assessed by auscultation and palpation. Palpation should be done below the thyroid cartilage and not adjacent to the thyroid cartilage, the location of the carotid sinus. The carotid pulse waveform can indicate specific clinical diagnoses, as shown in Figure 2-2. It is the pulse that most reliably reflects the condition of the aortic valve. For instance, when a systolic murmur is heard yet the carotid upstroke is normal, significant aortic stenosis is unlikely. In the converse, in the same circumstance, if the carotid has a shudder or a slow upstroke, significant aortic stenosis is very likely. Idiopathic hypertrophic subaortic stenosis (IHSS) is associated with a characteristic fast upstroke and low volume, while aortic insufficiency is associated with bounding pulses.

During auscultation, carotid bruits may be heard between the upper end of the thyroid cartilage to just below the angle of the jaw. Most bruits are heard during systole, but some may occur during diastole and systole. Venous hums are differentiated from carotid bruits because they are more prominent in diastole, while a patient is sitting. Bruits are often associated with PVD and are associated with coronary atherosclerosis as well. They must also be differentiated from cardiac murmurs that transmit from the precordium. Asymptomatic carotid bruits are common for middle-aged adults (about 2%) and older adults (8%), with the prevalence increasing after age 75.

All accessible *peripheral pulses* should be assessed for amplitude, contour, and rhythm. Bilateral comparison of pulses is extremely important in the identification of discrepancies in pressure between them. This is particularly the case for the brachial artery when aortic dissection is suspected. Irregular rhythm occurs with atrial fibrillation and arrhythmias, especially premature ventricular contractions. The amplitude (volume) will be affected by heart rhythm, local vessel diameter, and cardiac output. As with the carotid pulse, pulsus alternans and pulsus paradox

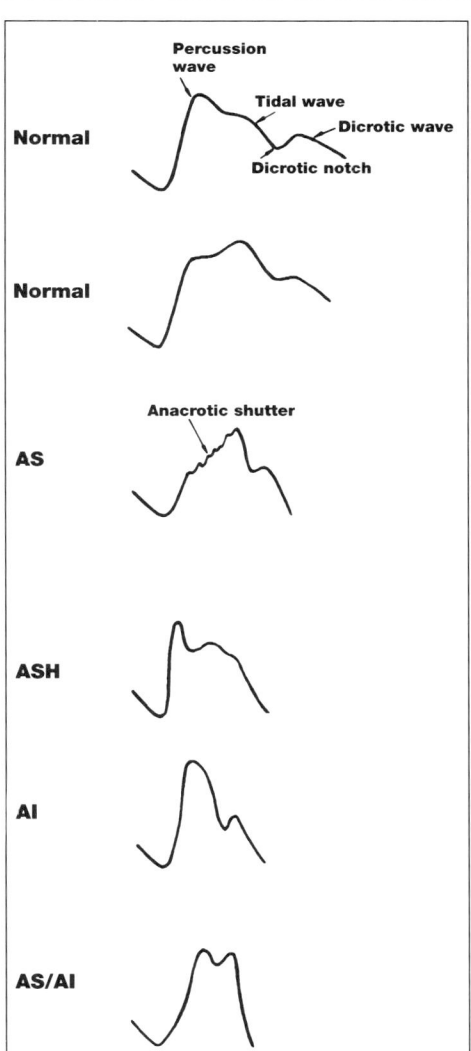

Fig. 2-2. The carotid pulse contour in health and disease. Two normal contours are illustrated, with either dominant tidal or dominant percussion waves. AS = aortic stenosis with a slow upstroke and a palpable vibration on it; ASH = asymmetric septal hypertrophy, with a fast rise and delayed completion of the waves (this is sometimes best appreciated during Valsalva's maneuver); AI = aortic insufficiency and stenosis, with a double-humped pulse (bisferiens).

must be recognized. Specific pulses to be assessed include the radial, brachial, femoral, popliteal, dorsalis pedis, and posterior tibial. If PVD is suspected from the history or physical examination, then bruits should be listened for at the pulse site. The normal contour of the peripheral pulses is affected by reflected pulse waves such that the systolic peak becomes greater, the total volume (or width of the pulse) becomes less, and the diastolic pressure is lower. In coarctation of the aorta, the femoral systolic pressure is lower than the brachial, whereas normally it is greater. In combined valvular lesions sometimes the brachial pulse better describes the major lesion by its contour.

7. Thyroid: Thyroid disease can exacerbate heart failure and is associated with cholesterol abnormalities and atrial fibrillation; nodules or enlargement should be noted.

8. Cardiac examination: The major components of the physical examination of the cardiovascular system including inspection, palpation, and auscultation are presented in detail below.

PHYSICAL EXAMINATION OF THE CARDIOVASCULAR SYSTEM

Inspection

General

The signs of COPD, edema, skin turgor, breathing pattern, and emotional state can all be assessed and integrated into the final analysis of the patient.

Jugular Venous Pulse Wave

An important part of inspection is the jugular venous pulse [7]. Care should be taken to distinguish the internal from the external jugular vein, though the external can be helpful because it is more easily seen. The examiner should be sure the jugular veins are filling from below rather than above by milking them upward and blocking retrograde filling by pressure with a finger. Another trick for their recognition consists of abdominal pressure, which makes them rise. The internal jugular vein should be assessed for its level above the right atrium, which is an estimate of right atrial pressure. Since normal central venous pressure is less than 5 mm Hg and about 1.4 cm H_2O equals 1 mm Hg, the estimate should not be more than 7 cm above the right atrium. The jugular venous pulse is easily seen normally when the individual is reclined below 45 degrees. If it is apparent when the patient is in a position from 45 degrees to sitting, the venous pressure clearly is elevated. If seen with the patient standing, then there is no question that the pressure is elevated.

The contour of the pulse should be assessed for abnormal movements, particularly the "CV" wave of tricuspid regurgitation and the cannon "A" waves of complete heart block or ventricular tachycardia. The A wave is due to the retrograde pulse wave of right atrial contraction and occurs with S_1 preceding the carotid upstroke. Large A waves occur with pulmonary high BP or biventricular failure. The "X" descent is due to atrial relaxation. The CV wave occurs during the filling of the right atrium but becomes the only wave seen when tricuspid insufficiency is present.

Apical Impulse

The intensity, duration, and location of the LV apical impulse should be noted by inspection, though this will be less sensitive than palpation or percussion. The location should be approximately at the intersection of the midclavicular line and the fifth intercostal space; it should only be of brief duration and no larger than a quarter.

Palpation

As previously described, peripheral pulses should be checked for strength and contour. Brisk pulses and a wide pressure should lead one to listen longer for aortic insufficiency. As illustrated in Figure 2-2, the contour of the carotid pulses provides valuable information. The combination of a harsh crescendo-decrescendo early systolic murmur that radiates upward and a carotid pulse with a shudder or slow ascension is highly associated with significant aortic stenosis. The brisk upstroke and then flattened dome of IHSS or ASH are also characteristic.

Palpation of the precordial movements of the heart gives valuable information enabling appreciation of cardiac dilation or hypertrophy, aneurysm, and right ventricular overload. These movements are due to the anterior twisting motion of the heart during the first half of systole. Confounders that make the assessment difficult or impossible include obesity, increased anteroposterior diameter due to COPD, pectus excavatum, and breast size. Precordial movements cannot even be appreciated in all normal subjects.

The palpable LV apical impulse is generally analyzed in terms of its location, area or size, amplitude, duration, and association with a definite presystolic hump ("a" wave) or distention (atrial kick). The apical impulse moving rapidly with a large area (>2 cm) and amplitude is described as "hyperdynamic," and an apical impulse with a longer-than-normal duration is described as "sustained." The hyperdynamic impulse is usually associated with LV volume overload states such as mitral or aortic regurgitation. The sustained impulse is generally associated with LV hypertrophy as seen with hypertension, aortic stenosis, and hypertrophic cardiomyopathy. The extent to which the character of the apical impulse is altered by LV dysfunction in the absence of pressure or volume overload is not clearly known. Although the association between LV dysfunction and sustained apical impulses has been noted, the extent of alteration in relation to different degrees of LV dysfunction has not been demonstrated. The impulse should not exceed the size of a quarter, just rise to tap the fingers, and not be lateral to the midclavicular line in the fifth intercostal space. However, it can exceed these limits on occasion in healthy athletes.

In a clinical study, physical examination and two-dimensional echocardiography were used to determine the relationship between the location of the apex and LV end-diastolic volume [8]. With the patient in the supine position, an apical impulse lateral to the midclavicular line or larger than 10 cm from the midsternal line was sensitive, but not specific, as an indicator of LV enlargement. An apical diameter larger than 3 cm with the patient in the left lateral decubitus position was 90% sensitive and specific for an enlarged LV. The location of the apical impulse in relation to the midclavicular line or the midsternal line was not a reliable indicator of increased LV end-diastolic volume. However, an apical impulse larger than 3 cm was an accurate indicator of LV enlargement.

A similar study was performed in 103 patients referred for ultrafast CT of the heart [9]. The distance of percussion dullness from the midsternal line in the left fourth through sixth intercostal spaces, distance of the apical impulse from the midsternal line, and apical impulse diameter with the patient in the left lateral decubitus position were measured and compared with LV end-diastolic volume, mass, and wall thickness. Percussion dullness distance in the left fifth intercostal space was the best discriminator of LV volume, percussion dullness distance in the left sixth intercostal space was the best discriminator of LV mass, and percussion dullness distance of more than 10.5 cm in the left fifth intercostal space detected increased LV volume and mass with a sensitivity of 91% and a specificity of 30%. In patients in the left lateral decubitus position in whom an impulse was palpated, an apical impulse diameter of more than 3.0 cm detected increased LV volume and mass with a sensitivity of 100% and a specificity of 40%. However, an impulse was palpable in only 53% of patients and the results showed only slight interobserver reproducibility. Percussion of the precordium was concluded to be an accurate and moderately reproducible maneuver for excluding cardiomegaly due to increased LV volume or mass. Although measurement of apical impulse diameter was useful for excluding cardiomegaly, poor reproducibility and lack of a palpable impulse in many patients place limits on its utility in clinical practice.

Parasternal impulses such as lifts or heaves can be associated with right ventricular enlargement. Palpable heart sounds and murmurs (thrills) can also rarely be appreciated.

Auscultation

Cardiac auscultation is experiencing renewed interest because of simple amplification and recording devices [10] and because of its cost-efficiency [11].

Heart Sounds
Below is an outline of the heart sounds:

I. First heart sound—S_1
   a. Mitral and tricuspid valve closure
   b. Sound caused by vibratory motion of valve
   c. Intensity due to
      1. Contractile state of the ventricles
      2. Position of valve leaflets at onset of ventricular systole
      3. Certain disease states (atrial fibrillation, hyperthyroidism)
   d. Intensity patterns
      1. Loud S_1—mitral stenosis (increased LV contractility due to increased end-diastolic pressure)
      2. Faint S_1—decreased LV function
      3. Varying intensity—atrial fibrillation and heart block
   e. Splitting—normal (M_1 and T_1, M_1 loudest); accentuated split with right bundle-branch block, tricuspid valve closure delayed

II. Second heart sound—S_2
   a. Closure of aortic and pulmonic valves and loudest at base
   b. Sound caused by rapid vibrations of valve
   c. Intensity derived from LV and valve condition and blood viscosity
   d. Splitting—normal and wider on inspiration due to decreased pulmonary (physiologic) vascular impedance, which delays pulmonic valve closure, or because of increased preload, which causes longer right ventricular ejection
      1. Delayed P_2 usually accentuated by right bundle-branch block and mitral regurgitation (even wider split on inspiration)
      2. Delayed A_2 usually associated with a paradoxical split—decreased on inspiration, increased expiration—and possibly due to
         a. Mechanical—LV dysfunction, aortic stenosis, or regurgitation
         b. Electrical—left bundle-branch block, Wolff-Parkinson-White syndrome, right ventricle pacemaker
         c. Atrial septal defect with a wide fixed split
   e. Intensity
      1. Soft S_2—aortic stenosis, pulmonic stenosis
      2. Loud S_2—pulmonary hypertension
III. S_3 gallop
   a. Low-frequency sound, early diastole, after S_2—use bell of stethoscope
   b. Sound due to sudden cessation of the distention of the ventricle at end of the rapid filling phase during early diastole; occurs as the ventricle ends relaxation and starts tensing
   c. Determinants of S_3
      1. Stiffness of ventricle
      2. Velocity of inflow (preload)
      3. Completeness of ventricular relaxation
   d. Clinical situations
      1. High velocity of filling—increased atrial pressure, aortic regurgitation, volume overload, high-output states
      2. Resistance to filling due to increased LV stiffness—dilated cardiomyopathy, myocardial fibrosis, large MI, constrictive pericarditis
      3. Very common in bradycardic healthy young aerobic athletes

    4. Common in patients with mitral regurgitation, but do not necessarily reflect LV systolic dysfunction or increased filling pressure

    5. Uncommon in patients with aortic stenosis, but usually indicate the presence of systolic dysfunction and elevated filling pressure

    6. An indicator of LV dysfunction in patients with CHF; if present, the EF is less than 30%; when heard, digoxin is usually effective

IV. S_4 gallop

   a. Ventricular filling sound resulting from atrial contraction in late diastole

   b. Heard when LV end-diastolic pressure (pressure overload) is increased, and is a clue for diastolic dysfunction

   c. Clinical situations—LV hypertrophy due to high BP, aortic stenosis, hypertrophic cardiomyopathy, or CHF

   d. Maneuvers

     1. Squat, hand grip, leg elevation—increased preload and increased S_4

     2. Standing—decreased preload, decreased S_4

   e. Low pitched—use bell of stethoscope

   f. Common in everyone over 50 years old

   g. Most clinically meaningful when a precordial "a" impulse is felt before the "e" wave in the precordial cardiac impulse

TIMING OF CARDIAC SOUNDS.   For a complete listing of the timing of all cardiac sounds, see Table 2-1. Pericardial friction rubs can have up to three components (in relation to the normal atrial and ventricular movements), sound extracardiac, and are best described as similar to the sound of rubbing fingers across a rubber balloon. The rub occurring with atrial contraction in diastole can sometimes be so harsh as to simulate a systolic murmur. Mitral valve clicks can be singular or multiple occurring in midsystole. They are very variable in intensity, being affected by position and volume status of the patient.

THE RULE OF SIXES.   Auscultation of the heart sounds is aided by the "rule of sixes." A_2 and P_2 should separate by 6 msec with inspiration while the subject is sitting, an opening snap of mitral stenosis should follow S_2 by 6 msec, and follow S_3 by another 6 msec. Gallops and opening snaps are best heard over the apex with the subject in the left lat-

Table 2-1.   Timing of Cardiac Sounds

Cardiac Cycle	Sound
Begin systole	S_1
Early systolic	Ejection click
	Aortic prosthetic valve opening sound[a]
Mid/late systolic	Midsystolic click
	Rub
Begin diastole	S_2
Early diastolic	Opening snap
	S_3
	Mitral prosthetic valve opening sound[b]
	Tumor plop[c]
Middiastolic	S_3
	Summation gallop[d]
Late diastolic (sometimes called *presystolic*)	S_4
	Pacemaker sound

[a]Opening and closure of the prosthetic aortic valve are heard with many prosthetic valves. The opening is comparable to an ejection click; the closing is a "prosthetic" S_2.
[b]Opening and closure of the prosthetic mitral valve are heard with many prosthetic valves. The opening is comparable to an opening snap; the closing is a "prosthetic" S_1.
[c]An atrial myxoma that is pedunculated may "plop" in and out of the mitral annulus, simulating the signs of mitral stenosis.
[d]At fast heart rates, the diastolic period shortens. If S_3 and S_4 are present, the sounds may be "summated" into a single sound called a summation gallop.

eral decubitus position. An increased intensity of S_1 is the earliest sign of mitral stenosis and should lead to closer auscultation for this abnormality, including auscultation timed to the carotid pulse after running in place. An increased S_2 occurs with hypertension, but an increased second component along with tachycardia suggests a pulmonary embolus or other lung disease. An S_4 is most often actually a split S_1 and has little prognostic value unless it is accompanied by a presystolic palpable "a" wave kick in the precordial impulse or unless it is brought out by exercise. An S_3 occurring with aortic stenosis is more indicative of LV dysfunction and a poor prognosis than is an S_3 occurring with mitral regurgitation.

The relationship of the heart sounds to the carotids, jugular venous pulse, ECG, and the M-mode echocardiogram is illustrated in Figure 2-3. Figure 2-4 lists the diagnoses suggested by different patterns of the second heart sound's response to respiration.

AUSCULTATION DURING BIGEMINY. A not uncommon error is to be fooled into thinking that the heart sounds from a coupled beat are part of a single contraction. Palpitation

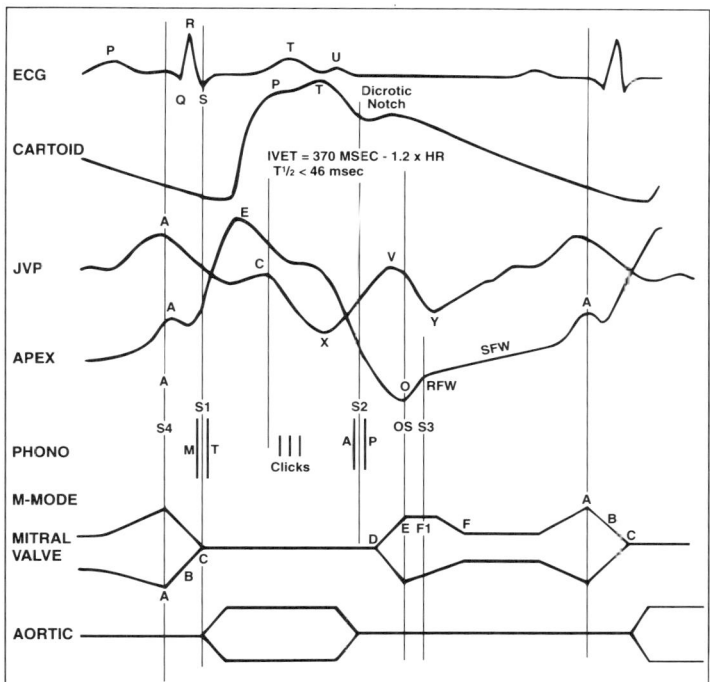

Fig. 2-3.   A modern cardiovascular hemodynamic diagram illustrating the temporal relationship of the cardiac events, including those represented by the valve movements as seen with the M-mode echocardiogram. JVP = jugular venous pulse; apex = apical impulse of the left ventricle; phono = phonocardiography; LVET = left ventricular ejection time.

can sometimes help if the coupled beat is effective as with a premature atrial contraction. However, sometimes an ECG is required to confirm the bigeminy.

MURMURS.   Heart murmurs are caused by noise produced by turbulent blood flow. This can be due to obstruction, increased velocity of flow, or regurgitant flow. Murmurs are described according to their timing (systolic, diastolic, continuous, early, late), location, radiation, quality (harsh, soft, blowing, rumbling), and configuration (crescendo, decrescendo, diamond, plateau). Murmurs are graded, with grade 1 being the faintest with auscultation and grade 6 the loudest heard without a stethoscope.

SYSTOLIC MURMURS.   Systolic murmurs can be classified as either midsystolic ejection or pansystolic regurgitant.

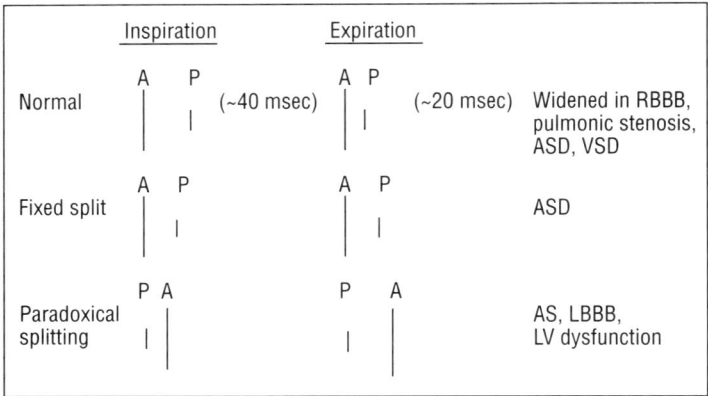

Fig. 2-4.   Auscultation of the second heart sound, showing the normal response of the second heart sound to respiration while the subject is sitting upright. Abnormal movements of the two components of the second heart sound are illustrated for various conditions. RBBB = right bundle-branch block; ASD = atrial septal defect; VSD = ventricular septal defect; AS = aortic stenosis; LBBB = left bundle-branch block; LV = left ventricle.

The midsystolic ejection murmur or aortic overflow is diamond shaped and the intensity is related to peak flow velocity during ejection. Conditions that increase stroke volume such as exercise, long diastolic pause after premature ventricular contraction, or anxiety will increase the intensity whereas conditions that decrease stroke volume (CHF, beta-blockers) will decrease intensity. Examples of this type of murmur are the innocent murmur, systolic ejection murmur due to high cardiac output states (functional), mitral valve prolapse (MVP), aortic stenosis, and hypertrophic cardiomyopathy. Pansystolic regurgitant murmurs are produced by retrograde flow from a high-pressure chamber to a lower-pressure chamber. They are usually holosystolic, high pitched, blowing, and plateau shaped. These murmurs do not vary with cardiac output. Mitral regurgitation is the best example and maneuvers that increase LV pressure (handgrip, squatting) will potentiate the intensity.

Characteristics that can be helpful in separating the two most common forms of systolic murmur are presented in Table 2-2.

DIASTOLIC MURMURS.   Diastolic murmurs are always pathologic and are caused from either structural abnor-

Table 2-2. Differentiation of the Two Most Common Forms of Systolic Murmur

Characteristics of Systolic Murmur	Aortic Outflow Ejection	Mitral Regurgitant
Onset, offset	After S_1, before S_2 (usually mid)	From S_1 to S_2 (throughout or late)
Shape	Diamond	Even
Maximal location	Parasternal, third intercostal space	Apical
Radiation	To neck	To axilla

malities of the atrioventricular (AV) and semilunar valves or increased flow across anatomically normal AV valves. Diastolic filling murmurs cause a rumbling, low-frequency sound. They tend to occur during early and late diastole because of the two phases of rapid ventricular filling (early diastole and presystole). Mitral stenosis is a diastolic rumble that is introduced by an opening snap. Diastolic regurgitant murmurs result from retrograde flow across an incompetent semilunar valve. In aortic regurgitation, a high-pitched blowing murmur results, but fades as the gradient between the two chambers declines.

The patient should always be auscultated in several positions, including the left lateral decubitus position. While sitting, the patient should be instructed to take a deep breath in, to let it out while leaning forward, and then to hold it out. This is an important maneuver to listen for aortic insufficiency. Table 2-3 illustrates the characteristics of the murmurs associated with the most prevalent valvular lesions. The two hardest murmurs to appreciate are mitral stenosis and aortic insufficiency; in fact, they are often missed unless highlighted by clues. *A wide pulse pressure and a loud first heart sound are clues for aortic insufficiency and mitral stenosis, respectively.* If a wide pulse pressure is noted, the patient should be carefully examined while sitting, leaning forward during expiration. This maneuver should also be instituted if the patient has any of the physical findings of aortic insufficiency (hyperdynamic pulse manifestations), if the patient has a systolic murmur (aortic insufficiency often accompanies calcific aortic stenosis and if heard, ensures that the systolic murmur is pathologic and not functional), or if a patient has a prosthetic aortic valve (perivalvular leaks are heard as an aortic insufficiency murmur). If a loud first

Table 2-3. The Major Cardiac Murmurs

Type	Description	Location	Associated Cardiovascular Findings	Maneuvers
Major Systolic Murmurs				
Aortic stenosis	S¹ ——— S² (diamond-shaped murmur)	On diagonal line from aortic area to apical area	Radiates to carotids Decreased carotid pulses (slow upstroke) PMI laterally displaced S₄, if severe Soft, paradox split S₂ Soft S₁	Decrease with Valsalva's maneuver Increase with expiration
Mitral regurgitation	S¹ ——— S² (holosystolic murmur)	Apical area to lower left sternal border	Radiates to axilla Decreased carotids Parasternal heave Possible S₃, S₄ Soft S₁	Increase with handgrip, expiration, and squatting Decrease with standing, Valsalva's maneuver, and inspiration
Mitral valve prolapse	S¹ ——— S² (late systolic murmur with Clicks)	Apical area to lower left sternal border	Radiates to axilla Carotids normal Clicks	Decrease with handgrip, expiration, and squatting Increase with Valsalva's maneuver and standing

Major Diastolic Murmurs

	S_1 S_2			
IHSS		Lower left sternal border	Radiates to carotids PMI laterally displaced S_4 Paradoxically split S_2 Quick carotid upstroke, fast drop off	Increase with Valsalva's maneuver and standing Decrease with squatting and handgrip
Aortic regurgitation		Aortic area, right sternal border	Soft S_1 Paradoxically split S_2 Possible S_3 High-pitched blow	Decrease with Valsalva's maneuver Increase with expiration, squatting, and handgrip
Mitral stenosis		Apical area	Loud S_1 No S_4 Opening snap Low-frequency rumble harsh it sounds systolic	Increase with expiration, handgrip, and exercise Be sure to time systole by carotid pulse because diastolic murmur is so

OS = opening snap; PMI = point of maximal impulse on chest wall over the heart; IHSS = idiopathic hypertrophic subaortic stenosis.

heart sound is noted, or if the patient has a history of rheumatic fever, then the patient should exercise (running in place will suffice) and then be auscultated in the left lateral decubitus position while the carotid artery is palpated. Palpation allows one to appreciate that the mitral rumble is in diastole; its volume is so great that it seems to be occurring in systole. For most people, the rheumatic fever occurred decades ago; therefore, things they may remember are painful, swollen joints and purposeless arm, leg, or tongue movements.

Figure 2-5 summarizes the cardiac physical examination, illustrating the location of the various findings. Keep in mind that the location of murmurs is often "misplaced" in the elderly; that is, an outflow murmur may be loudest toward the apex and a regurgitant mitral murmur may be loudest parasternally.

Physiologic Versus Pathologic S_3 Gallops

Although the S_3 gallop sound has long been used clinically as an indicator of LV systolic dysfunction, the mechanism responsible for its production remains controversial. The same sound is often found in young healthy individuals, and whether a similar mechanism is responsible is also unknown. The relationship of the S_3 gallop sound to the dynamics of LV filling was compared in healthy young athletes and older subjects with cardiac disease [12]. Healthy normal subjects without an S_3 were included as control subjects. Phonocardiographic, two-dimensional echocardiographic, and Doppler echocardiographic analyses of LV inflow were evaluated. The S_3 in both groups always occurred close to peak early filling velocity (E), during early flow deceleration. Mean E deceleration rate was higher in the subjects with an S_3 than in the control subjects. The athletes underwent examination both before and immediately after 30-degree head-up tilt. The E deceleration rate dropped significantly with the head-up tilt, while concurrently the S_3 disappeared or was diminished in amplitude. Similar changes were seen in subjects with cardiac disease. It appears that both the pathologic and physiologic S_3 sounds are related to abnormally rapid deceleration of early diastolic LV inflow. Although the presence of the S_3 is not dependent on the state of LV systolic function, diastolic filling is characterized by a predominance of early inflow with a rapid flow deceleration rate. In clinical practice, the most useful distinction is the accompanying heart rate: the athlete's S_3 occurs

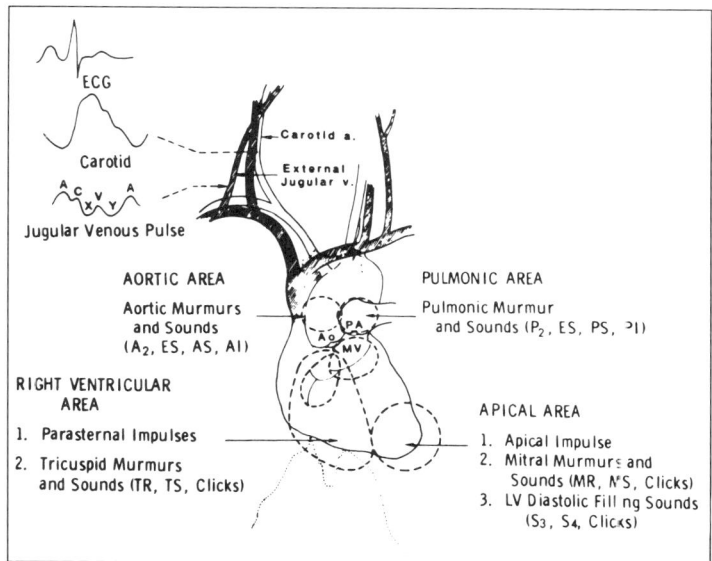

Fig. 2-5. The major aspects of the cardiac examination. TR = tricuspid regurgitation; TS = tricuspid stenosis; LV = left ventricle; AS = aortic stenosis; AR = aortic regurgitation; MS = mitral stenosis; MR = mitral regurgitation; ES = ejection click; PS = pulmonic stenosis; PI = pulmonic insufficiency.

with a bradycardia while a pathologic S_3 occurs with a tachycardia.

Auscultatory Aids

Various aids including respiratory and positional maneuvers, pharmacologic agents, and intrinsic changes in cycle length have been used to assist in cardiac auscultation [13]. These are all summarized in Table 2-4.

RESPIRATION (OR CARVALLO'S MANEUVER).   The murmur of tricuspid regurgitation, occurring with severe right-sided heart failure, usually increases during sleep inspiration, with postinspiratory apnea, or even during normal inspiration in some patients. Respiration has also been used to differentiate right-sided from left-sided murmurs. Right-sided gallops can also be increased with inspiration. Remember that the normal splitting of S_2 with inspiration is most evident in the sitting position and fixed splitting can be normal during the supine position.

HEPATOJUGULAR REFLUX.   The hepatojugular reflux is commonly used for detecting CHF. The first observation

Table 2-4. Effects of Auscultatory Maneuvers

Maneuver	Venous Return (VR), Systemic Vascular Resistance (SVR), Cardiac Output (CO), LV Ejection Velocity (LVEV)	Accentuates	Diminishes
Valsalva's (phase II)	↓ VR →↓ SVR →↓ CO →↑ LVEV	HOCH (IHSS, ASH) Mitral valve prolapse	Mitral regurgitation Aortic stenosis Aortic regurgitation
Inspiration	↑ VR	Tricuspid regurgitation-stenosis Pulmonic stenosis Pulmonic regurgitation	Mitral regurgitation
Expiration	→↓ VR ← Pulmonary venous return	Mitral stenosis Mitral regurgitation Aortic regurgitation Aortic stenosis	Mitral valve prolapse Tricuspid regurgitation
Squatting	↑ VR ←↑ SVR ←↑ CO	Mitral regurgitation Pulmonic flow murmur Tricuspid stenosis (? regurgitation) Aortic regurgitation	HOCM (IHSS, ASH) Mitral valve prolapse

Maneuver	Physiologic change	Increases murmur intensity	Decreases murmur intensity
Standing	↓ VR, ↓ CO, ↓ LVEV	HOCM (IHSS, ASH) Mitral valve prolapse	Tricuspid regurgitation Pulmonic flow murmurs Mitral regurgitation HOCM (IHSS, ASH)
Handgrip	↑ SVR, ↑ CO	Mitral regurgitation Ventricular septal defect Aortic regurgitation Mitral stenosis	HOCM (IHSS, ASH)
Post PVC (long RR interval)	↓ SVR, ↑ LVEV	HOCM (IHSS, ASH) Aortic stenosis	No change mitral regurgitation
Amyl nitrite	↑ VR, ↓ SVR, ↓ LV volume, ↑ LVEV	Mitral stenosis Mitral valve prolapse HOCM (IHSS, ASH) Aortic stenosis Pulmonic stenosis-regurgitation Tricuspid stenosis-regurgitation	Aortic regurgitation Mitral regurgitation Ventricular septal defect

HOCM = hypertrophic obstructive cardiomyopathy (also known as IHSS = idiopathic hypertrophic subaortic stenosis or ASH = asymmetric septal hypertrophy); PVC = premature ventricular contraction.

of the effect of abdominal compression on the filling of the neck veins was reported by Pasteur in 1885 as a manifestation of tricuspid regurgitation. This technique augments the tricuspid regurgitation murmur, especially in conjunction with passive leg raising. In applying hepatojugular reflux, the examiner should exert firm, sustained pressure inward and cephalad below the right costal margin. The patient should breathe normally so as to avoid an inadvertent Müller or Valsalva maneuver. A positive response is an increase in the height of the jugular venous pulse. The failing right ventricle is unable to receive the increased preload without increasing venous pressure.

Because hepatojugular reflux and Carvallo's sign (i.e., increase with inspiration) do not occur in normal patients, they have a specificity of 100%. Nearly all patients had a positive response to one or the other maneuver (combined sensitivity, 93%). Thus, an increase in a murmur with hepatojugular reflux or with inspiration is helpful in the diagnosis of tricuspid regurgitation.

MÜLLER'S MANEUVER.   Müller's maneuver (deep inspiratory effort against a closed glottis) decreases intrathoracic pressure increasing both venous return and right ventricular stroke volume. The increased venous return and the consequent increased right ventricular stroke volume may be associated with an increase in the intensity of right-sided heart murmurs. Also, the increase in LV transmural pressure may be associated with a decrease in the outflow gradient across the aortic valve in patients with asymmetric septal hypertrophic cardiomyopathy (ASH).

VALSALVA'S MANEUVER.   During Valsalva's maneuver, venous return is decreased so that LV volume declines. This should cause the murmur of ASH or IHSS to increase while all other systolic murmurs should decrease. Valsalva's maneuver also has been used to distinguish left-sided from right-sided murmurs because after release of this maneuver, left-sided heart murmurs take longer than right-sided ones to recover their maximal intensity.

SQUATTING.   Prompt squatting causes a sharp increase in venous return, which may increase the intensity of most cardiac murmurs except for the systolic murmur of ASH. The ASH murmur should diminish because the increase in LV volume reduces the degree of dynamic outflow obstruction. Squatting also increases the peripheral arterial resistance, which should increase the intensity of aortic insufficiency and mitral regurgitation murmurs.

STANDING.   Prompt standing has been recommended to evaluate both ASH and MVP. Rapid standing causes an initial decrease in the stroke volume secondary to venous pooling; thus, a decrease in the murmurs of aortic or pulmonic stenosis and of mitral or tricuspid regurgitation should occur. In contrast, decreased LV chamber size may increase obstruction and be associated with an increase in the intensity of the murmur of ASH. In MVP, a decrease in LV volume while standing may accentuate the degree of mitral prolapse, increasing the intensity and duration of the murmur.

ISOMETRIC HANDGRIP EXERCISE.   Isometric exercise is a sustained muscle contraction that maintains the same muscle length. Handgrip causes an increase in heart rate, systolic and diastolic BPs, and cardiac output. The use of handgrip to differentiate aortic stenosis from mitral regurgitation presumes that an increase in LV afterload will increase that degree of regurgitation, but this is not a consistent finding.

CYCLE LENGTH.   Changes in cardiac cycle length can be an aid in distinguishing aortic outflow murmurs (increase after long diastole) from mitral regurgitation (no change with variable cycle length). Variations in cycle length cause several hemodynamic alterations in patients with atrial fibrillation and aortic stenosis. After longer cycle lengths, LV outflow gradient increases. The intensity of the aortic stenosis murmur, in turn, varies directly with the amplitude of the LV-aortic pressure gradient. After long cycle lengths in patients with ASH, LV systolic pressure increases and arterial pressure decreases, causing an increase in the LV-aortic pressure gradient. Also, longer cycle lengths are associated with increased contractility that increases the obstruction with ASH.

AMYL NITRITE.   Amyl nitrite causes a decrease in vascular resistance and systemic arterial pressure, as well as a reflex increase in heart rate, LV ejection velocity, and cardiac output. Systemic arterial pressure drops within the first 15 to 30 seconds of inhalation. Subsequently, there is a reflex tachycardia and increases in both cardiac output and venous return. The decrease in systemic vascular resistance reduces the impedance to forward flow out of the LV, thus lessening regurgitant blood flow. Therefore, left-sided regurgitant murmurs due to aortic insufficiency, mitral regurgitation, or ventricular septal defect (with a left-to-right shunt) should decrease with amyl nitrite. The reflex tachycardia and the increases in LV ejection velocity and pressure gradient may contribute to an increase in the LV outflow murmurs of valvular aortic stenosis and ASH. The increases in heart rate and venous return with amyl nitrite can accentuate right-sided murmurs and mitral stenosis. The murmur of aortic stenosis should increase in intensity, whereas the murmur of mitral regurgitation should decrease with amyl nitrite administration.

**Conclusions: Who Should See
a Cardiologist for a Murmur?**
Despite the tradition surrounding these aids for cardiac auscultation, their diagnostic efficacy is limited. While a practitioner can "look good" when the echocardiogram corroborates his or her hypothesis based on the findings using these maneuvers, the echocardiogram will just as often prove him or her wrong. Many of the aids help to differentiate and recognize rare abnormalities in the outpatient setting though, affecting your threshold for ordering echocardiography.

Patients with hypertrophic cardiomyopathies including ASH and IHSS, which have associated mitral regurgitation and outflow obstruction, have murmurs that vary greatly from examination to examination because of changes in vascular volume, positions, and sympathetic tone. *Such patients always need cardiology follow-up because it is difficult to control their symptoms and to judge prognosis. Therefore, a patient with any systolic murmur that increases with Valsalva's maneuver requires referral. Any diastolic murmur is pathologic and requires referral. A patient with any holosystolic murmur requires referral as well as one with any loud systolic murmur accompanied by delayed, abnormal carotid pulses.*

Remember to carefully listen for aortic insufficiency by having the patient exhale and lean forward and hold out his or her breath when there is a wide pulse pressure or any physical findings of aortic insufficiency, when subacute bacterial endocarditis is suspected, when a systolic ejection murmur is present, or when the patient has a prosthetic aortic valve.

A patient with aortic regurgitation findings should be referred to a cardiologist. A functional murmur thus is an isolated systolic murmur without any of the above-mentioned associated findings and it usually does not require referral.

HISTORY AND PHYSICAL EXAMINATION
FOR THE KEY FEATURES (SEE APPENDIX F)
History for Myocardial Dysfunction
Historical Features of Myocardial Dysfunction

A definite history of MI suggests some degree of myocardial dysfunction. However, the damage can be minimal if Q waves or other ECG abnormalities are not present. Multiple infarcts or large infarctions complicated by shock or CHF clearly indicate considerable loss of ventricular muscle, which leads to myocardial dysfunction. Also, a history of hypertension, myocarditis, or alcoholism would support a diagnosis of myocardial dysfunction. In general, individuals who have had a true episode of CHF also have some degree of myocardial dysfunction. One must be careful because bouts of pneumonia or other respiratory problems are often called CHF, particularly in the elderly. Other conditions that can simulate CHF are right ventricular infarction, constrictive pericarditis, and cardiac tamponade.

Patients can present with right-sided symptoms, left-sided symptoms, or biventricular failure. Right-sided symptoms are caused by venous congestion, which causes the patient to present with peripheral edema, abdominal swelling, ascites, abdominal discomfort, and nausea. Because of decreased myocardial performance, left-sided symptoms are primarily due to low cardiac output. Heart rate rises, fluid retention occurs, and poor perfusion persists. Patients complain of DOE, PND, orthopnea, cough, nocturia, night sweats, fatigue, lethargy, weight gain, and disorientation. The practitioner should identify whether symptoms are new or chronic. If they are chronic, questions should be directed at identifying the severity of the exacerbation and its time frame.

In dilated cardiomyopathy, the myocardium has been damaged from ischemia, chronic overload, or scarring or myocyte damage secondary to numerous processes. This causes the LV to dilate, resulting in a low cardiac output and a large end-diastolic volume. The most common cause of dilated cardiomyopathy is MI (ischemic cardiomyopathy). Other causes include alcohol abuse, previous viral infection, diabetes mellitus, and unknown factors (idiopathic). Myocardial damage can also occur from toxins, infections, autoimmune responses, and antitumor drugs. Contractility can be suppressed by beta-blockers, calcium antagonists, or antiarrhythmics like disopyramide (Norpace). Both the type of cardiomyopathy and the age of the diagnosis are important. Noncompliance with medication regimen, increased sodium and fluid intake, and overmedication can cause an exacerbation of heart failure symptoms.

In contrast to systolic dysfunction, diastolic dysfunction occurs with a normal-size heart that is stiff due to an infiltrative process or hypertrophy causing an increased end-diastolic pressure and limited filling. Cardiac tamponade can simulate CHF but this is usually an acute presentation of an enlarged cardiac silhouette, increased neck veins, distant heart sounds, and falling BP without rales or other signs of pulmonary edema. It usually follows a viral upper respiratory tract infection or occurs in a patient with a malignancy or chronic renal failure.

Cardiac Versus Pulmonary Causes of Dyspnea
The spectrum and frequency of diseases presenting as unexplained dyspnea can be used to develop a logical diagnostic approach to such patients [14]. Seventy-two consecutive physician-referred patients had dyspnea for more than 1 month unexplained by the initial history, physical examination, chest x-ray, and spirometry findings [15]. Patients underwent a standard diagnostic evaluation. A definite cause for dyspnea was recognized in 58 patients, and no answer was found in 14. Twenty-two diseases were recognized in the patient group. Dyspnea was due to pulmonary disease in 26 (36%) patients, cardiac disease in 10 (14%), hyperventilation in 14 (19%), and extrathoracic disease in only 3 (4%). Miscellaneous causes were found in 5 (7%) patients. Age younger than 40 years, intermittent dyspnea, and normal alveolar-arterial oxygen pressure difference $(P(\text{A-a})O_2)$ at rest breathing room air were strongly predictive of bronchial hyperreactivity or hyperventilation. No patient diagnosed as having disease of the lung parenchyma or vasculature had a $P(\text{A-a})O_2$ less than or equal to 20 mm Hg.

The differential diagnosis to explain dyspnea in patients with nondirective histories, normal findings from physical examinations, normal-appearing chest x-ray films, and normal spirograms is extensive. The patient's age and pulmonary function at rest help to formulate a diagnostic approach. Correctable causes such as hypersensitivity and allergic pulmonary reactions definitely should not be missed, so clearly diffusion capacity should be measured. If the pulmonary function is normal except for diffusion capacity, hypersensitivity or allergic pulmonary reactions should be considered as causes. The conditions can be reversed by a course of steroids, stopping a medication such as nitrofurantoin (Furadantin), or removing some pollutant or allergen from the patient's environment. Both cardiac and pulmonary disease can often be present, making the diagnosis and treatment more difficult.

Physical Examination for Myocardial Dysfunction
Any or all of the signs of CHF usually indicate myocardial dysfunction. An abnormal precordial movement is one of the best markers. A large dilated heart with a diffuse precordial movement and a parasternal lift suggest dilated cardiomyopathy. Weak carotid pulses and neck vein distention are also signs of poor myocardial function. Patients with dilated cardiomyopathy can present with tachypnea, tachycardia, and decreased BP with a narrow pulse pressure. Paradoxical pulse (greater-than-normal drop in systolic BP with inspiration, i.e., >10 mm Hg) can occur due to low cardiac output, and pulsus alternans (alternating strength of the pulse waves) may be present. Carotid pulses will be diminished due to low stroke volume. Jugular neck vein distention with probable positive hepatojugular reflux, accompanied by weight gain and lower edema, indicates worsening heart failure. If tricuspid regurgitation is present, V waves may be visible in the jugular venous pulse. Possible heart sound changes include a soft S_1, S_3, S_4, and a systolic murmur of mitral regurgitation or tricuspid regurgitation. Rales and possibly effusions due to fluid overload can be present. Ascites, right-upper-quadrant tenderness, and hepatomegaly can be present, depending on the degree of right-sided symptoms. Often right and left ventricular failure can be distinguished by physical examination; however, it is very common to see biventricular failure. On the basis of ischemia alone, bouts of CHF are possible and indicate considerable muscle in jeopardy.

Right and left ventricular failure should be distinguished by physical examination. Right ventricular involvement means that the lungs have succumbed to elevated LV filling pressure and increased right-sided (pulmonary artery) pressure. Elevated jugular venous pressure, positive hepatojugular reflux, peripheral edema, and an S_3 heard best on inspiration, but without rales or weakened pulses, suggest pure right ventricular dysfunction. On the other hand, rales, a consistent S_3, weak pulses, and abnormal precordial movements are consistent with LV dysfunction. However, biventricular failure or dysfunction must always be considered.

The sensitivity, specificity, and utility of the cardiovascular examination in predicting cardiac hemodynamics in patients with advanced chronic CHF have been investigated [16]. The history, the cardiovascular physical signs present at bedside examination, and the hemodynamic measurements obtained by right-sided heart catheterization in 52 patients with chronic CHF undergoing in-hospital evaluation for possible heart transplantation were recorded. In addition, chest radiographs and multigated nuclear scans for the evaluation of LV function were obtained. Pulmonary rales, a LV third heart sound, jugular venous distention, and a positive result on the hepatojugular test indicated higher right-sided heart pressures and lower measures of cardiac performance. The presence of jugular venous distention, at rest or inducible, had the best combination of sensitivity, specificity, and predictive accuracy (about 80%) for elevation of the pulmonary capillary wedge pressure (≥18 mm Hg). The probability of an elevated wedge pressure was very high when either variable was present.

The most common clinical occurrence of isolated diastolic dysfunction is when systolic dysfunction is in a compensated state due to treatment. The main characteristic of diastolic dysfunction is that cardiac size is not increased and, while right-sided symptoms are less prominent than with systolic dysfunction, the other physical findings of CHF can be present.

Lungs Versus Heart—Forced Expiratory Time

Since COPD is frequently confused clinically with CHF, clarification of differential physical findings of pulmonary disease by the physical examination would be helpful. While hyperresonance and a low diaphragm can be subjective markers, forced expiration can be standardized by timing. To evaluate the test characteristics of forced expiratory time (FET) in the diagnosis of obstructive airway disease, more than 400 subjects were evaluated by a physician and the results were compared with the spirometric findings [17]. The highest number of subjects with obstructive airway disease were correctly diagnosed using the FET maneuver with a cutoff value of 6 seconds. The FET maneuver was more discriminating for subjects 60 years or older than for younger subjects. The positive likelihood ratio for COPD when the FET was 4 to 6 seconds was low, whereas when the FET was 6 to 8 seconds the likelihood was doubled and when the FET was greater than 8 seconds COPD was four times as likely. *In clinical practice, the distinction between the heart and the lungs as the cause of DOE is usually easily resolved by the physical examination and pulmonary function testing including diffusion capacity.*

Estimations of Ejection Fraction
To determine whether a simpler method of evaluating ejection fractions was reliable, nuclear-derived ejection fractions were compared with those estimated by a cardiologist's examination of 125 hospitalized patients [18]. Of the physician estimates, 56% were accurate to within 7.5%, while 17% were underestimates and 27% were overestimates. The variables that were most predictive of reduced LV ejection fraction included cardiomegaly and pulmonary venous congestion on chest x-ray films and S_3 gallop, hypotension, and sustained LV apex beat on examination. Prior hypertension was correlated with an increased LV ejection fraction. Variables associated with physician error in LV ejection fraction estimation included a history of hypertension, bronchodilator therapy, and right bundle-branch block seen on the ECG.

Presentation of CHF: Systolic Versus Diastolic Dysfunction
It is important to recognize symptomatic heart failure with preserved LV systolic function. To determine its frequency and identify clinical features that make the bedside diagnosis likely, patients admitted for decompensated heart failure were classified by echocardiographic results [19]. Female gender and diastolic BP higher than 105 mm Hg predominated in those with normal systolic function and CHF. Jugular venous distention was identified more frequently in those with systolic dysfunction. No other differences were noted in age, duration of symptoms, history of hypertension, ischemic heart disease, and heavy alcohol drinking or physical findings. The combination of diastolic BP higher than 105 mm Hg and an absence of jugular venous distention had a high specificity and positive predictive value for identifying CHF patients with normal systolic function (i.e., CHF due to diastolic dysfunction).

The Framingham Criteria for CHF
The subjectivity of the clinical diagnosis of CHF can be lessened by using standardized criteria. The Framingham criteria for CHF consist of a listing of historical and physical findings; a definitive diagnosis of CHF relies on the concurrent presence of two major or one major and two

minor criteria. The **major criteria** include PND or orthopnea, neck vein distention, rales, cardiomegaly, acute pulmonary edema, S_3, and hepatojugular reflux. The minor **criteria** include ankle edema, night cough, DOE, hepatomegaly, pleural effusion, and tachycardia of more than 120 bpm.

Confounders of Myocardial Dysfunction

PERICARDIAL EFFUSION. A pericardial effusion is frequently found in the setting of CHF. It can also be a confounder of the diagnosis of CHF and lead to cardiac tamponade. Cardiac tamponade can simulate CHF but usually is an acute presentation of an enlarged cardiac silhouette, increased neck veins, distant heart sounds, and falling BP without rales or other signs of pulmonary edema. It usually follows a viral upper respiratory tract infection or occurs in a patient with a malignancy or chronic renal failure.

The following etiologies must be considered:

1. Serous effusate: CHF (which is the most common cause), radiation, virus, tuberculosis, bacteria
2. Blood effusate (hematocrit > 10%): iatrogenic (cardiac operation or catheterization, trauma, anticoagulation, chemotherapy), neoplasm, trauma, acute MI, cardiac rupture, rupture of aorta or artery, coagulopathy, uremia
3. Lymph or chyle effusate: neoplasm, iatrogenic (cardiothoracic surgery), congenital, idiopathic, nonneoplastic obstruction of thoracic duct

RADIATION HEART DISEASE. Radiation heart disease can be a confounder of the diagnosis of CHF. In the earlier days of radiation therapy, the major dose was delivered to the skin. Now with the linear accelerator, megavoltage x-rays spare the skin and larger doses hit the deeper structures, including the heart. Radiation therapy is being widely used in the treatment of Hodgkin's disease and lung and breast cancers.

Most of what is known about the histopathology of radiation damage comes from animal models (rabbits). There are three stages. The acute phase occurs within a few days, involving all three layers of the heart. Neutrophilic infiltrates with inflammation around small and medium-size arterioles are seen. During the latent phase, no clinical signs are apparent until 2 to 3 months later. There is evidence of damage to the capillary endothelial cells, with extensive division, with a 45% net reduction in the ratio of capillary cells to myocytes. The delayed phase is seen 3 to 12 months after therapy; there are isolated reports of presentation up to several years later.

In humans, acute pericarditis occurring during treatment can be associated with pleuritic chest pain, pericardial friction rub, fever, and effusions. It is seen most commonly in patients with tumors contiguous to the heart, and therefore may be due to a reaction to tumor necrosis rather than to the radiation itself. These patients respond to a short hiatus from therapy and no deaths have been reported.

The delayed acute phase is seen in a reported 3 to 30% of patients being treated for Hodgkin's disease. Fever, chest pain, and a rub may be seen. The chest x-ray film may show a widened cardiac silhouette and pleural effusion. ECG may show diminished QRS voltage and nonspecific ST abnormalities. Most patients recover by treatment with aspirin, nonsteroidal anti-inflammatory drugs (NSAIDs), or steroids. Some progress to tamponade, which is more common than progression to constrictive pericarditis. Both tamponade and constrictive pericarditis cause dyspnea, orthopnea, tachycardia, and hepatic engorgement, and must be distinguished from each other by physical examination, Swan-Ganz catheterization, and echocardiography.

A pericardial effusion presenting months to years after treatment may present a diagnostic dilemma in that differentiation from recurrent tumor can be difficult. Chronic pericardial effusions are usually benign and asymptomatic.

Pancarditis was usually due to poor techniques or attempts to retreat Hodgkin's disease patients. The consequences were severe restrictive cardiomyopathy with intractable cardiac failure. The chest x-ray film revealed a small cardiac silhouette and echocardiography showed decreased LV end-diastolic volume and ejection fraction. There was no effective treatment for this disease. Also in the past, a subclinical cardiomyopathy was seen by a diminished ejection fraction; this is no longer a risk with current therapy techniques. Conduction system defects such as left atrial P-wave abnormalities, decreased QRS voltage (associated often with effusions), intraventricular conduction defects, and an increased incidence of right bundle-branch block in those receiving mantle radiation for Hodgkin's disease do occur but have no clinical significance.

There is a higher incidence of coronary disease in patients who receive radiation treatment, because of intimal proliferation and endothelial damage caused by the radiation.

ATHLETES' HEART SYNDROME.   Some of the loudest third heart sounds heard are in healthy aerobically trained athletes, such as distance runners, bicyclers, and swimmers. These athletes often also have laterally displaced, hyperdynamic cardiac impulses and functional systolic murmurs. Their ECGs can also exhibit LV hypertrophy, right bundle-branch block, right-axis deviation, and early repolarization or T-wave inversion. This syndrome is not indicative of disease but can often be mistaken for hypertrophic cardiomyopathy (refer to Chapter 5). Nonaerobically trained athletes, such as weightlifters, do not experience such changes but may develop concentric cardiac hypertrophy.

History for Myocardial Ischemia

The history of classic angina pectoris has a high probability for underlying significant coronary artery disease. Angina pectoris is usually described as a pain, though some patients will deny having pain and instead only admit to a pressure or strange sensation or discomfort substernally. It is usually brought on by exercise, but variations are walk-through angina, which lessens after an initial warm-up phase, and pain that occurs within 3 to 4 minutes after exercise. It also can be brought on by anger or emotional upset. It is usually worse after meals, in the morning, and in the cold. Other historical items increasing the probability of the presence of myocardial ischemia include past MI, coronary artery bypass grafting, or percutaneous transluminal coronary angioplasty. While an infarction usually is complete and does not leave muscle in jeopardy, this is not so in about a third of the survivors, and though procedural revascularization can be complete, there can be residual ischemia. Establishing the frequency, duration, timing, and stability of angina is critical for its management. Review of the family history for coronary disease, risk factors, and associated vascular problems including Raynaud's syndrome and claudication can increase the suspicion for coronary disease and myocardial ischemia. Aortic stenosis can cause angina due to myocardial ischemia without atherosclerosis.

Angina

Angina pectoris is a syndrome first described by John Heberden in the eighteenth century. He experienced it but his angina was due to syphilitic aortitis rather than coronary atherosclerosis. The words originate from the Greek meaning "seizure of the chest." Realizing that anger brought it on, he said, "My life is in the hands of any scoundrel who raises my ire." True to his words, he died after an argument.

The following list gives the standard definitions for types of angina.

1. *Typical angina* pectoris is chest pain or a pressure/squeezing sensation located in the substernal area, brought on by exertion or anger, lasting constantly for 2 to 15 minutes and relieved by rest or NTG. It is aggravated by cigarette smoking, cold weather, or a heavy meal. It is associated with a high probability for the presence of obstructive coronary artery disease. The Coronary Angiography and Surgery Study (CASS) classification of *definite angina* is comparable to this.

2. *Atypical angina* is present when the presenting symptoms do not include all the classic features of angina, for instance, a location of the pain or sensation other than substernal (neck, jaw, teeth). Dyspnea or epigastric pain as part of atypical angina is sometimes called an anginal equivalent. The CASS classification of *probable angina* is comparable to this.

3. *Unstable angina* occurs when there is increased coronary arterial obstruction due to thrombus formation or plaque rupture defined as (a) rest angina, (b) new angina (recent onset), or (c) angina of increased frequency or severity.

4. *Rest angina* is angina occurring at rest, either due to increased arterial obstruction (unstable angina) or coronary arterial spasm (variant angina).

UNSTABLE ANGINA AND VARIANT ANGINA. Angina at rest implies unstable angina or variant angina. The Braunwald classification of unstable angina has been shown to have prognostic power. Subgroups are based on four categories: severity, clinical circumstances, ECG changes (present or not), and intensity of treatment. Severity classes are as follows: I—accelerated or new onset without pain at rest, II—angina at rest but not within the last 48 hours (subacute at rest), and III—angina at rest within the last 48 hours (acute at rest). Clinical circumstances are categorized as follows: A—secondary to extracardiac condition, B—absence of noncardiac condition, and C—after an MI. Intensity of treatment ranged from none or one antianginal agent (minimal) to including intravenous nitrates (maximal). For the severity category, prognosis was best for class II, intermediate for class I, and worst for class III. In a Dutch study, prognosis was surprisingly good with medical management [20].

Variant angina is a relatively rare syndrome related to coronary artery spasm. The chest pains usually occur at rest. They are often cyclic, occurring at the same time of day. The angina is also frequently marked by ST-segment elevation (or depression) and dysrhythmias, including heart block and even ventricular tachycardia. The spasm can occur in normal coronary vessels or in proximity to fixed lesions. Unstable angina and variant angina are two higher-risk forms of myocardial ischemia.

ROSE QUESTIONNAIRE.   The Rose Questionnaire was developed for epidemiologic studies but the many studies of its validity showed it to be a useful diagnostic tool. The diagnosis of angina pectoris using the Rose Questionnaire requires the patient to answer the following questions:

Questions	Answers		
1. Have you ever had any pain or discomfort in your chest?	Yes	No	
2. Do you get it when you walk uphill or hurry?	Yes	No	Never hurry
3. Do you get it when you walk at an ordinary pace on the level?	Yes	No	
4. What do you do if you get it while you are walking?	Stop or slow down	Carry on	
5. If you stand still, what happens to it?	Relieved	Not relieved	
6. How soon?	10 minutes or less	More than 10 minutes	
7. Will you show me where it was?	Sternum (upper or middle)	Sternum (lower)	
	Left anterior chest	Left arm	Other
8. Do you feel it anywhere else?	Yes	No	

Questions	Answers
9. Did you see a doctor because of this pain (or discomfort)?	Yes No
10. If yes, what did he say it was?	

The following responses to questions 1 through 6 indicate a diagnosis of angina pectoris:

1, 2, or 3. Yes
4. Stop or slow down
5. Relieved
6. 10 minutes or less

PROGNOSIS. Clinical measures of ischemia can predict infarct-free survival in patients with angina and angiographic coronary artery disease. In the study by Califf et al [21] the following variables were chosen in descending order of predictive power: more than 1 mm of resting ST-segment depression or T-wave inversion, frequency of angina, unstable angina, typical angina, and duration of symptoms. An angina score was derived from the Cox coefficients and when entered into a model with catheterization data, the following variables were chosen in descending order of ability to predict survival: ejection fraction, number of diseased vessels, left main coronary artery stenosis, angina score, and age and sex. This score helped predict prognosis even when the catheterization data were considered. Figure 2-6, considering these simple variables, can be used to estimate infarct-free survival in patients with coronary disease and angina.

Pericarditis—A Confounder for Myocardial Ischemia
Pericarditis can be the cause of a rather frightening pain. However, it is usually sharp and related to respiration and position, which distinguishes it from angina. A frequent physical finding is a pericardial friction rub. Since pericarditis can be a confounder of angina, the following causes of pericarditis must be considered in the patient's chest pain history: infections (viral, bacterial, tuberculous, fungal, parasitic), neoplasm (primary pericardial tumors, metastatic or contiguous spread from extracardiac neoplasms), radiation-induced injury, uremia, rheumatic fever, autoimmune diseases (rheumatoid arthritis, systemic lupus erythematosus, scleroderma), acute MI, autoimmune cardiac injury, Dressler's syndrome, post-

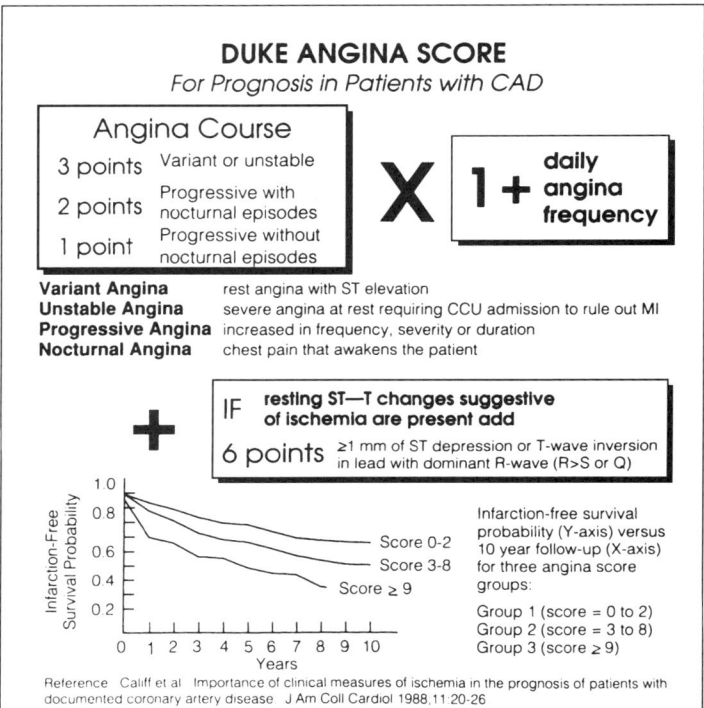

**Fig. 2-6.   The Duke Clinical Ischemia Prognostic Score. CAD =
coronary artery disease; MI = myocardial infarction.**

pericardiotomy syndrome, trauma and iatrogenic injury
(cardiac   catheterization,   pacemaker   penetration),
pseudoaneurysm rupture, dissecting aortic aneurysm,
anticoagulants, drugs (procainamide, hydralazine, isoniazid, penicillin, methysergide, daunorubicin), myxedema,
cholesterol pericarditis, and chylopericardium.

In the outpatient setting, the most common presentations of pericarditis are in association with viral illnesses,
malignancies, and renal disease. Often groupings of occurrences of pericarditis will occur with a particular strain of
viral pneumonia. A confusing form can occur a month or
two after an MI has occurred, and can cause dysphagia or
simulate ischemic pain. The pain of pericarditis is nicely
controlled with ibuprofen and other NSAIDs. Remember
that pericarditis is frequently recurrent, suggesting that
often it is an autoimmune process or that tissue damage
occurs and results in relapses of the inflammation.

Physical Examination for Myocardial Ischemia
The best chest pain history can often be obtained when ischemia occurs during the physical examination. Also Levine's sign may only be appreciated at that time (i.e., when the patient describes the pain with a squeezing closed left fist). Typical myocardial ischemia is most frequently associated with a sympathetic release, and therefore patients rarely exhibit indifference on its occurrence. The pain causes a person to lie still rather than to squirm. Xanthelasma and tendon xanthoma are markers of familial hypercholesterolemia, which increases the probability of coronary artery disease. Signs of PVD such as bruits also imply that the coronaries are diseased. Earlobe creases and premature arcus senilis are not strongly associated with coronary heart disease. Gallops, papillary muscle dysfunction, and bulges can sometimes be appreciated during acute ischemia.

History for Valvular Heart Disease
A history of rheumatic fever alerts the physician to the possibility of rheumatic heart disease. The physician should inquire about the usual findings of rheumatic fever (e.g., painful joints) as well as identify purposeless movements of the arms and legs or tongue. Due to its frightening nature, this manifestation of the disease tends to hold a prominent place in patients' memories. The finding (Syndeham's chorea) is highly specific for acute rheumatic fever. Patients should be questioned for murmurs observed during screening for the military or for sports. Other etiologies include Marfan's syndrome and degenerative, congenital, calcific, and autoimmune diseases. A history of intravenous drug usage should be sought. Secondary causes of valvular disease include a torn chordae tendineae, papillary muscle dysfunction, and valve root dilation causing tricuspid, mitral, or aortic regurgitation.
    Episodes of syncope, angina, and CHF may be associated with aortic stenosis. Episodes of irregular heart beat could result from atrial fibrillation or ventricular ectopy due to valvular disease. Fatigue and dyspnea on exertion are associated with the CHF that comes with decompensated valvular disease.

Physical Examination for Valvular Heart Disease
The classic auscultatory findings of valvular disorders are illustrated in Table 2-3. An abnormal precordial movement is often helpful for identifying the patient whose

heart has hypertrophied or dilated in response to the valvular lesion. Also, a parasternal lift may indicate right-sided heart involvement.

The presence of third heart sound in patients with valvular heart disease is often regarded as a sign of heart failure, but its meaning depends on the type of valvular disease present. The prevalence of third heart sound is higher in patients with mitral regurgitation (46%) or with aortic regurgitation (28%) than in those with aortic stenosis (11%) or mitral stenosis (8%) [22]. *The LV ejection fraction is lower when third heart sound is detected in patients with aortic stenosis or mixed aortic valve disease. However, the ejection fraction is only slightly lower in patients with mitral regurgitation and third heart sound.* The pulmonary capillary wedge pressure is higher in patients with aortic stenosis who have third heart sound. There is no association between the wedge pressure and third heart sound in patients with mitral regurgitation. The prevalence of third heart sound increases with the severity of mitral regurgitation. In patients with mitral regurgitation, third heart sound is common but does not necessarily reflect LV systolic dysfunction or increased filling pressure. In patients with aortic stenosis, third heart sound is uncommon but usually indicates the presence of systolic dysfunction and elevated filling pressure.

History for Poor Exercise Capacity
Patients will present with varying complaints of symptoms that affect functional capacity, most commonly angina, fatigue, dyspnea, claudication, and decreased exercise tolerance. General activity undertaken either daily or weekly should be reviewed, including the frequency of exercise, the speed of the activity, and the time needed for completion. The practitioner should identify a pattern change indicating a decreased functional capacity and note the limiting factor. Lifestyle patterns such as dietary consumption, fluid intake, tobacco use, and alcohol intake must be reviewed. Occupational history should include exertion and type of activity required. As functional status can be altered by other illnesses beside cardiac disease, neuromuscular disease including stroke, muscular sclerosis, arthritis, and other general problems including COPD and obesity should be identified for differential or contributing diagnoses.

Though possibly confused by patients who exaggerate or deny having symptoms, a history of the usual levels of daily activity provides a good estimate of the patient's exercise capacity. Specific questions relating to work, climbing stairs, and recreational activities give a rough estimate of the functional capacity. From another point of view, the patient is as functional as need be if he or she is satisfied by the curent level of activities.

One of the major potential shortcomings of the older functional classifications (New York Heart Association [NYHA] functional classification and the Canadian Cardiovascular Society classification of angina pectoris, see Tables C-1 and C-2 in Appendix C) is their reliance on what is referred to as ordinary activity. The definition of ordinary activity might change as a patient's disease progresses; the patient becomes accustomed to progressively more limitations, and thus voluntarily restricts and reduces "ordinary" activities so as to reduce symptoms. Because of the shortcomings of the functional classification systems, Goldman et al [23] devised the Specific Activity Scale (SAS) (see Table C-3 in Appendix C). The SAS is based on precise questions that refer to activities requiring known amounts of metabolic equivalents of oxygen consumption. Patients are categorized in the class that corresponds to the most strenuous activity that they can perform to completion, regardless of whether or not symptoms may be provoked.

The SAS appears to have several distinct advantages over previous classification systems. First, it has a significantly higher interobserver reproducibility than does the NYHA classification system, and it is significantly more predictive of objective exercise performance by treadmill testing than either the NYHA classification system or the Canadian system. Second, reliance on the precise questions in the SAS corrects a bias in the NYHA system. By relying on objective criteria rather than on the subjective definition of ordinary activity or degree of compromise, the SAS more accurately estimates true exercise tolerance. Some patients are not reliable historians, and even if they are, they may not perform activities during their daily living that stress them to their maximal exercise tolerance. The explicit questions included in the SAS appear to be a practical way of assessing the benefit of a variety of interventions used in the practice of medicine, and in many cases these questions may replace sequential exercise tests. The Duke Activity Scale Index and Veterans Specific Activity Questionnaire appear to be effective as well (see Table C-4 and Figure C-1, respectively, in Appendix C).

Physical Examination for Poor Exercise Capacity

In general, the physical findings for functional capacity are indirect and identify underlying causes for the limiting factor. The effects of surgeries, arthritis, or injuries often are apparent on physical examination, and must be taken into account as a major limitation on activities. Decreased peripheral pulses and femoral bruits are associated with PVD and possible limitation by claudication rather than cardiac disease. Obesity can indicate a decreased exercise capacity or suggest that the individual is not interested in exercise performance. Debilitating diseases and severe illnesses such as anemia and cancer should be screened for during examination.

Increased heart rate after minimal exertion can imply a deconditioned state or possibly decreased cardiac output from heart failure. Elevated neck veins are associated with heart failure. Lungs should be assessed for wheezing (COPD) and rales (CHF). Heart sounds identifying myocardial dysfunction and valve disease should be addressed.

History for Arrhythmias

Indicators of atrial or ventricular arrhythmias include a history of palpitations, the feeling of "skipped beats" or "a fish flopping in the chest," and syncope, while an episode of cardiac arrest or sudden death is limited to a ventricular arrhythmia origin. The patient who feels his or her arrhythmias but is not put at risk by them poses a difficult problem because the treatment can be more dangerous than the symptoms. Arrhythmias can be caused by structural heart disease, medications, and electrolyte problems. Atrial arrhythmias should be distinguished from ventricular arrhythmias, particularly because atrial arrhythmias are relatively benign. Rare causes of life-threatening arrhythmias include MVP (in its severe forms), IHSS, and right ventricular dysplasia. While a common faint is associated with prodromal symptoms, AV block and ventricular tachycardia are not; that is, they occur without warning.

Physical Examination for Arrhythmias

Arrhythmias are often noted during palpation of the pulses, and a determination can be made as to their efficacy by simultaneous auscultation (i.e., do pulses occur with all heart beats?). Wide splitting of both heart sounds often occurs with ventricular tachycardia and AV dissociation (atrial contraction against a closed tricuspid valve). An abnormally irregular pulse is classically due to atrial fibrillation but can also result from other rhythms.

REFERENCES

1. Peterson MC, et al. Contributions of the history, physical examination, and laboratory investigation in making medical diagnoses. *West J Med* 1992;156: 163–165.
2. Gillespie DJ, Staats BA. Unexplained dyspnea. *Mayo Clin Proc* 1994;69:657–663.
3. Hart GT. Evaluation of syncope. *Am Fam Physician* 1995;51:1941–1948, 1951–1952.
4. Williams CC, Bernhardt DT. Syncope in athletes. *Sports Med* 1995;19:223–234.
5. Fifth report of the JNCR on HBP detection. *Arch Intern Med* 1993;153:154–183.
6. Cavallini MC, et al. Association of the auscultatory gap with vascular disease in hypertensive patients. *Ann Intern Med* 1996;124:877–883.
7. Cook DJ, Simel DL. Does this patient have abnormal CVP? *JAMA* 1996;275:630–635.
8. Eilen SD, Crawford M, O'Rourke R. Accuracy of precordial palpation for detecting increased left ventricular volume. *Ann Intern Med* 1983;99:628–630.
9. Heckerling PS, et al. Accuracy and reproducibility of precordial percussion and palpation for detecting increased left ventricular end-diastolic volume and mass. *JAMA* 1993;270:1943–1948.
10. Tavel M. Cardiac auscultation. *Circulation* 1996;93: 1250–1253.
11. Shaver JA. Cardiac auscultation: a cost effective diagnostic skill. *Curr Probl Cardiol* 1995;20: 442–532.
12. Downes TR, et al. Mechanism of physiologic and pathologic S3 gallop sounds. *J Am Soc Echocardiogr* 1992;5:211–218.
13. Rothman A, Goldberger AL. Aids to cardiac auscultation. *Ann Intern Med* 1983;99:346–353.
14. Sherman DL, Ryan TJ. Differentiating cardiac and pulmonary causes of dyspnea. *ACC Curr J Rev* 1995;3:64–67.
15. DePaso WJ, et al. Chronic dyspnea unexplained by history, physical examination, chest roentgenogram, and spirometry. Analysis of a seven-year experience. *Chest* 1991;100:1293–1299.

16.   Butman SM, et al. Bedside cardiovascular examination in patients with severe chronic heart failure: importance of rest or inducible jugular venous distention. *J Am Coll Cardiol* 1993;22:968–974.

17.   Schapira RM, et al. Forced expiratory time for obstructive airways disease. *JAMA* 1993;270:731–736.

18.   Eagle KA, et al. Left ventricular ejection fraction. Physician estimates compared with gated blood pool scan measurements. *Arch Intern Med* 1988;148:882–888.

19.   Ghali JK, et al. Bedside diagnosis of preserved versus impaired left ventricular systolic function in heart failure. *Am J Cardiol* 1991;67:1002–1006.

20.   Van Miltenburg-Van Zijl A, et al. Incidence and follow-up of Braunwald subgroups in unstable angina pectoris. *J Am Coll Cardiol* 1995;25:1286–1292.

21.   Califf RM, et al. Importance of clinical measures of ischemia in the prognosis of patients with documented coronary artery disease. *J Am Coll Cardiol* 1988;11:20–26.

22.   Folland ED, et al. Implications of third heart sounds in patients with valvular heart disease. *N Engl J Med* 1992;327:458–462.

23.   Goldman L, et al. Comparative reproducibility and validity of systems for assessing cardiovascular function class: advantages of a new specific activity scale. *Circulation* 1981;64:1227–1234.

Basic Tests for Evaluation: The Electrocardiogram and the Chest X-Ray Film

The testing methods most commonly used for cardiac patients are the ECG and the chest x-ray film. These tests are commonly obtained during the work-up of the cardiac patient; therefore, they are discussed separately from the specialized tests. However, as tests they do have a limited sensitivity and specificity for their associations with findings and are not required for all patients.

THE ECG

With more than 100 million performed per year at an annual cost of $5 billion, the ECG is the most frequently utilized cardiovascular laboratory test. Reimbursement has decreased partially because of the impact of computer interpretation. The most common abnormality is inverted or low amplitude T-waves but these changes are very nonspecific.

The ECG contains important information because of its association with pathophysiologic findings. However, it only represents the electrical activity of the heart and cannot be absolutely equated to pathologic or anatomic features. For instance, a large anterior infarct can be simulated by an ice pick wound of the heart, and the ECG does not actually differentiate hypertrophy from dilation.

Basic ECG principles that should be mastered include the leads, their placement, and the myocardial segments that they represent. A systematic approach should be followed for ECG interpretation, including consideration of the patterns caused by common errors (e.g., right/left arm reversal). The order should initially consider heart rate and rhythm, then axis, intervals, amplitudes, and durations of the component waveforms.

Computer analysis of the ECG is now available in most ECG machines, and most manufacturers have their own analysis program. These programs use mathematical constructs of all 12 leads that make very accurate measurements. They require physician overreading for verification but are comparable to cardiologists. The programs read normal ECGs well but exaggerate interpretation and do not consider clinical data. The available programs have problems with arrhythmias and pacemaker spikes because P waves are not recognized and because digitalization can miss narrow, high-frequency complexes. These computer-assisted machines allow for varied presentations in addition to the standard three-lead by four-second segments. Serial averaged beats can be compared, and additional channels can display 10 seconds of continuous rhythm data.

Indications
Indications for an ECG include the following:

Chest or epigastric pain or sensation
CHF signs or symptoms including dyspnea
Abnormal pulse and palpitations
Hypotension or hypertension
Unexplained weakness
Altered mental state (coma, cerebrovascular
   accident [CVA])
Drug overdose
Chest trauma
Syncope or near syncope
Systemic illness
Metabolic disease

Systematic Approach
The first basic principle of ECG interpretation is to follow a systematic approach (Fig. 3-1). Determine the rate as fast (>100 bpm), normal (60–100 bpm), or slow (<60 bpm). Computers calculate heart rate well, except in the presence of arrhythmias. Heart rate calculation can be done in three ways:

1. Number of QRS complexes in 3 seconds (1 mm = 0.04 second, 5 mm = 0.2 second; therefore, fifteen 5-mm boxes = 3 seconds)
2. Divide 300 by the number of 5-mm (large) blocks in one R wave to R-wave interval
3. Divide 1,500 by the RR interval in millimeters

The following should then be considered in order:

1. Rhythm should be determined as sinus, atrial, or ventricular, and the presence of blocks should be noted.
2. The durations of the P wave (≤100 msec) and QRS complex (≥120 msec) should be measured.

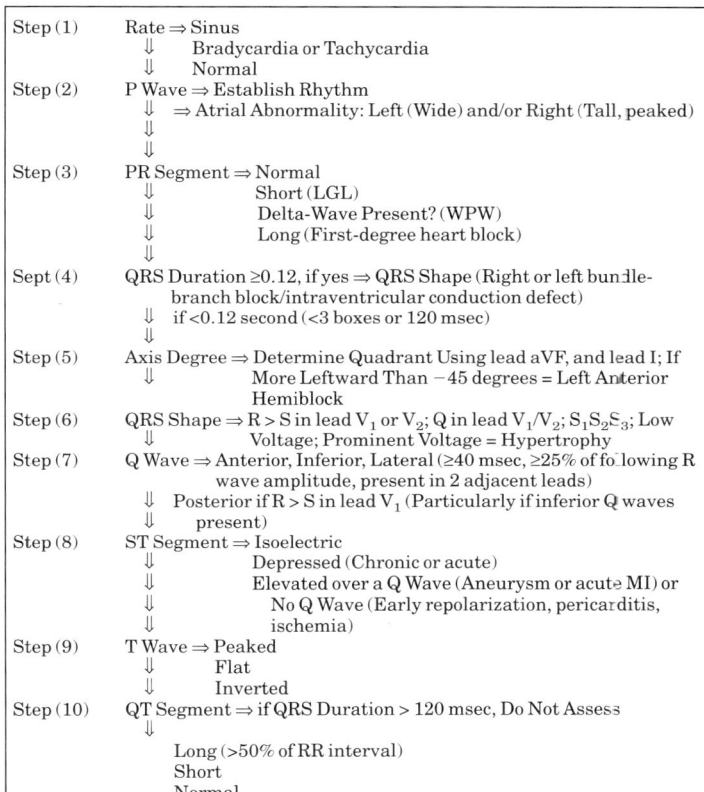

Step (1)   Rate ⇒ Sinus
⇓   Bradycardia or Tachycardia
⇓   Normal
Step (2)   P Wave ⇒ Establish Rhythm
⇓   ⇒ Atrial Abnormality: Left (Wide) and/or Right (Tall, peaked)
⇓
⇓
Step (3)   PR Segment ⇒ Normal
⇓   Short (LGL)
⇓   Delta-Wave Present? (WPW)
⇓   Long (First-degree heart block)
⇓
Sept (4)   QRS Duration ≥0.12, if yes ⇒ QRS Shape (Right or left bundle-branch block/intraventricular conduction defect)
⇓   if <0.12 second (<3 boxes or 120 msec)
⇓
Step (5)   Axis Degree ⇒ Determine Quadrant Using lead aVF, and lead I; If
⇓   More Leftward Than −45 degrees = Left Anterior Hemiblock
Step (6)   QRS Shape ⇒ R > S in lead V_1 or V_2; Q in lead V_1/V_2; $S_1S_2S_3$; Low
⇓   Voltage; Prominent Voltage = Hypertrophy
Step (7)   Q Wave ⇒ Anterior, Inferior, Lateral (≥40 msec, ≥25% of following R wave amplitude, present in 2 adjacent leads)
⇓   Posterior if R > S in lead V_1 (Particularly if inferior Q waves
⇓   present)
Step (8)   ST Segment ⇒ Isoelectric
⇓   Depressed (Chronic or acute)
⇓   Elevated over a Q Wave (Aneurysm or acute MI) or
⇓   No Q Wave (Early repolarization, pericarditis,
⇓   ischemia)
Step (9)   T Wave ⇒ Peaked
⇓   Flat
⇓   Inverted
Step (10)   QT Segment ⇒ if QRS Duration > 120 msec, Do Not Assess
⇓
Long (>50% of RR interval)
Short
Normal

Fig. 3-1. Flow diagram of the systematic approach to ECG interpretation. MI = myocardial infarction; LGL = Lown-Ganong-Levine; WPW = Wolff-Parkinson-White.

3. Axis should be defined as normal, rightward, or leftward. The most simple way to determine axis is to consider the direction of the major QRS deflection in limb leads I and aVF. If the deflection is positive or upright in both I and aVF leads, the axis is normal (i.e., to the left and downward). If the deflection is positive in lead I and negative lead in aVF, left-axis deviation is present; if the deflections are equal or more negative than positive in lead II, then the axis is leftward −45 degrees or more, possibly consistent with left anterior hemiblock (LAHB). If the deflections are negative in lead I and positive in lead aVF, right-axis deviation is present. If the axis is indeterminate, which frequently

occurs when $S_1S_2S_3$ is present, pulmonary disease is suggested. Axis determination is done simply by determining the net QRS amplitude voltage in the leads representing the X (lead I) and Y (lead aVF) axes, as shown in Figure 3-2:

Net positive in leads I and aVF = normal quadrant (0 to 90 degrees)

Net positive in lead I and net negative in lead aVF = left quadrant (0 to -90 degrees)

Net positive in lead aVF and net negative in lead I = right quadrant (90 to 180 degrees)

The ECGs in Figures 3-3 and 3-4 illustrate rightward and leftward axes, respectively.

4. Intervals should be determined for the PR segment, QRS complex, and the QT interval.

5. Amplitudes of the P wave, QRS waves, ST segment, and the T wave should be measured.

6. Criteria for P-wave and QRS abnormalities should be applied and patterns consistent with specific diseases should be noted.

7. Compare the current ECG to previous ECGs when available.

Fig. 3-2.   Define the axis by determining the net QRS amplitude voltage in the leads representing the X (lead I) and Y (lead aVF) axes. $-$I = net negative in I, $+$I = net positive in I, $-$AVF = net negative in AVF, $+$AVF = net positive in AVF.

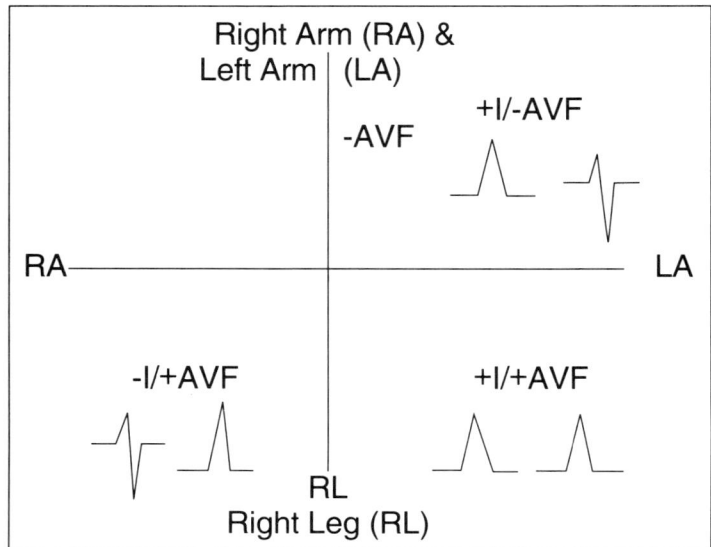

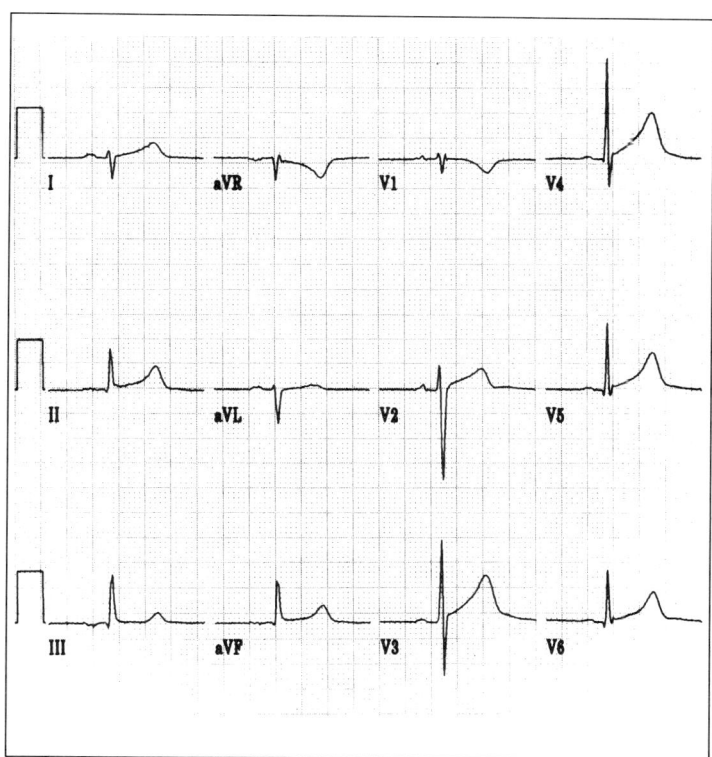

Fig. 3-3.   ECG showing rightward axis deviation.

8. Consider the clinical context or setting in which the ECG is obtained (e.g., emergency department versus clinic).

9. Be careful to obtain the correct data. Check the calibration square wave for amplitude (1 mV = 10 mm high for normal amplitude, 5 mm for half amplitude with hypertrophy, 5 mm wide for normal paper speed) and duration (indicates paper speed [5 mm = 25 mm/sec]). Common lead errors include arm reversal and V_1 and V_3 reversal (Fig. 3-5). Right-sided chest leads are often obtained when an inferior infarction occurs, in order to see if there is right ventricular involvement (Fig. 3-6).

10. Check for pacemaker spikes, electrical interference, wandering baseline, and tremor artifact (which may suggest the diagnosis of parkinsonism).

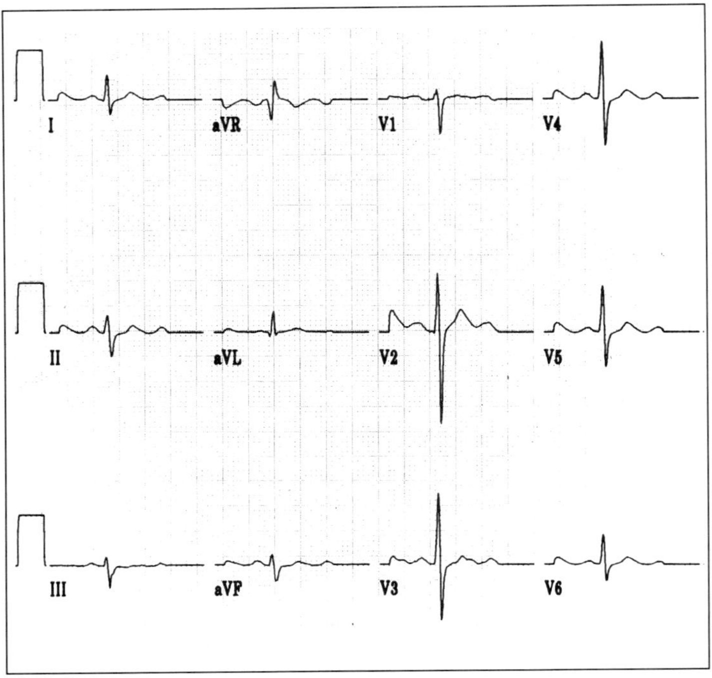

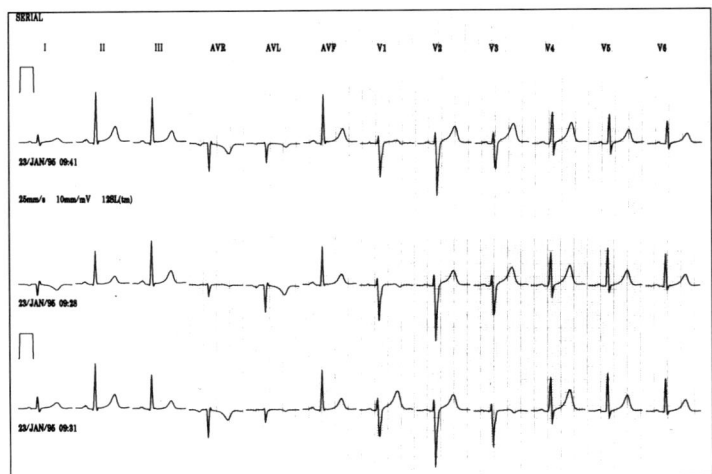

Fig. 3-4.   ECG showing leftward axis deviation.

Fig. 3-5.   Common lead errors: arm lead reversal (middle) and V_1 and V_3 reversal (bottom). The top line shows normal lead placement.

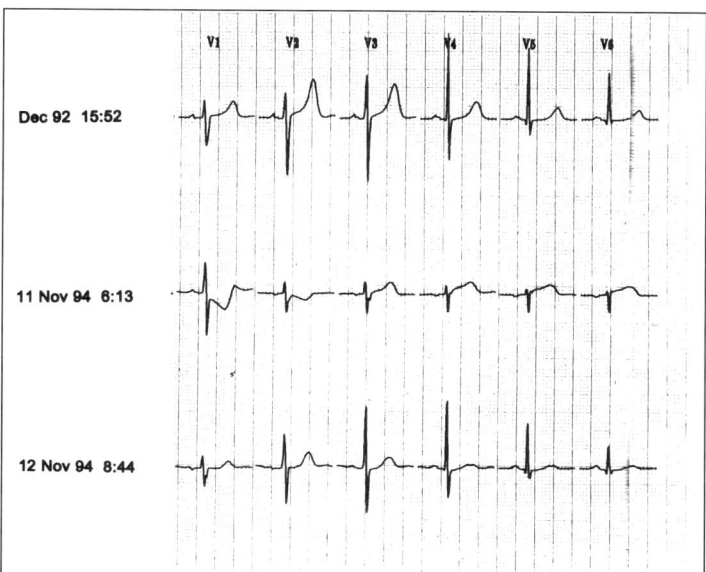

Fig. 3-6. Right-sided chest leads (middle) are usually obtained with inferior myocardial infarctions to check for right ventricular involvement. The bottom line and the top line show normal left chest lead placement.

A Cause of Marked Axis Deviation: The Hemiblocks
The left bundle can be thought of as consisting of two fascicles, anterior and posterior. The loss of the anterior fascicle (left anterior fasicular or hemiblock [LAHB], Fig. 3-7) results in marked left-axis deviation (>45 degrees) and loss of the posterior fascicle (left posterior fasicular or hemiblock [LPHB]) results in right-axis deviation. Neither should result in prolongation of QRS duration, and LPHB is a diagnosis of exclusion of all other causes of right-axis deviation (i.e., lung disease). When axis deviation accompanies right bundle-branch block, it is assumed that one of these fascicles is involved and bifascicular block (i.e., two of the three fascicles, the right bundle plus one of the two left fascicles) is said to be present.

Hemiblocks are determined largely by axis:

Normal QRS duration (if width is prolonged, then it is a nonspecific intraventricular conduction defect)
Left anterior fascicular: left-axis deviation (≥45 degrees) and small Q wave in lead aVL
Left posterior fascicular: right axis not due to lung disease

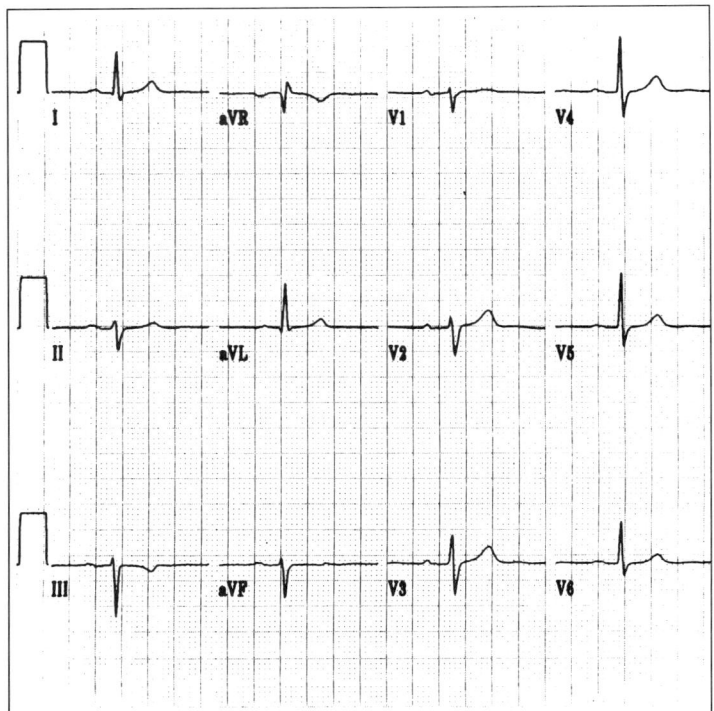

Fig. 3-7. Left anterior fascicular block.

There are no data to suggest that these patterns are ominous as a precursor to more severe conduction disease.

ECG Interpretation Rules and Characteristics for Pattern Reading of Normal

ECGs can be confusing and complicated for the novice and for the physician who reads them only occasionally. Two rules make pattern reading much easier. These two rules are convenient pneumonic devices to assist in pattern recognition of P-wave, QRS, and T-wave components of the normal ECG. Variations from these patterns alert the physician that an abnormality may be present. They can help teach ECG interpretation to medical students and to other health professionals.

Diagonal Rule
The diagonal rule (Fig. 3-8) allows easy recognition of the normal 12-lead ECG, as recorded on the three-channel

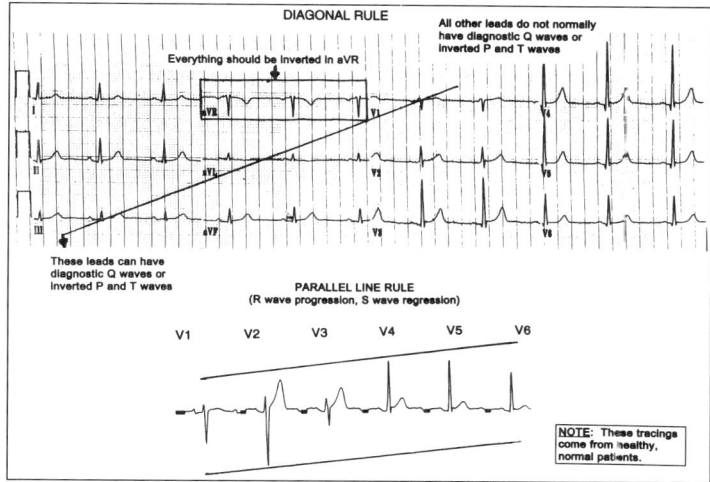

Fig. 3-8.   The diagonal rule and the parallel line rule.

ECG machine. The three-channel ECG records three leads simultaneously, creating a matrix with leads I, II, and III in the first column; aVR, aVL, and aVF in the second column; and V_1 to V_6 in the last two columns. A diagonal line is drawn from lead III through aVL to V_1. All the leads crossed by this line (III, aVL, V_1) can have upright, inverted, or biphasic P or T waves in a normal tracing. Significant Q waves (>0.04 second in duration or >25% of the R wave) can be seen in these leads as well. A box around aVR is a reminder that the P and T waves are inverted, and a significant Q wave is always present in this lead on a normal ECG record. aVR is a view that looks down the long axis of the left ventricle. *All other leads should have upright P or T waves as well as the absence of a significant Q wave.*

Parallel Line Rule
The parallel line rule for the precordial leads describes the normal pattern exhibited in the frontal plane leads going from V_1 to V_6, as depicted in Figure 3-8. The R wave should increase in amplitude while the S wave decreases from the right-sided leads (V_1 to V_2) of the chest to the left-sided leads (V_5 to V_6). However, the largest R wave is usually seen in V_5 with a decrease in V_6.

An understanding of the characteristics of poor R-wave progression and normal (nondiagnostic) Q waves also helps with pattern reading of the normal ECG.

POOR R-WAVE PROGRESSION.   Failure for the R-wave deflections to increase in relative amplitude from V_1 to V_5, as in the parallel line rule, most often is a normal variant. It can occur with pulmonary disease and right ventricular dilation, left ventricular hypertrophy, anterior infarction, pectus excavatum, and incorrectly placed leads.

NORMAL Q WAVES.   Because the septum depolarizes before the rest of the left ventricle after the left bundle is activated, normal, nondiagnostic Q waves can be seen, particularly in the lateral leads (I, V_5, V_4). Their absence has been called septal fibrosis but this is without anatomic correlation. Absence of these small Q waves is more frequent in the elderly.

Abnormal ECG Pattern Grouping
The following pattern groupings are very helpful for interpretation of the ECG. The order follows the systematic approach by focusing first on the P waves, which are important in determining rhythm, and then QRS duration, which affects the interpretation of all the other patterns:

Atrial abnormalities
QRS duration
Q waves in V_1 and V_2
R wave of greater absolute amplitude than S wave in V_1 or V_2
Q-wave infarction patterns
Hypertrophy patterns
Disease patterns: pulmonary disease, chronic CHF
Low QRS amplitude
Electrolyte abnormalities
ST-segment elevation
ST-segment depression
Long QT interval
T-wave changes
Serial changes

Atrial Abnormalities
Anatomic correlates (Fig. 3-9) that serve as memory aids for atrial patterns are that the normal two humps to the P wave are composed of a right and left atrial component:

1. The right atrial notch comes first (because the sinus node is in the superior vena cava [SVC] above the right atrium) representing the depolarization of the right atria. The right atria makes up the right border of the heart (thus, pulling the P-wave vector to the right).

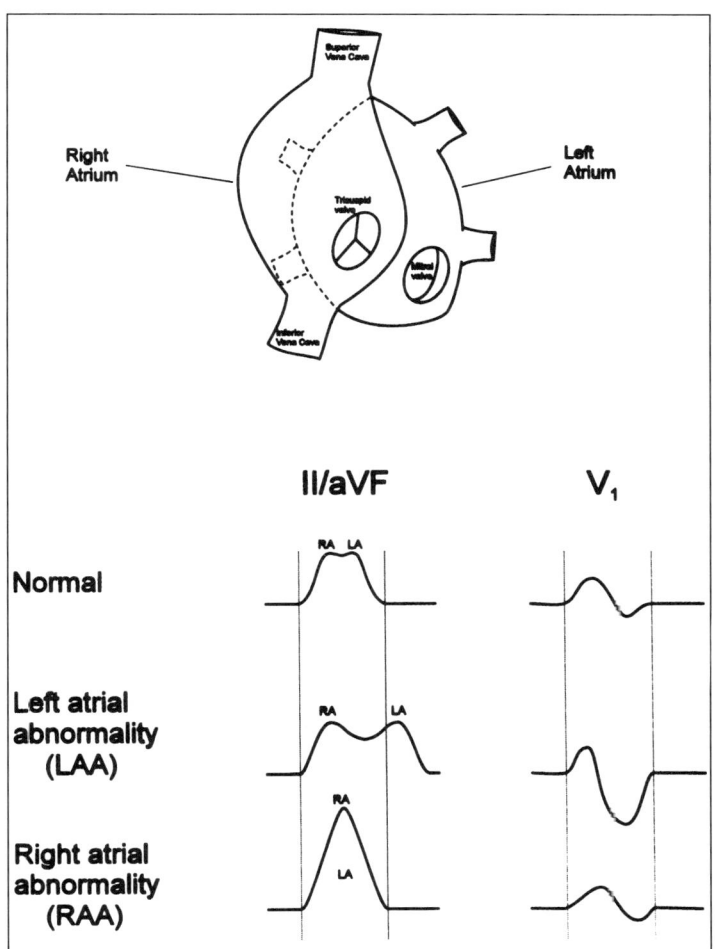

Fig. 3-9.   Atrial abnormalities: anatomic location and ECG findings.

2. The left atrial notch comes second with the subsequent depolarization of the left atrium. The P wave can have a negative component in V, because the left atrium makes up the posterior border of the heart.

The two types of atrial abnormalities are:

Right atrial abnormality or P-pulmonale (Fig. 3-10): tall, peaked P waves (>2.5 mm high or 0.25-mV amplitude) with a vertical axis (seen in leads II, III,

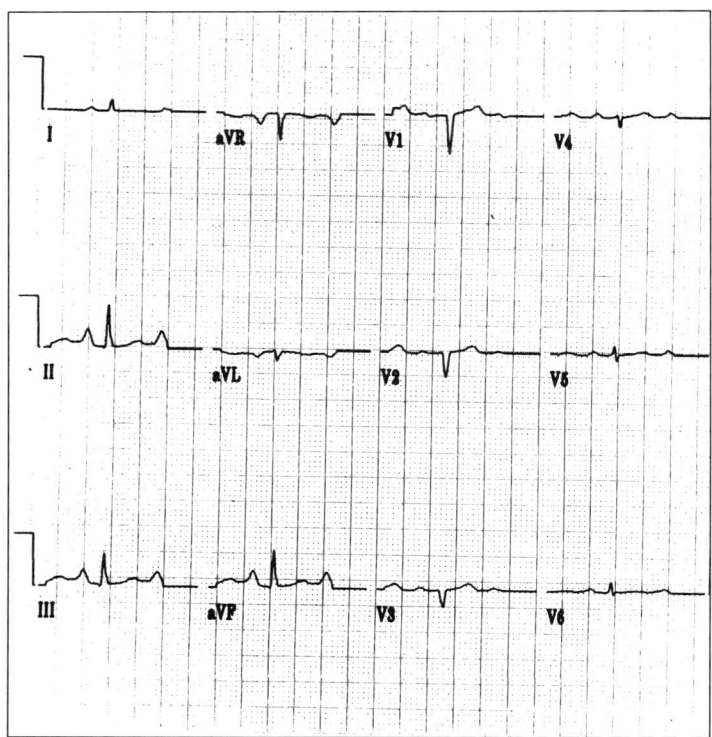

Fig. 3-10.   ECG showing right atrial abnormality: right atrial enlargement with chronic obstruction pulmonary disease.

and aVF)—associated with lung disease, pulmonary embolus, or other causes of pulmonary hypertension.
Left atrial abnormality or P-mitrale (Fig. 3-11): broad, notched P waves in leads II and aVF (>2.5 mm wide or 100-msec duration) with a negative component in V_1 or V_2 (that exceeds 1 mm × 1 mm, e.g., 40 msec × 0.1 mV)—associated with mitral regurgitation, congestive heart failure (CHF) or any clinical condition that elevates left ventricular filling pressure. It can even be transient with the occurrence of CHF.

QRS Prolongation Longer Than 120 Milliseconds
The following conditions are associated with a QRS complex duration greater than 120 milliseconds.

1. Ventricular origin: premature ventricular contractions (Fig. 3-12), ventricular tachycardia, or ventricular elec-

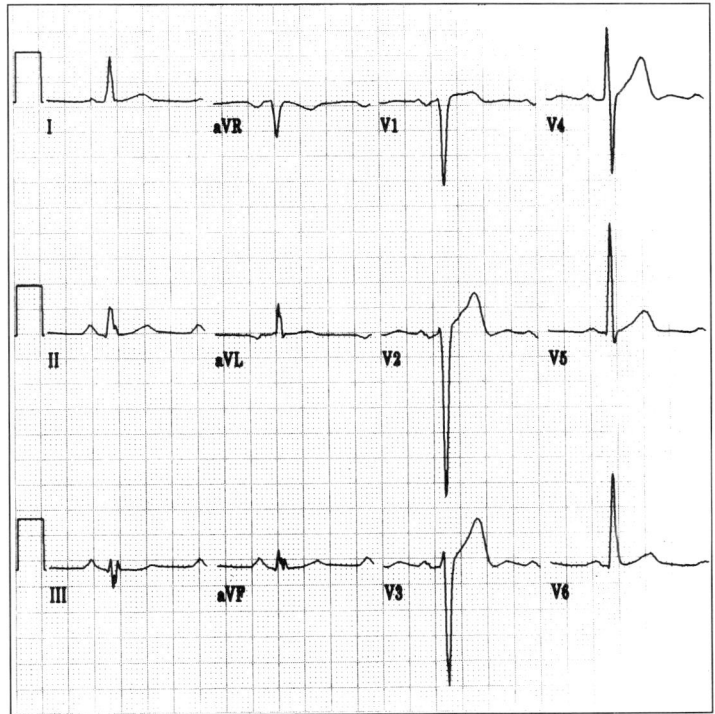

Fig. 3-11.   ECG showing left atrial abnormality. Echocardiography confirmed left atrial enlargement of 5.5 cm.

tronic pacemaker (Fig. 3-13). The absence of associated preceding P waves and the presence of retrograde P waves are critical for confirming premature ventricular contractions or ventricular tachycardia, whereas identification of the electrical spike is critical for recognizing an electronic pacemaker.

2. Supraventricular tachycardia with aberrancy. *If the answer to all four of the following questions is no, then the diagnosis is supraventricular tachycardia rather than ventricular tachycardia:*

   Is there an absence of an RS complex in all precordial leads? (Only QS, QRS, QR, or R or rSR complexes are present.)

   Is the R to S interval longer than 100 msec in any one precordial lead?

   Is there atrioventricular (AV) disassociation?

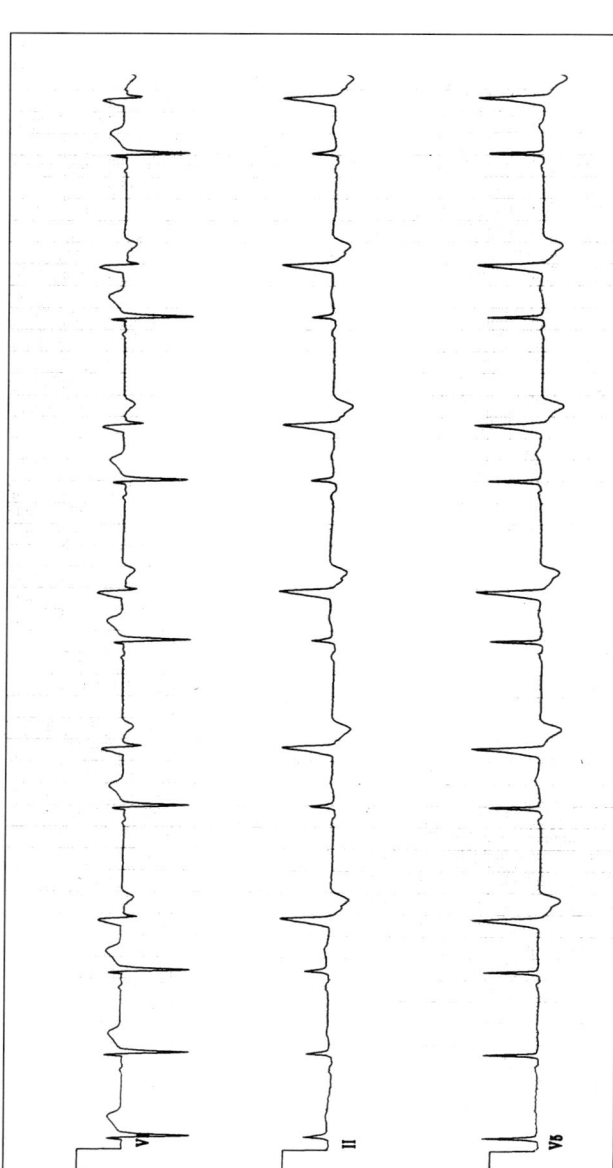

Fig. 3-12.   QRS prolongation of ventricular origin: premature ventricular contractions. Notice the bigeminy that develops during the course of the rhythm strip.

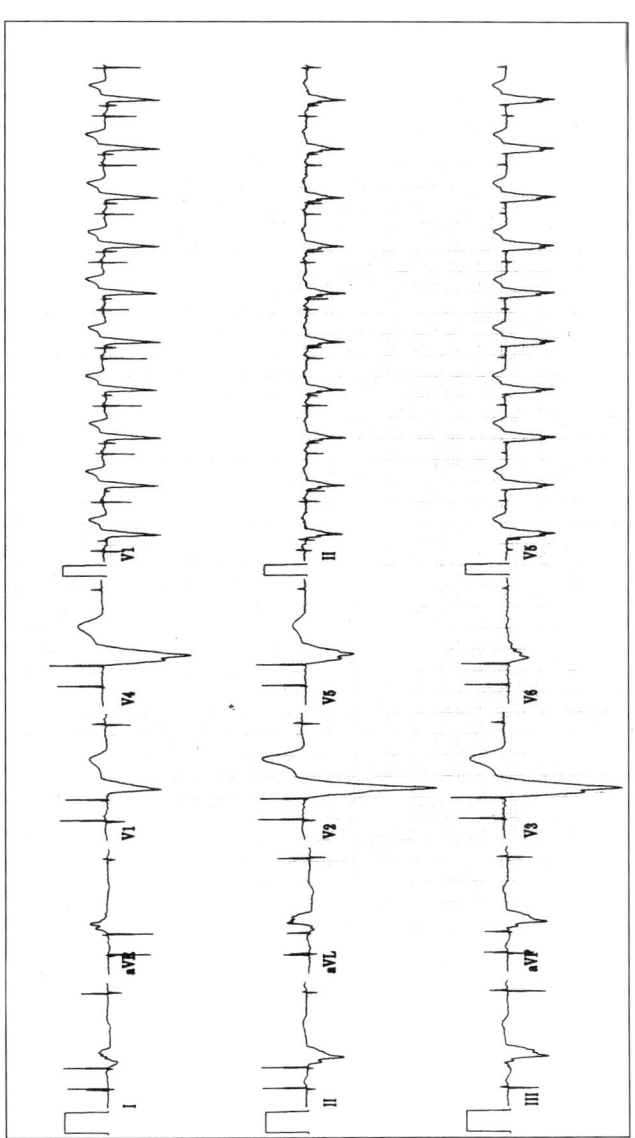

Fig. 3-13. QRS prolongation of ventricular origin: ventricular electronic pacemaker. Dual chamber pacer with average beat format on left half and half paper speed (10 mm/sec) on the right half of the page.

Are there morphology criteria for ventricular tachycardia present both in V_1 to V_2 and V_6?

(However, the pretest probability for a wide complex tachycardia to be ventricular is 85% [1, 2].)

3. Bundle-branch block:

Right (Fig. 3-14)—"rabbit ears" (rSR pattern) on the right side (V_1, V_2), and the R-wave complex looks normal if the terminal S wave on the left side (V_4, V_5, V_6) is disregarded.

Left (Fig. 3-15)—"rabbit ears" on the left side (V_5, V_6) and lead I and Q waves in V_1 to V_3. LBBB is usually associated with an EF of 30% in patients with symptoms of CHF.

4. Wolff-Parkinson-White (Fig. 3-16): short PR interval and delta wave present.

Fig. 3-14. QRS prolongation: right bundle-branch block. Notice the "rabbit ears" on the right side—lead V_1.

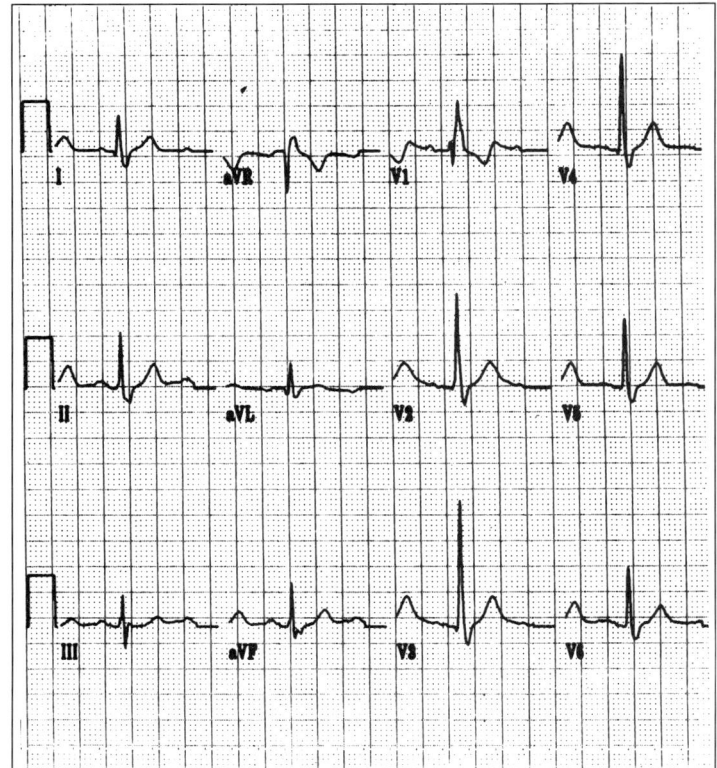

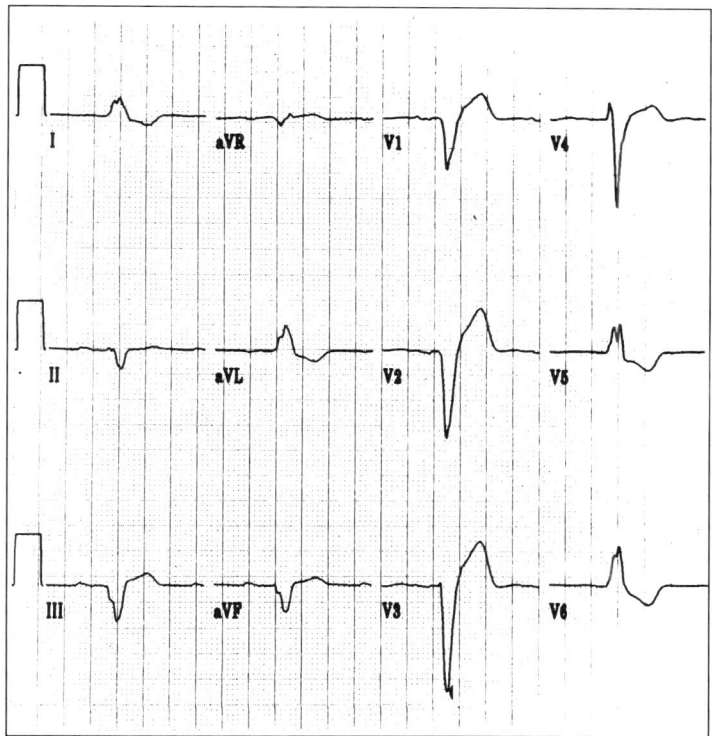

Fig. 3-15. QRS prolongation: left bundle-branch block. Notice the "rabbit ears" on the left side—leads V_5, V_6, and I.

5. Intraventricular conduction block or peri-infarction block (Fig. 3-17): looks like a bundle-branch block but cannot be distinguished as characteristic of left or right.

   DIFFERENTIATION OF WIDE COMPLEX TACHYCARDIA.   The clinical probability of a wide complex tachycardia being ventricular tachycardia is 85%. When confronted with a patient with such an arrhythmia and there is no time to carefully make a distinction, remember that intravenous verapamil is not appropriate therapy for ventricular tachycardia while adenosine is acceptable for either supraventricular or ventricular tachycardia. Also, if the patient is hemodynamically unstable, restore the normal cardiac rhythm with direct current (DC) electrocardioversion. The hemodynamic response to the tachycardia does not help differentiate (i.e., whether or not hypotension

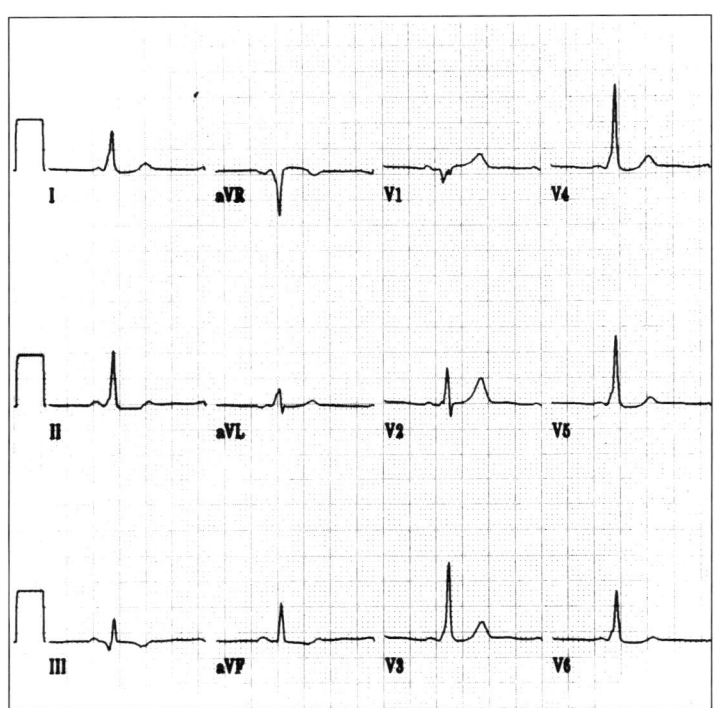

Fig. 3-16.   QRS prolongation: Wolff-Parkinson-White syndrome.

develops). An easy summary of the above rules follows: (1) It most likely is a supraventricular tachycardia if right bundle-branch block is present and the rate is more than 170 bpm and (2) the tachycardia most likely is ventricular if left-axis deviation is present with a QRS duration longer than 140 msec, with no RS in any precordial lead, with AV dissociation, or with an RS interval longer than 100 msec. The differences are outlined in Table 3-1.

Q Wave in V_1 and V_2
With the exception of errors of techniques, the genesis of the QS pattern in leads V_1 and V_2 in individuals without myocardial infarction or other forms of myopathy is due to altered orientation of the initial septal vector. The conditions that alter the main vector include (1) spurious change of order of septal depolarization; (2) change in anatomic orientation due to rotation, displacement, or both; and (3) abnormalities of intraventricular conduction [3].

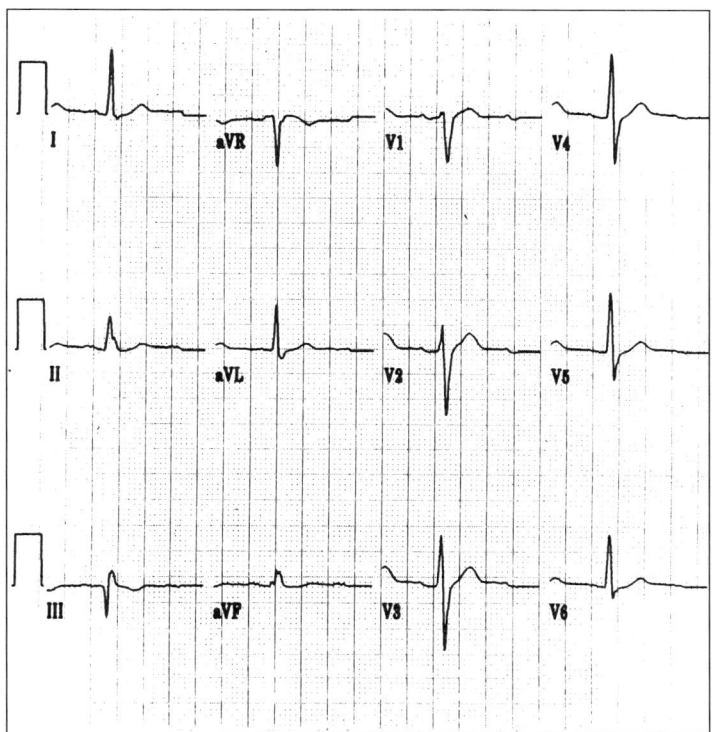

Fig. 3-17.   QRS prolongation: intraventricular conduction block.

Table 3-1.   Differential Characteristics of Wide Complex Tachycardia

Ventricular (Pre-analysis Probability of Ventricular Origin = 85%)	Supraventricular (Pre-analysis Probability of Supraventricular Origin = 15%)
1. AV dissociation	1. No AV dissociation
2. Any of the following: Rr in lead V_1, QR or QS in lead V_6	2. None of these morphologies
3. No RS complex in precordial leads	3. RS complex present in all precordial leads
4. QRS > 140 or RS > 100 msec	4. RS complex > 100 msec in all precordial leads
5. Ventricular response < 170 bpm	5. RBBB and >170 bpm
6. LAD	
7. Presence of fusion or capture beats	

AV = atrioventricular; LAD = left-axis deviation; RBBB = right bundle-branch block.

ORDER OF SEPTAL DEPOLARIZATION.   Septal activation may be directed inferiorly and perpendicular to the lead axis of leads V_1 and V_2, inscribing an isoelectric early component of the QRS complex and thus a QS pattern.

LEAD MISPLACEMENT.   Placing the V_1 and V_2 electrodes in a higher interspace than the fourth can cause Q waves in V_1 and V_2. The ECG should be repeated with anatomically correct electrode placement.

CHANGE IN ANATOMIC POSITION.   ECG of a patient with chronic obstructive lung disease provides a common example of a QS pattern in leads V_1 and V_2 due to a change in anatomic position, with the heart assuming a vertical position and rotating clockwise. Other ECG findings with lung disease should be present.

ABNORMALITIES OF INTRAVENTRICULAR CONDUCTION.   Intraventricular conduction defects may be responsible for a QS pattern in leads V_1 and V_2. Of these, LAFB, left bundle-branch block (LBBB), and Wolff-Parkinson-White syndrome (WPW) are most common.

In summary, whereas usually a QS pattern in leads V_1 and V_2 is due to myocardial infarction, there are patients in whom this pattern appears in the absence of any heart disease. The possibility that a QS pattern in leads V_1 and V_2 is due to altered direction of septal forces or is due to faulty recording technique should be considered when the pretest likelihood for infarction is low and there is no supporting evidence for myocardial infarction [4]. The ECG should be carefully examined for other patterns that explain the Q waves.

R Wave of Greater Absolute Amplitude
Than S Wave in V_1 or V_2
The following conditions are associated with an R wave of greater absolute amplitude than the S wave in V_1 or V_2.

- Right bundle-branch block
- Posterior infarction (usually also has inferior wall diagnostic Q waves, i.e., Q waves in lead II, aVF, or III >40 msec and >25% the amplitude of the following R wave)
- WPW
- Right ventricular hypertrophy
- Normal variant
- V_1 to V_3 lead reversal

Q-Wave Infarction Patterns
Inferior infarcts (Fig. 3-18) are associated with diagnostic Q waves in at least two of the inferior leads: II, III, and

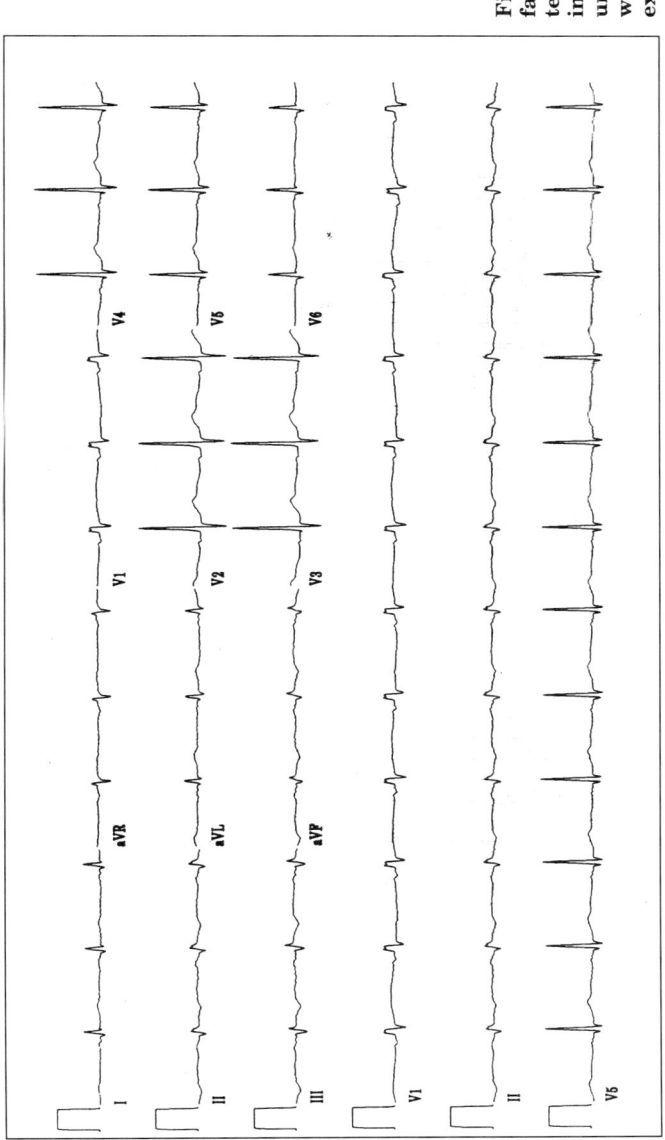

Fig. 3-18. Infarction patterns: inferior infarct, age undetermined, with posterior extension.

aVF (this is the most common myocardial infarction pattern). Anterior infarcts (Fig. 3-19) are associated with diagnostic Q waves in at least two of the anterior leads, V_2, V_3, and V_4. Septal infarcts (Fig. 3-20) are associated with diagnostic Q waves in V_1 and V_2. While a QS pattern in V_1 and V_2 usually is associated with a septal infarct, it can occur with anatomic changes (vertical axis) due to lung disease or left ventricular hypertrophy and with intraventricular conduction defects such as LAFB, LBBB, and WPW or with hypertrophic cardiomyopathy. Lateral infarcts are associated with diagnostic Q waves in at least two of the lateral leads, I, aVL, V_4, V_5, and V_6 (this is the least common myocardial infarction pattern). Non-Q-wave infarctions cannot be localized by their ST-T wave changes!

The diagnostic Q waves must be at least 40 msec in duration and at least 25% the amplitude of the following R wave. The waves must occur in two adjacent or contiguous leads. If not all criteria are met, the Q waves are nondiagnostic.

Q waves can be used for estimates of ventricular function. *If the ECG is entirely normal, there is a 95% probability that the ejection fraction is normal* (i.e., above 55%). Assigning Q wave values (30 for Q waves in V_2, V_3, or V_4; 10 for V_1 and V_2; 10 for II, III, or aVF; and 15 for I, aVL, or V_5) and subtracting the value from 60 approximates the ejection fraction.

Hypertrophy Patterns

RIGHT VENTRICULAR HYPERTROPHY. Attempts have been made to divide right ventricular patterns into volume and pressure abnormalities. Both have a vertical axis; pressure increases cause an R wave greater than the S wave in V_1 and V_2 or an R wave greater than 7 mm in V_1, and volume increases cause a loss of anterior forces and a counterclockwise rotation with large terminal S waves laterally. Figure 3-21 is an example of pressure overload.

LEFT VENTRICULAR HYPERTROPHY. Unfortunately, left ventricular dilation cannot be separated from hypertrophy by the ECG (Fig. 3-22). However, intrinsicoid deflection (time of ascent of the R wave) may be lengthened with hypertrophy. Goldberg's sign (the limb leads are <10 mm while the precordial leads are large) appears to be associated with left ventricular dilation. The thinned heart wall does not generate much electromotive energy, but the proximity to the chest wall results in increased voltage in the precordial leads.

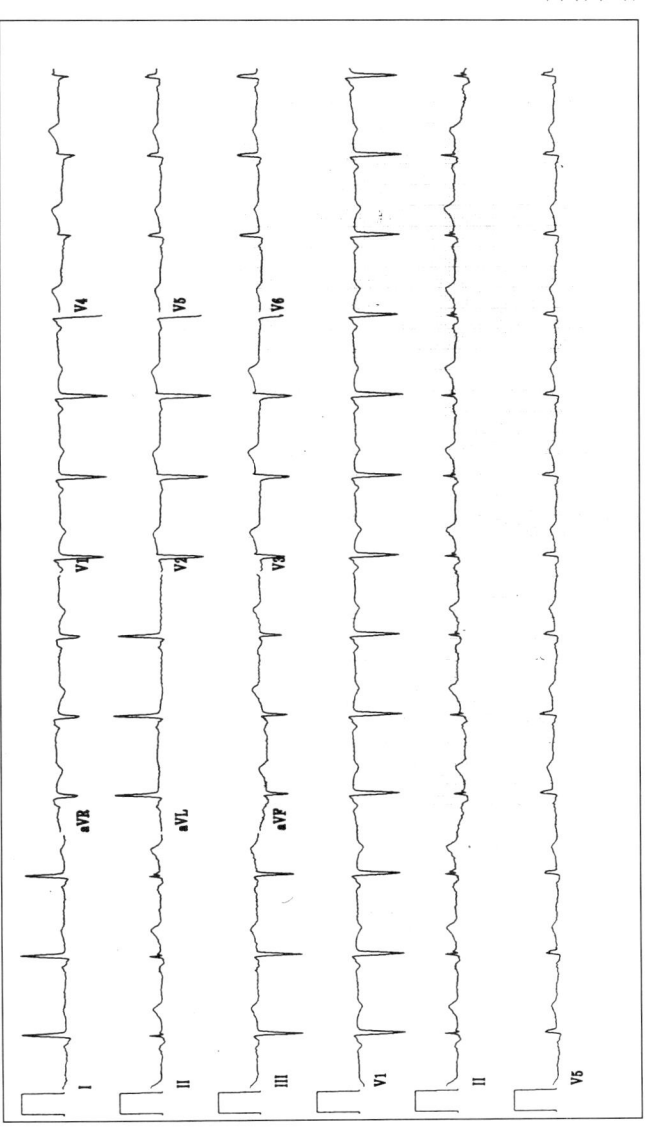

Fig. 3-19. Infarction patterns: anterior infarct.

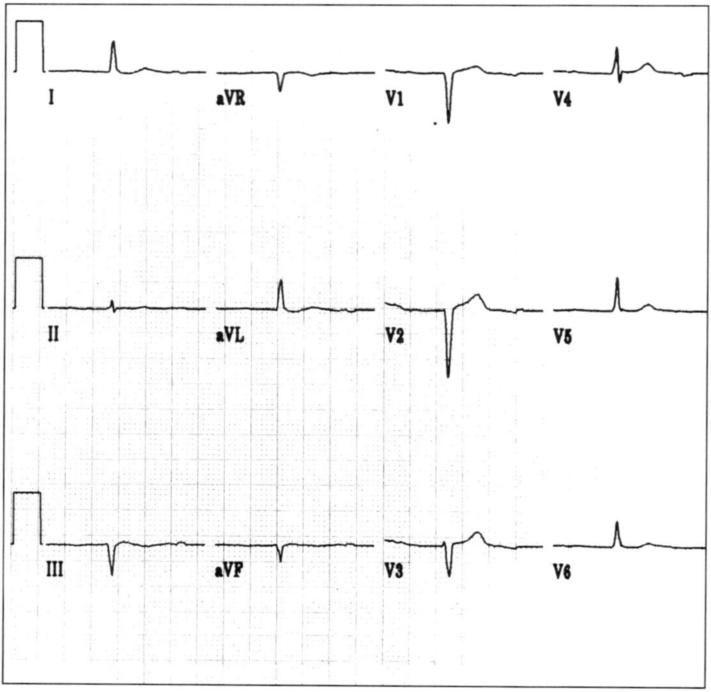

Fig. 3-20.   Infarction patterns: septal infarct. There seems to be inferior involvement as well. Notice the Q waves in leads II and aVF.

The following findings add to the probability of left ventricular hypertrophy:

- Sum of the largest S wave in V_1 to V_3 and the R wave in V_4 to V_6 exceeds 35 mm
- R wave in aVL greater than 11 mm
- Any other limb lead exceeds 15 mm
- Left atrial abnormality
- Left-axis deviation
- ST-segment depression ("strain")

The Cornell-Framingham Left Ventricular Mass Equation.   The Cornell ECG voltage, defined as the sum of voltages for the R wave of lead aVL and the S wave of lead V_3, correlates very closely with echocardiographically estimated left ventricular mass. Because the magnitude of this voltage varies with both age and obesity, an adjustment formula was estimated from the Framingham Heart Study cohort who was

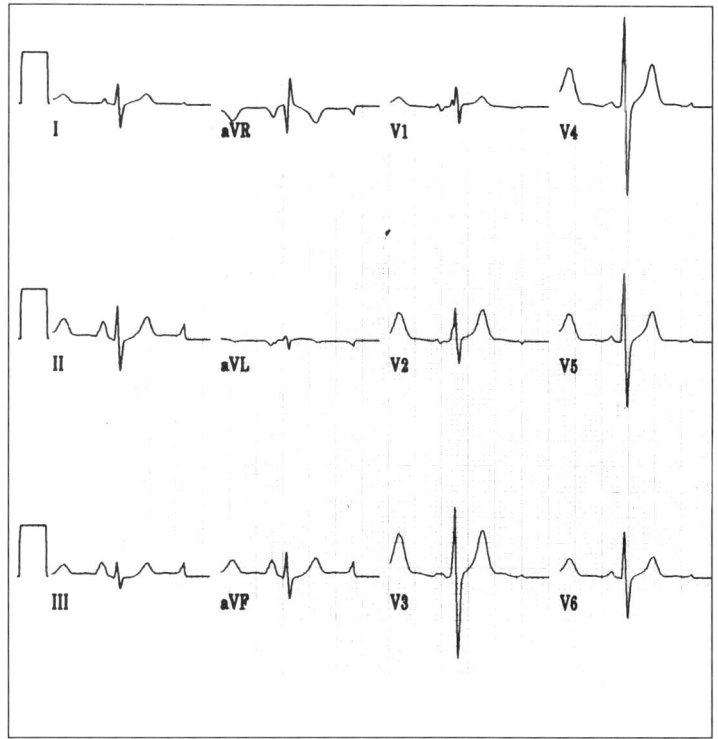

Fig. 3-21.   Right ventricular hypertrophy, and $S_1S_2S_3$ (pulmonary disease pattern).

free of myocardial infarction and who had both ECG and echocardiography during the same clinic examination [5]. When implemented in computerized ECG machines, such equations will provide a more accurate estimate of left ventricular mass than is currently possible.

Specific ECG Patterns Associated with Disease Conditions

LUNG DISEASE PATTERNS.   The $S_1S_2S_3$ pattern (S waves in leads I, II, and III) or an indeterminate frontal plane axis is pathognomonic of lung disease (see Fig. 3-21). Lung disease also causes generalized low voltage and poor R-wave progression across the precordium (Fig. 3-23). Naturally, lung disease must also be considered when right-axis deviation or right ventricular hypertrophy is present. All or some of the findings listed below may be present in patients with lung disease:

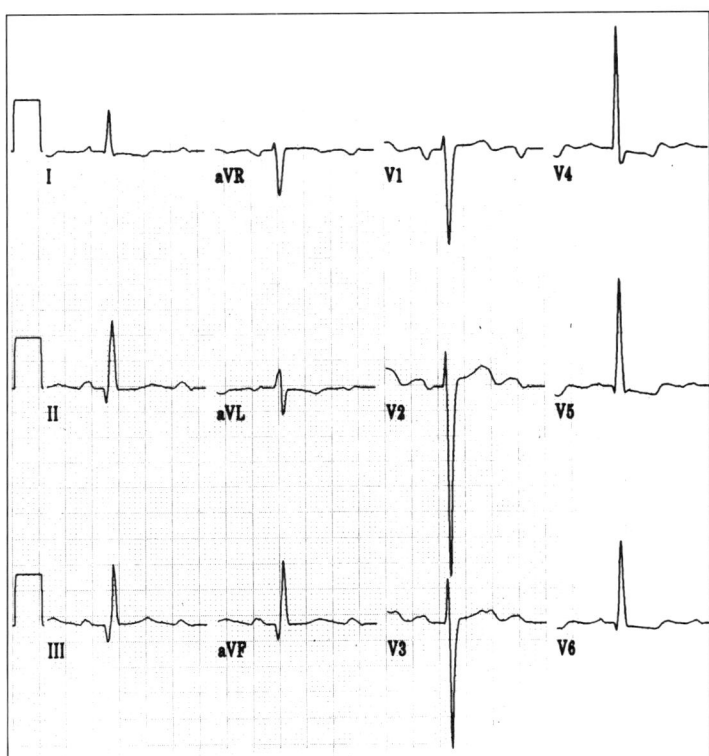

Fig. 3-22.   Left ventricular hypertrophy with QRS widening and repolarization abnormality.

- Right atrial abnormality
- $S_1S_2S_3$ = S waves in leads I, II, and III or indeterminate frontal plane axis
- Right-axis deviation or right ventricular hypertrophy
- Poor R-wave progression from V_1 to V_6
- Low voltage

ACUTE PULMONARY EMBOLUS.   Some of the findings listed below may be present when a pulmonary embolus (Fig. 3-24) occurs:

- Tachycardia
- Right-axis deviation or shift
- Right bundle-branch block
- Right atrial abnormality
- Right ventricular strain pattern

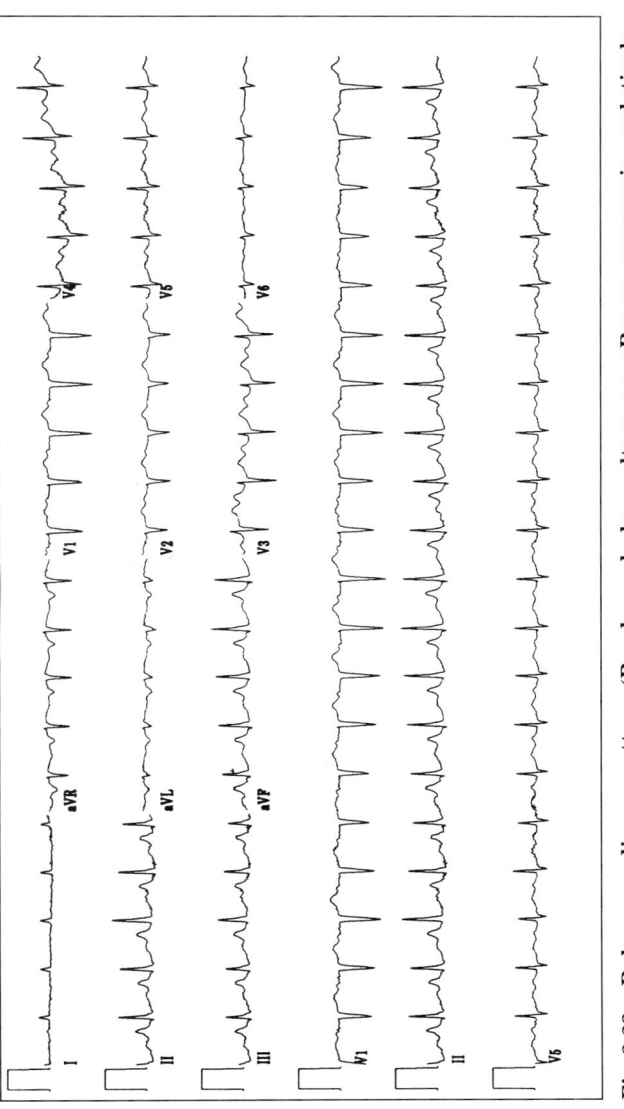

Fig. 3-23. Pulmonary disease pattern. (P-pulmonale, low voltage, poor R wave progression, relatively large S wave laterally).

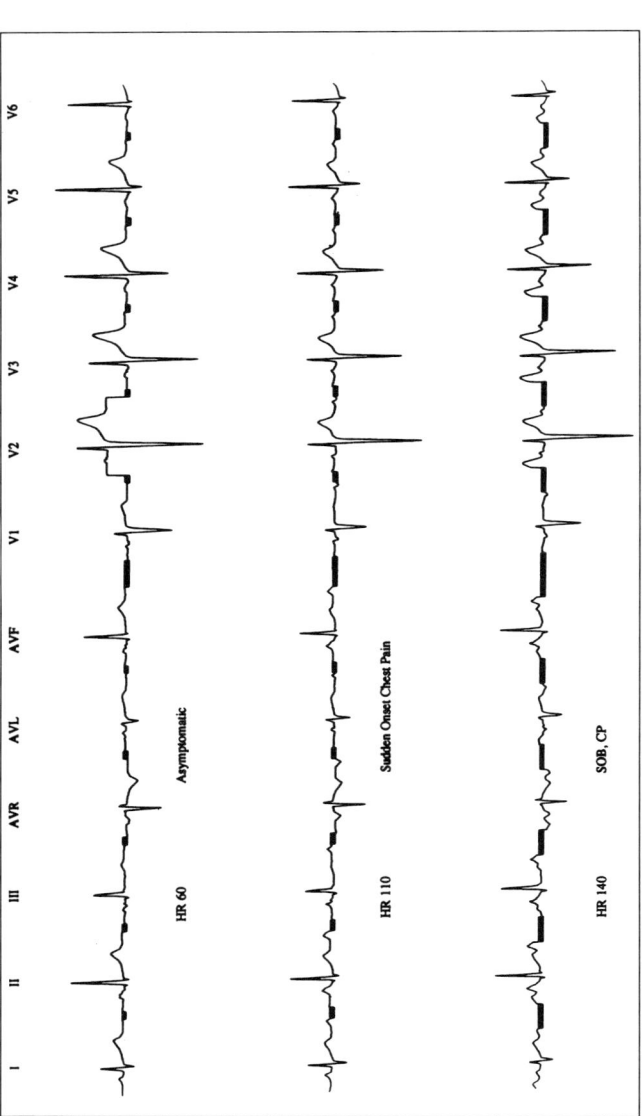

Fig. 3-24.   Pulmonary embolus. SOB, CP = shortness of breath, chest pain. Serial changes of right ward axis, tachycardia and P-pulmonale.

CONGESTIVE HEART FAILURE. Some or all of the following are seen in patients with CHF; some of these findings may worsen acutely and improvements may be seen after treatment.

* Atrial fibrillation/flutter
* Left atrial abnormality
* Q waves, particularly anterior and/or lateral
* Bundle-branch block (particularly LBBB)
* Left ventricular hypertrophy with strain
* Low voltage

Generalized Low Voltage

The differential diagnosis includes hypothyroidism, obesity, pleural or pericardial effusion, acute bronchitis and chronic obstructive lung disease, cardiomyopathy, and infiltrative heart diseases such as amyloidosis (Fig. 3-25). A decrease in QRS voltage that is a change from a previous ECG strongly suggests a new pericardial effusion or an exacerbation of lung disease.

Electrolyte Abnormalities

The ECG patterns associated with specific electrolyte abnormalities are listed below [6].

POTASSIUM. Hyperkalemia (Fig. 3-26) is indicated by tall, peaked T waves (as is ischemia), a shortened QT interval, a longer QRS duration, and atrial arrest. Hypokalemia is indicated by low-amplitude T waves, prominent U waves, and slight QRS widening.

CALCIUM. Hypercalcemia is represented by a short QT interval, and hypocalcemia (Fig. 3-27) by a long QT interval (as are quinidine usage and ischemia).

MAGNESIUM. Hypermagnesemia produces a short QT interval and hypomagnesemia a long QT interval.

ST-Segment Elevation

Acute ST-segment elevation can be due to severe transmural ischemia secondary to thrombus, spasm, or a tight fixed coronary artery lesion or a combination of these situations. It can be the first ECG manifestation of an evolving myocardial infarction and it represents the ECG criteria for administration of thrombolysis (Fig. 3-28). However, if the pain pattern does not persist, it more likely is due to variant or unstable angina. The elevation localizes the ischemia and is very arrhythmogenic.

Chronic or persistent ST-segment elevation could be due to an aneurysm when it occurs over Q waves or to chronic

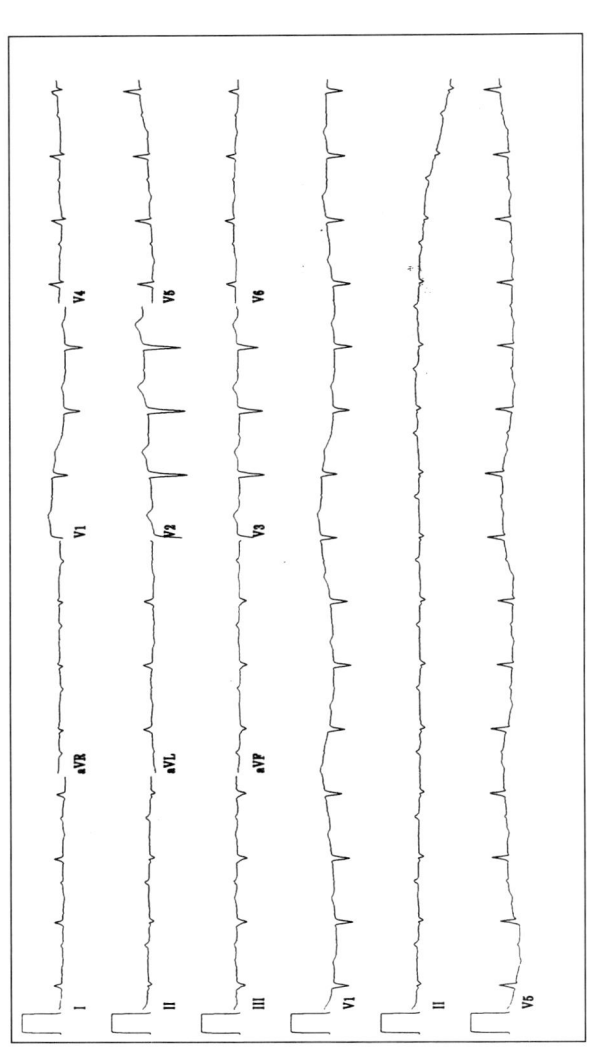

Fig. 3-25. Low QRS voltage. Echocardiography confirmed amyloid heart disease.

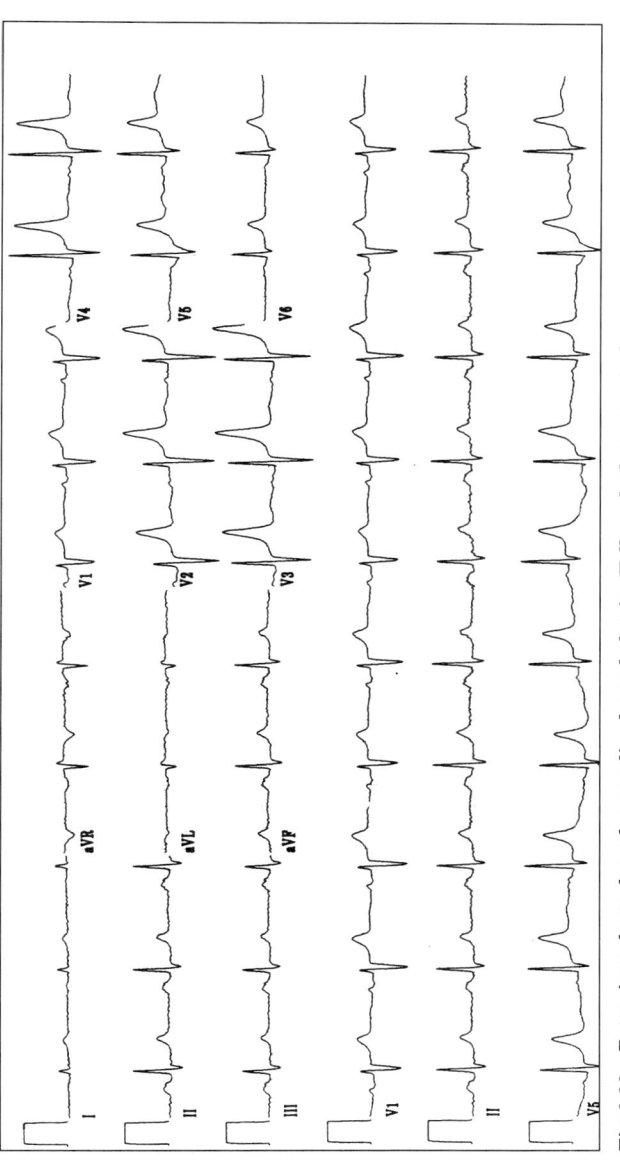

Fig. 3-26. Potassium electrolyte abnormality: hyperkalemia. (Tall, peaked symmetrical waves).

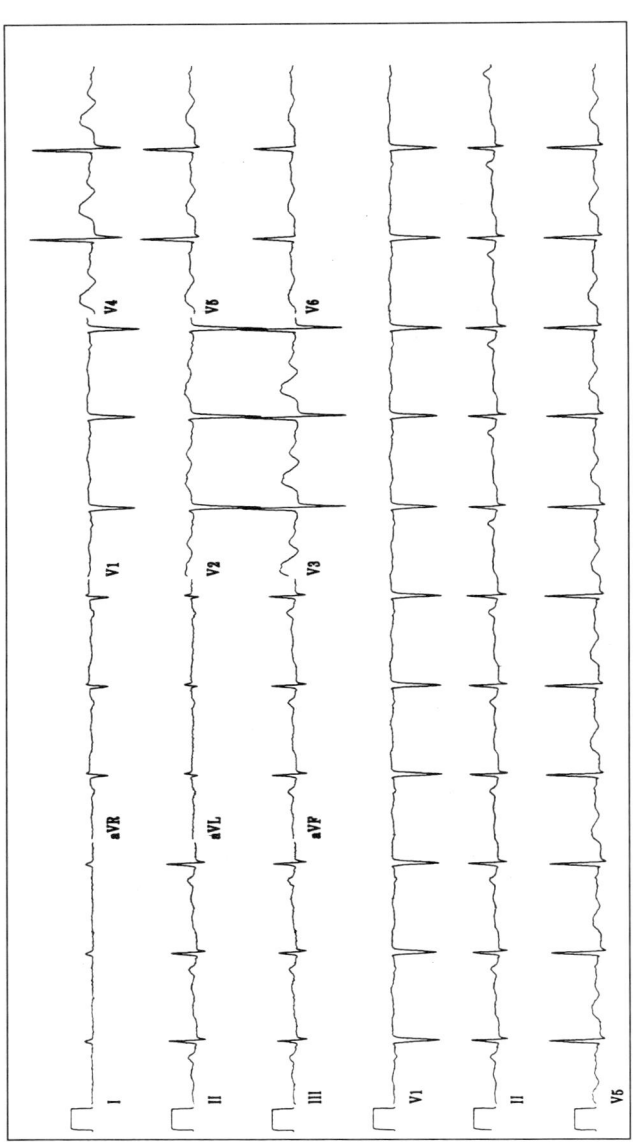

Fig. 3-27.   Calcium electrolyte abnormality: hypocalcemia; prolonged QT interval.

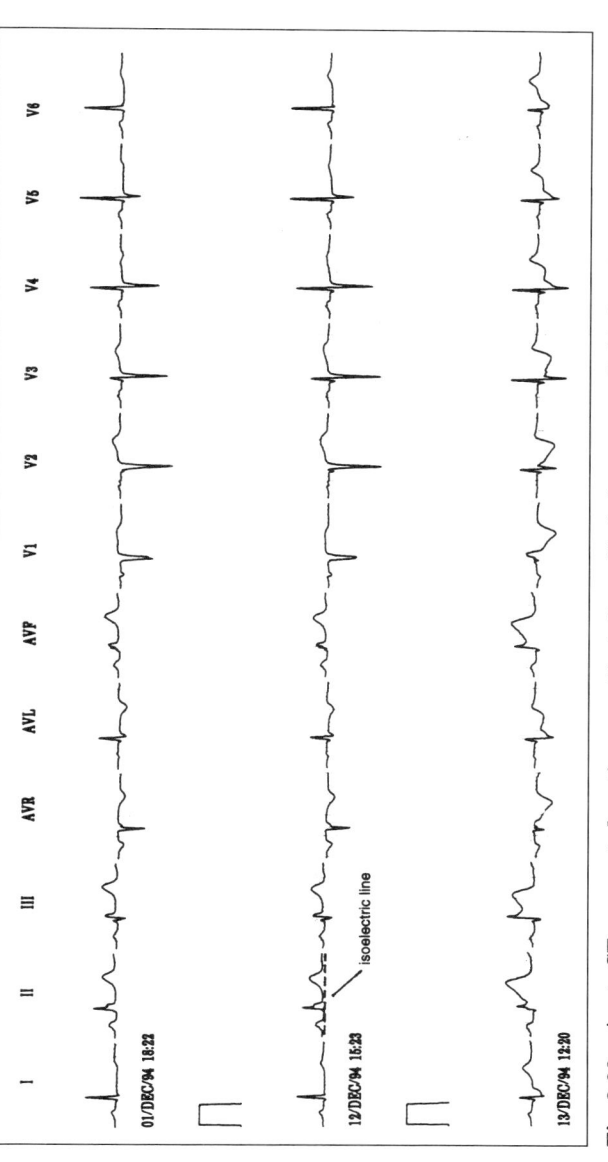

Fig. 3-28.   Acute ST-segment elevation: manifestation of inferior myocardial infarction. Notice the elevation in the inferior leads and reciprocal depression in the precordial leads. There is also an old anteroseptal infarct pattern present in leads V_1 to V_3 and RBBB.

pericarditis (i.e., with uremia), but it most commonly occurs with a normal ECG pattern and is known as early repolarization (Fig. 3-29). It may actually be due to late depolarization and is a very normal finding even to 3 to 4 mm in amplitude.

The differential diagnosis of resting ST-segment elevation is shown in Table 3-2.

ST-Segment Depression

Acute ST-segment depression can be associated with ischemia, hyperventilation, standing, and usage of certain drugs. An ECG should be obtained in any patient with chest pain of uncertain etiology because an acute ST shift can confirm that it is due to ischemia. The amount of ST-segment depression is measured from the PR segment (the isoelectric line).

Fig. 3-29.   Chronic ST-segment elevation: early repolarization in a healthy young male athlete.

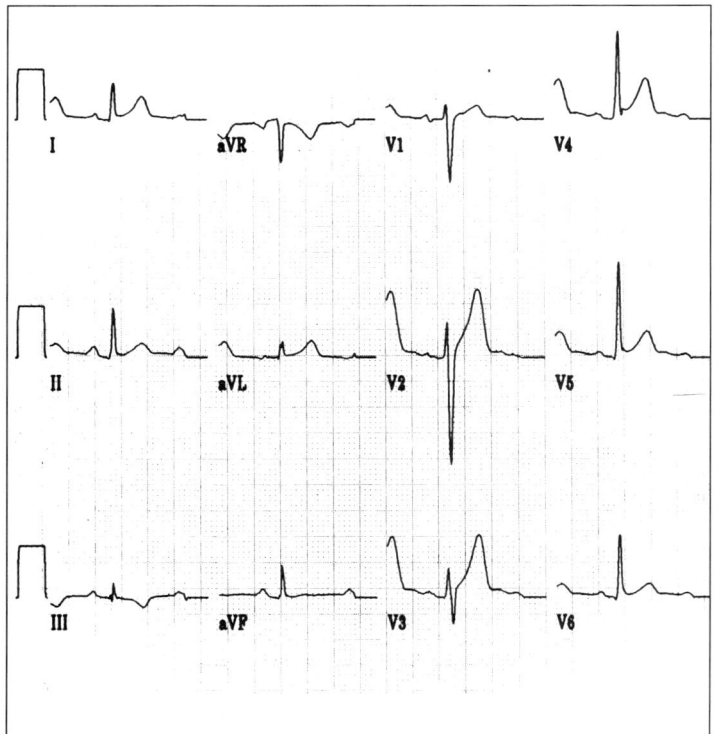

Table 3-2. Differential Diagnosis of Resting ST-Segment Elevation

	Early Repolarization	Acute MI	Pericarditis	Variant AP	Left Ventricular Aneurysm
Time pattern	Constant except with tachycardia	Less than an hour until Q waves appear	Hours to several days	Transient with pain (minutes)	Immediately after MI and for months
Chest pain	None or noncardiac	Typical AP	Positional, pleuritic	Cyclic, at rest, typical AP	None
Other history	Young, athletic	At risk for CAD	Recent URI, pneumonia	Migraines, Raynaud's syndrome	History of MI
PR depression	Rarely in inferior leads	None	Often generalized	None	None
Q wave	Nondiagnostic size	Enlarges as ST elevation lessens	Nondiagnostic size	Can be present	Diagnostic Q waves
ST elevation pattern	Generalized	Localizes to occlusion	Generalized	Localizes to spasm	Localizes to wall motion abnormality

MI = myocardial infarction; AP = angina pectoris; CAD = coronary artery disease; URI = upper respiratory tract infection.

Chronic ST-segment depression is a nonspecific marker for cardiac disease, but is associated with subsequent CHF or death. It can be due to electrolyte abnormalities and usage of drugs, particularly digoxin. It may be associated with subendocardial damage, as opposed to Q waves, which are associated with transmural damage due to infarction. There is some controversy over whether or not resting ST-segment depression ever represents chronic ischemia associated with hibernating myocardium.

Long QT Syndrome
Prolongation of the QT interval is seen in the presence of congenital syndromes, electrolyte/metabolic abnormalities, intrinsic cardiac disease, medication usage, CNS disorders, and systemic illnesses.

Recognition of a prolonged QT interval is complicated by the inaccuracy of Bazlet's formula for correcting for heart rate. Judging the QT interval by changes in length or using the criterion that it exceeds 50% of the RR interval may be preferable. A prolonged QT interval can be due to rare hereditary abnormalities [7], to type Ia antiarrhythmics such as quinidine, to nonsedating antihistamines (such as Seldane) administered along with antifungals or antibiotics, and to hypocalcemia or hypomagnesemia; it is associated with torsades de pointes (turning of the points), a type of ventricular tachycardia. On the other hand, a short QT interval can also result from hypercalcemia, hypermagnesemia, digoxin, or thyrotoxicosis.

T-Wave Changes
In general, T-wave changes are very nonspecific. They can occur with hyperventilation, anxiety, drinking hot or cold beverages, and positional changes. Dramatic T-wave inversions are often seen with athletes' heart syndrome (a constellation of findings not associated with any pathology), and the dramatic T-wave inversions associated with CNS events are very rare. Hyperkalemia (hyperpotassemia) can cause tall, peaked T waves. Hypokalemia and ischemia can cause low-amplitude or inverted T waves.

Serial ECG Changes
Any temporal change in the ECG usually has more significance than a constant, isolated finding. A recent decline in voltage could signify a sudden pericardial effusion. Normalization of ST-segment depression during chest pain could be due to ischemic ST-segment elevation, resulting in a more "normal" ECG than without ischemia. Compari-

son of serial ECGs is critical to proper ECG interpretation. New computer and printing formats are especially helpful for noticing serial changes.

THE CHEST X-RAY FILM

Figure 3-30 illustrates the margins of the cardiac silhouette that present abnormalities on the chest x-ray film and what they indicate. The interpretation of the chest x-ray findings should consider the following.

Technical Factors

1. The heart appears larger on anteroposterior than posteroanterior views.
2. Expiration simulates pulmonary edema and the heart appears larger.
3. One should check side markers for dextrocardia.
4. One should check the clavicles for angulation.
5. Overpenetrated film may miss heart failure.

Extracardiac Structures

1. Rib notching indicates coarctation of the aorta.
2. Pectus excavatum simulates cardiac enlargement.
3. Straight back is associated with mitral valve prolapse and aortic insufficiency.
4. Right-sided pleural effusion occurs with CHF.

Physiologic Analysis of the Pulmonary Vasculature

Though the chest x-ray findings can lag behind hemodynamic changes, the following patterns can predict pulmonary artery wedge pressure:

Grade 0: normal—pulmonary artery wedge pressure less than 12 mm Hg

Grade 1: pulmonary venous hypertension, pulmonary vascular redistribution (venous markings into the upper lobes), and loss of the right hilar angle—pulmonary artery wedge pressure 12 to 19 mm Hg

Grade 2: interstitial edema (Kerley's B lines), hilar haze or blurriness, peribronchial vascular thickening—pulmonary artery wedge pressure 20 to 25 mm Hg

Grade 3: generalized or perihilar alveolar edema—pulmonary artery wedge pressure higher than 25 mm Hg

Cardiovascular Anatomy

Evaluation of the cardiovascular anatomy includes assessment of heart and chamber size as well as the position and size of the great vessels.

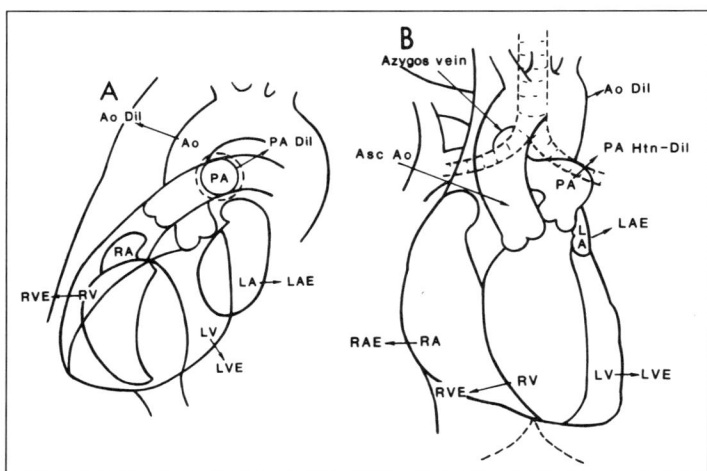

Fig. 3-30. Schematic representations of the cardiac silhouette in the lateral (A) and anteroposterior (B) projections. Ao Dil = aortic dilation; Asc Ao = ascending aorta; PA Htn-Dil = pulmonary artery bulging due to pulmonary hypertension; LAE = left atrial enlargement; RVE/LVE = right/left ventricular enlargement; RAE = right atrial enlargement; PA Dil = pulmonary artery dilation.

Posteroanterior Projection

In the frontal view, the upper right border is formed by the SVC and the lower cardiac border is formed by the right atrium. The left border has three well-defined segments: The uppermost is formed by the aortic arch, the main pulmonary artery lies immediately below the aortic knob, and the lower left cardiac border is formed by the left ventricle and the apex. The left atrial appendage lies between the pulmonary artery segment and the left ventricle and is usually not seen as a separate bulge.

Lateral Projection

In the lateral view, the right ventricle is the most anterior cardiac chamber and is in direct contact with the lower sternum. There should be a clear space (lung tissue) between the sternum, the right ventricular outflow tract, and the root of the pulmonary artery, but pectus excavatum as well as right ventricular enlargement can impinge on this space. The posterior cardiac border is made up of the left atrium above and the left ventricle below.

Chamber Enlargement

ENLARGEMENT OF THE LEFT ATRIUM.   The left atrium is the most posterior of the cardiac chambers and lies in the midline below the carina of the trachea and the mainstem bronchus. The left atrium has two distinct components—a body and an appendage. The body of the left atrium is centrally placed and does not form a border on the frontal view. The left atrial appendage is to the left of the body, immediately beneath the pulmonary artery segment, and above the left ventricle. Chest x-ray studies are most accurate in detecting enlargement of the left atrium compared to the other three chambers. The most common findings are a double density of the right cardiac shadow, bulging of the atrial appendage along the middle of the left cardiac border on the frontal view, and a posterior bulge of the upper cardiac border on the lateral view.

ENLARGEMENT OF THE LEFT VENTRICLE. The left ventricle forms the apex of the heart on the frontal view. With dilation, the cardiac apex is displaced downward toward the diaphragm and to the left. With hypertrophy, the apex becomes rounded.

ENLARGEMENT OF THE RIGHT SIDE. The right atrium forms the right lateral cardiac border. The right ventricle is normally an anterior midline chamber located directly behind the sternum. Enlargement fills in the space behind the sternum [8].

The echocardiogram is much more specific for identifying structural abnormalities and chamber enlargement. The echocardiogram also is very important for distinguishing hypertrophy from dilation and recognizing pericardial effusions.

ECG AND CHEST X-RAY FINDINGS FOR THE KEY FEATURES
ECG Findings with Myocardial Dysfunction
With normal voltage, no abnormal Q waves, and no ST-segment abnormalities, there is a 95% probability of normal ventricular function (i.e., an ejection fraction > 50%). Point systems based on scores for R and Q waves have been used to derive equations to predict ejection fraction, but there is a wide scatter. In general, the size of Q waves, particularly their anterolateral extent, are associated with left ventricular dysfunction. The ECG criteria for left ventricular hypertrophy can be due to hypertrophy or dilation, so the ejection fraction may be good or bad, respectively. In general, LBBB in the older population implies left ventricular dysfunction and a poor prognosis. Low voltage in the limb leads with increased voltage in the precordial leads has been associated with dilated cardiomyopathy.

Chest X-Ray Findings with Myocardial Dysfunction

A large heart on chest x-ray films supports the diagnosis of systolic myocardial dysfunction. A lateral view is often helpful to check for right-sided failure. If the space behind the sternum is filled in, right-sided heart failure and right ventricular dilation are possible. However, echocardiography is most useful for identifying enlargement of a specific chamber and separating dilation from hypertrophy. Increased vascular markings in the upper lobes are secondary to increased filling pressure of about 13 to 18 mm Hg. Interstitial edema (Kerley's B lines) suggests a left ventricular end-diastolic pressure of 19 to 25 mm Hg, and alveolar infiltrates (pulmonary edema) are consistent with a left ventricular end-diastolic pressure higher than 25 mm Hg. Blunting of the margins is due to effusion. The chest x-ray can help rule in or out other causes of dyspnea such as pulmonary fibrosis or chronic obstructive pulmonary disease.

ECG Findings with Myocardial Ischemia

Evidence of old infarction or left ventricular hypertrophy implies underlying coronary artery disease or an imbalance between myocardial oxygen supply and demand, respectively. Resting ST-segment depression has not been consistently associated with ischemia. The ECG findings may point to pericarditis rather than ischemia as the cause of chest pain. While dynamic ST-segment elevation and depression during chest pain should be considered as due to ischemia, they could be due to hyperventilation or a change in heart rate.

Chest X-Ray Findings with Myocardial Ischemia

Special x-ray imaging (fluoroscopy or CT) can demonstrate coronary artery calcification, but this is an uncertain marker. It has not had the test characteristics that were originally anticipated because calcification of the arterial walls is not necessarily associated with luminal occlusion, particularly in older individuals.

ECG Findings with Valvular Dysfunction

Most valvular abnormalities of significance result in evidence of left ventricular hypertrophy with strain, except for mitral stenosis, which shows signs of right ventricular hypertrophy.

Chest X-Ray Findings with Valvular Dysfunction

Signs of CHF and chamber enlargement can be detected

using the chest x-ray studies. Valvular calcification can sometimes be seen.

ECG Findings with Exercise Capacity Status
Sinus bradycardia occurs with athletic training. Fixed-rate pacemakers limit cardiac output. ECG findings consistent with chronic obstructive pulmonary disease and CHF can support a specific cause for decreased exercise capacity. Left ventricular hypertrophy is frequently seen with valvular heart disease.

Chest X-Ray Findings with Poor Exercise Capacity
Signs of pulmonary disease can suggest a noncardiac limitation to exercise and a large heart could suggest cardiac disease. Signs of CHF can offer the possibility of a cardiac cause for a change in exercise capacity.

ECG Findings with Arrhythmias
The resting ECG, particularly accompanied by a rhythm strip, can help in the diagnosis of dysrhythmias. Wide complexes and rhythms that P waves can be seen to march through indicate ventricular arrhythmias. Signal averaging during the resting ECG enables identification of late action potentials and may have value in evaluating the risk for ventricular arrhythmias and sudden death. Heart block can be recognized by a dissociation between the P waves and the QRS complexes. This is most clear when the P waves are faster than the QRS complexes. Otherwise, it is often difficult to recognize and classify the heart block. A long QT interval is usually arrhythmogenic and associated with a number of abnormalities. Absence of P waves with a chaotic ventricular response or fibrillation or flutter waves is atrial fibrillation or flutter.

Chest X-Ray Findings for Arrhythmias
X-ray films are of little use in the diagnosis of arrhythmias. However, finding problems that are often associated with arrhythmias, such as cardiac enlargement and lung disease, should alert the physician to the possibility of arrhythmias. The straight back syndrome or pectus excavatum was thought to be associated with mitral valve prolapse and arrhythmias.

REFERENCES
1. Brugada P, et al. A new approach to the differential diagnosis of a regular tachycardia with a wide QRS complex. *Circulation* 1991;83:1649–1659.

2.   Wellens JJ, Bär WHM, Lie KI. The value of the electrocardiogram in the differential diagnosis of a tachycardia with a widened QRS complex. *Am J Med* 1978; 64:27–33.

3.   Fisch C. Abnormal ECG in clinically normal individuals. *JAMA* 1983;250:1321–1323.

4.   Fisch C. The electrocardiographic QS pattern in leads V1 and V2. *ACC Curr J Rev* 1993;2:72–73.

5.   Norman JE, et al. Improved detection of echocardiographic left ventricular hypertrophy using a new electrocardiographic algorithm. *J Am Coll Cardiol* 1993; 21:1680–1686.

6.   Fisch C. The electrocardiogram and electrolytes. *ACC Curr J Rev* 1994;3:29–30.

7.   Sanguinetti MC, et al. A mechanistic link between an inherited and an acquired cardiac arrhythmia: HERG encodes the I_{kr} potassium channel. *Cell* 1995;81: 299–307.

8.   Shuford WH. Detection of cardiac chamber enlargement with the chest roentgenogram. *Heart Dis Stroke* 1992;2:341–347.

Use and Interpretation of Specialized Tests

TEST EFFICACY
The efficacy of a test should be determined by answering four questions:

1. How well does the test identify those with and those without disease? (That is, what are the sensitivity, specificity, and range of these characteristics, represented by range of characteristic [ROC] curves, for various cutoff points?)
2. Does the test result change the thinking of the physician?
3. Does the test result change therapy?
4. Does the test result change patient outcome?

These questions must be considered when determining cost-efficiency of a testing procedure.

BAYES' THEOREM AND THE PREDICTIVE MODEL
An understanding of the concepts of the predictive model and of baysian statistics is important for the proper use and interpretation of tests [1–3]. Bayes' theorem simply states that the posttest likelihood of disease is determined by both the pretest likelihood and the characteristics of the test. The predictive model describes how the predictive value of a test depends on the prevalence of the disease in the population tested. These concepts are two ways of explaining the diagnostic value of a test, and both terms depend on the sensitivity and specificity of the test.

SENSITIVITY AND SPECIFICITY
Sensitivity is the percentage of abnormal responses when those with disease are tested. *Specificity* is the percentage of normal responses when those without disease are tested—a definition quite different from the conventional use of the word "specific." These two values are inversely related and are determined by the discriminate values or cutoff points chosen for the test that separate abnormal and normal [4].

CUTOFF POINTS OR
DISCRIMINATING VALUES

A basic step in applying any testing procedure for the separation of normal subjects from patients with a disease is to determine a test value that best separates the two groups. One difficulty lies in the considerable overlap of measurement values of a test in the groups with and those without disease. Consider two overlapping bell-shaped normal distribution curves, one representing a normal population and the other representing a population with disease (Fig. 4-1). Along the vertical axis is the number of patients, and along the horizontal axis could be the value for such measurements as Q-wave size, ST-segment depression, or creatinine kinase level. The optimal test would be able to achieve the most marked separation of these two bell-shaped curves and minimize the overlap.

Due to this overlap, problems arise when a certain value is used to separate these two groups (e.g., 1 mm of ST-segment depression, EF <50%, <5 METs, % fractional shortening <20). If the value is set far to the right (e.g., 2 mm of ST-segment depression) in order to identify nearly all the normal subjects as being free of disease, the test will have a high specificity. However, a substantial number of those with disease will be called normal. If a value far to the left is chosen (e.g., 0.5 mm of ST-segment depression) to identify nearly all those with disease as being abnormal, giving the test a high sensitivity, then many normal subjects will be identified as abnormal.

There may be reasons for wanting to adjust a test to have a relatively higher sensitivity or specificity. However, it is important to remember that sensitivity and specificity are inversely related. That is, when sensitivity is the highest, specificity is the lowest and vice versa. Any test has a range of inversely related sensitivities and specificities that can be chosen by selecting a certain discriminate or diagnostic value. Attempts have been made to use a series of tests to improve diagnostic power, but test interaction is complex and usually the combination exhibits the lowest specificity of the combination.

CRITERIA FOR DEMONSTRATING
DIAGNOSTIC CHARACTERISTICS

Guyatt's criteria [5] must be applied to judge the credibility and applicability of the results of studies evaluating diagnostic tests:

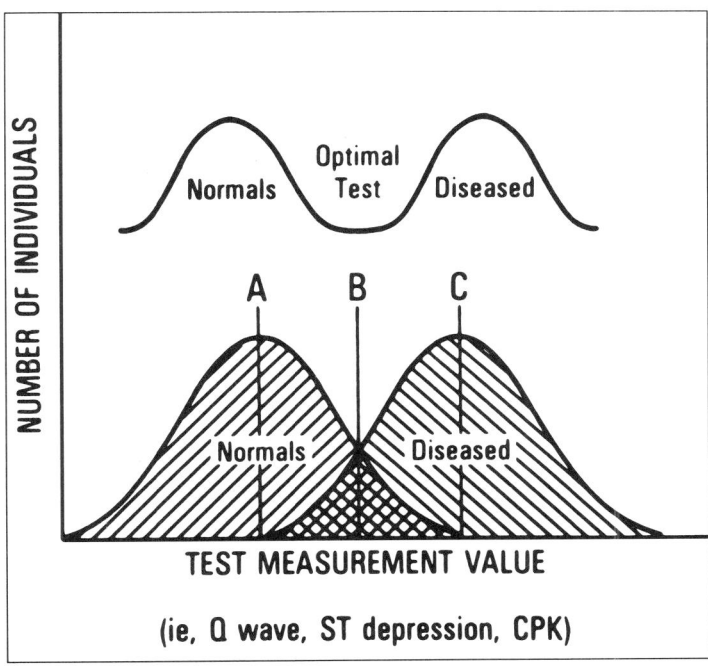

Fig. 4-1. Two overlapping bell-shaped normal distribution curves, one representing a normal population and one representing a population with disease, demonstrate how increasing sensitivity decreases specificity and vice versa. CPK = creatine phosphokinase.

1. The evaluation must include clearly defined comparison groups, at least one of which is free of the disease of interest.
2. The studies should include consecutive patients or randomly selected patients for whom the diagnosis is in doubt. This criterion avoids the two most common evaluation shortcomings: limited challenge and work-up bias.
3. Another issue is including patients who most certainly have the disease (e.g., post–myocardial infarction [MI] patients) in diagnostic samples. They may be included in studies to predict disease severity but should not be included in studies attempting to distinguish those with disease from those without disease.
4. The fourth "believability" criterion requires an independent "blind" comparison of the test with the perfor-

mance of a "gold standard." The gold standard should measure a clinically important state. For example, cardiac catheterization, an invasive test, is used as the gold standard for coronary artery disease rather than symptoms of chest pain alone or another indirect marker, such as nuclear perfusion.

5. Finally, if the gold standard result requires subjective interpretation (as would be the case even for coronary angiography), the interpreter of the gold standard result should not know the test result. Blinding the interpreters of the test to the gold standard and vice versa is necessary. Disagreements between the tests cannot be resolved after considering both test results.

**WORK-UP BIAS AND
LIMITED CHALLENGE**

If Guyatt's five criteria are met, the study can be used as a basis for performance of the test in clinical practice and to establish its diagnostic characteristics (e.g., sensitivity, specificity, and ROC curves for the test). Work-up bias and limited challenge are the two most common causes of inaccurate or nongeneralizable results. *Work-up bias* refers to the fact that most studies using angiography as the gold standard used the work-up (including the test in question) to decide who gets the catheterization. *Limited challenge* refers to the use of extreme groups (i.e., the most normal and the most ill) rather than consecutive patients presenting with the clinical problem or symptom. Any diagnostic test appears to function well if healthy normal subjects are compared with patients who obviously have the disease in question (such a selection is called limited challenge). In most cases clinicians do not need sophisticated testing to differentiate the normal population from the sick. Rather, we are interested in examining patients who are suspected but not known to have the disease of interest and in differentiating those who do from those who do not. If the patients enrolled in the study do not represent this "diagnostic dilemma" group, the test may perform well in the study, but it will not perform well in clinical practice.

PREDICTIVE VALUE

An additional term necessary to define how a diagnostic test performs is determined by the characteristics of the

**DEFINITIONS AND CALCULATION OF TERMS USED TO DEMONSTRATE
THE DIAGNOSTIC VALUE OF A TEST**

$$\text{Sensitivity} = \frac{TP}{TP + FN} \times 100$$

$$\text{Specificity} = \frac{TN}{FP + TN} \times 100$$

Predictive value of abnormal test =

$$\frac{TP}{TP + FP} \times 100$$

**Fig. 4-2. How relative risk and predictive value are calculated.
TP = true positives, or those with abnormal test results and
disease; FN = false negatives, or those with normal test results
and with disease; FP = false positives, or those with abnormal
test results and no disease; TN = true negatives, or those with
normal test results and no disease. Predictive value of an
abnormal response is the percentage of individuals with an
abnormal test result who have disease.**

population. This term is *predictive value*. Figure 4-2 shows
how this term is calculated. The predictive value of an
abnormal test result is the percentage of those persons
with an abnormal test result who have disease. Predictive
value cannot be estimated directly from a test's demonstrated specificity or sensitivity. Predictive value depends
on the prevalence of disease in the population tested. Figure 4-3 illustrates how a test with 70% sensitivity and 90%
specificity performs in a population with a 5% prevalence
of disease. If 5% of 10,000 men have disease, then 500 men
have disease. The middle column represents the number
of men with abnormal test results and the far right column, the number with normal test results. The test is 70%
sensitive; therefore, 350 of those with disease will have
abnormal test results and are true positives. The remaining 150 have normal test results and are false negatives.
As the test is 90% specific, 90% of the 9,500 without disease are true negatives, whereas the remainder are false
positives. To calculate the predictive value, the number of
true positives is divided by the number of those with an
abnormal test result. Figure 4-3 also shows the performance of a test with the same 70% sensitivity and 90%
specificity in a population with a 50% prevalence of disease. There are more false-positive responses when exercise testing is used in a population with a low prevalence of
disease than when it is used in a population with a high

Disease Prevalence	Subjects	Number with Abnormal Test Results	Test Performance	Number with Normal Test Results
5%	500 diseased	450 (TP)	90% sensitivity	50 (FN)
		350 (TP)	70% sensitivity	150 (FN)
	9,500 nondiseased	2,850 (FP)	70% specificity	6,650 (TN)
		950 (FP)	90% specificity	8,550 (TN)
50%	5,000 diseased	4,500 (TP)	90% sensitivity	500 (FN)
		3,500 (TP)	70% sensitivity	1,500 (FN)
	5,000 nondiseased	1,500 (FP)	70% specificity	3,500 (TN)
		500 (FP)	90% specificity	4,500 (TN)

	Predictive Value of Abnormal Test	
Disease Prevalence	5	50
Sensitivity/specificity		
70%/90%	27%	88%
90%/70%	14%	75%
90%/90%	32%	90%
66%/84%	18%	80%
50%/85%	14%	77%

Fig. 4-3.   How a test with various sensitivities and specificities performs in a population with a 5% prevalence of disease and a population with a 50% prevalence. Also shown are the results with a test with 50% sensitivity and 85% specificity, similar to the standard exercise ECG. TP = true positive; FN = false negative; FP = false positive; TN = true negative.

prevalence of disease. This fact explains the greater number of false positives found when the test is used as a screening procedure in an asymptomatic group as opposed to when it is used as a diagnostic procedure in patients with symptoms most likely due to coronary artery disease. Also in Figure 4-3 are the calculations for other test performance characteristics. The key point here is that predictive value is determined by the prevalence of disease in the population tested.

RANGE OF CHARACTERISTIC CURVES
Plots of sensitivity versus specificity for a range of measurement cutoff points allow for a comparison of test performance. They are particularly helpful when optimal cutoff points for discriminating those with disease from those

without disease are not established. An optimal cutoff point can be chosen along the plotted line. A straight diagonal line indicates that the measurement or test has no discriminating power for the disease being tested. The greater the area of the curve above the diagonal line, the greater its discriminating power. ROC curves make it possible to determine and then to choose the appropriate cutoff points for the desired sensitivity or specificity. An example of an ROC curve is given in Figure 4-4.

PROBABILITY ANALYSIS

The information most important to a clinician attempting to make a diagnosis is the probability of the patient having the disease once the test result is known. Such a probability cannot be accurately estimated from the test result and the diagnostic characteristics of the test alone. It also requires knowledge of the probability of the patient having the disease before the test is administered. Bayes' theorem states that the probability of a patient having the disease after a test is performed will be the product of the disease probability before the test and the probability that the test will provide a true result.

The probability of a test result being true can be shown as the likelihood ratio, which is the ratio of true results to false results. In the case of an abnormal test result, the positive likelihood ratio equals

$$\frac{\text{Percent with disease with abnormal test result}}{\text{Percent without disease with abnormal test result}} \quad or \quad \frac{\text{Sensitivity}}{1 - \text{Specificity}}$$

In the case of a normal test result the negative likelihood ratio equals

$$\frac{\text{Percent without disease with normal test result}}{\text{Percent with disease with normal test result}} \quad or \quad \frac{\text{Specificity}}{1 - \text{Sensitivity}}$$

Analysis of the statements in the equations on the left side reveals that they are equivalent to the numerators and denominators in the equations on the right.

The likelihood ratio is an indicator of how discriminating a test is for diagnosis; the higher it is, the greater the diagnostic impact of the test. With conventional techniques of analyzing ST-segment depression with a cutoff point of 0.1 mV, the maximal or near-maximal exercise test has a sensitivity of approximately 50% and a specificity of 85%. Therefore, the likelihood ratio for an abnormal test result is as follows:

Positive likelihood ratio = $0.50 / (1 - 0.85) = 3.3$

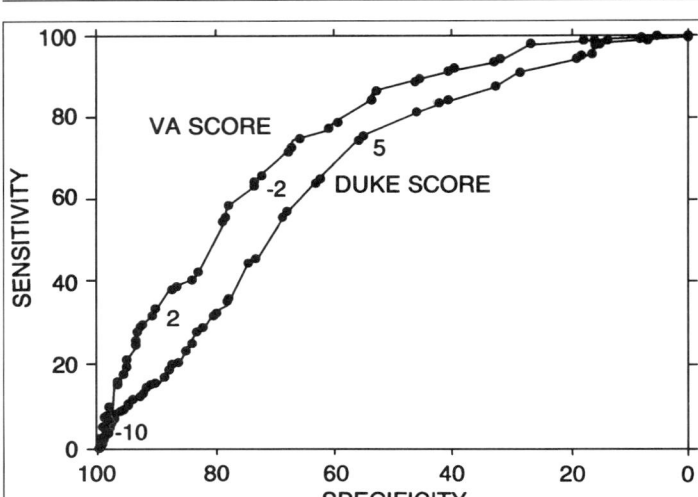

Fig. 4-4.   Example of a range of characteristic (ROC) curve. A straight 45-degree line would mean the test has an ROC area of 0.50, which indicates that it has no discriminating power. The area off the line actually equals the predictive accuracy or percentage of correct diagnoses. The ROC curve allows changing of the cutoff point or discriminating value to match the sensitivity or specificity needed.

The likelihood ratio for a normal test result equals:

Negative likelihood ratio = $0.85 / (1 - 0.50) = 1.7$

Bayes' theorem can be expressed in the following fashion:

Posttest odds of disease = Pretest odds of disease
$\times$ Likelihood ratio of the results

The clinician often makes this calculation intuitively when he or she suspects the abnormal result on an exercise test of a 30-year-old woman with atypical chest pain to be a false positive (low prior odds or probability). The same abnormal response would be accepted as a true result in a 60-year-old man with angina (high prior odds or probability).

Angiographic studies have been used to investigate the prevalence of significant coronary artery disease in patients with different chest pain syndromes. Because chest pain is the presenting complaint in the majority of patients referred for a diagnostic exercise test, the nature of the pain would seem a practical basis for estimating the prior probability of coronary artery disease. Approximately 90% of middle-aged men and postmenopausal women with typical angina pectoris have significant angiographic coronary disease. In similar patients presenting with atypical angina pectoris, approximately 50% have significant angiographic coronary disease. Atypical angina refers to pain that has an unusual location, prolonged duration, or inconsistent precipitating factors. Chest pain that is unresponsive to nitroglycerin is also classified as atypical. Table 4-1 demonstrates the calculation of the probability of coronary artery disease in patients with these different types of chest pain. Patients with multiple types of chest pain are categorized in the group with the most serious chest pain they have.

The 50-year-old male patient with typical angina pectoris has a 90% probability of having significant coronary artery disease. An abnormal exercise test result increases the probability of disease from 90% to 98%. Because such a patient still has a 75% probability of disease if the test result is normal, coronary angiography may yet be required to definitely rule out coronary disease or to ensure treatment is appropriate. The greatest diagnostic impact of testing would be on patients with atypical angina. An abnormal test result would increase the probability of disease to 90%, and for practical purposes, would establish the diagnosis. With a normal test result, the probability of coronary disease would be reduced to 25%.

To apply a valid diagnostic test properly to patients, the following must be considered. Most tests merely indicate an increase or decrease in the probability of disease. To apply imperfect tests appropriately, one must estimate the probability of disease before the test is done ("pretest probability"), then revise this probability according to the test

Table 4-1.   Probability of Coronary Disease for Middle-Aged Men and Postmenopausal Women Before and After the Available Noninvasive Tests for Ischemia

Chest Pain Character	Before the Test	After an Abnormal Test Result	After a Normal Test Result
Typical angina	90%	98%	75–80%
Atypical angina	50%	75–90%	25–40%
Nonangina	10%	25–45%	4–6%
None	2%	6–15%	<1–3%

result. The clinician's estimation of pretest probability is based on the patient's history (including age, gender, and chest pain characteristics), findings on physical examination and initial testing, and the clinician's own experience with this type of problem. Although forming accurate estimations from examination and experience may sound difficult, it is almost always implicitly performed. Lack of symptoms makes the pretest probability so low that a positive test result is most likely to be associated with no disease. Typical angina in a middle-aged man or a postmenopausal woman makes the pretest probability of disease so high that the test result does not have a significant effect. Atypical angina is a 50:50 probability and the test result plays an important role in the diagnostic decision process. The pretest probability is the basis for incorporating the test result. The clinician can use the pretest probability derived from a study as a guide, especially if the patients in that study were randomly selected from a defined group or a consecutive series and if the clinical setting was similar to the clinician's. Even then, the findings from the patient must be taken into account.

Establishing a diagnosis of the five key features of heart disease for patients with symptoms is essential. Identifying the cause of the symptoms and clarifying whether the symptoms are cardiac, pulmonary, neurologic, or psychological or due to disease in other organ systems makes it possible to logically decide if and how the symptoms should be treated. The same concern exists for routinely quantifying the five key features for determination of prognosis.

PROGNOSTIC APPLICATION OF TESTS

The two major uses of tests are for diagnosis and for prognosis. As discussed already, diagnosis relates to giving a probability value to whether or not an individual has a disease. Correct diagnosis is mandatory to determine whether treatment should be instituted to decrease symptoms. For instance, in a patient with chest pain, an abnormal exercise test result indicates that the patient has a high probability for coronary heart disease and could provide the basis for beginning an antianginal agent. Remember that a test can only generate a probability statement of an outcome! The results are not absolutes and the multifactorial nature of prognosis must be considered. For instance, the patient with poor left ventricular (LV) function who has good exercise capacity may do reasonably well. The prognosis predicted by any risk predictor can be modified by other predictors or by markers of outcome.

The following test results have reproducibly and consistently been associated with a good prognosis:

- Normal ejection fraction
- Normal ECG
- High MET level with exercise testing
- Normal nuclear perfusion test result

RATIONALE OF PROGNOSTIC TESTING

Of what use is the determination of prognosis? If treatments that alter prognosis are available, then certainly the key features can identify groups of patients for whom the treatment to alter prognosis may justify the inconvenience and risk of treating. However, few of the available treatments are as clearly beneficial as, for instance, beta-blockers are for altering the prognosis for MI. Most treatments are for symptomatic relief rather than for altering longevity. A good prognostic statement can reassure a patient, but most ethicists would say that the patient has a right to know the future impact of an illness, even if it is not reassuring. Such information enables the planning of life options accordingly. Does the patient want to continue in an unsatisfying job or to put money away for retirement? Should the payment of large life insurance premiums be a priority? These are some examples of the decisions that can be altered by prognostic determinations. The patient's need to know must be balanced by the psychological impact of the information on his or her current situation and mental health.

Therefore, there are two principal purposes of prognosis estimation. The first is to provide accurate answers to patients' questions regarding the probable outcome of their illness. Most patients find this information useful in planning their affairs regarding work, recreational activities, personal estate, and finances. The second reason to determine prognosis is to identify the patients in whom interventions might improve outcome.

Pathophysiology of the
Five Key Empirical Features

The basic pathophysiologic features of the first two key features, myocardial ischemia and myocardial dysfunction, are most commonly caused by coronary artery disease. The clinical variables and stress test responses that are due to myocardial ischemia include angina, ST-segment depression, ST-segment elevation over ECG areas without Q waves, thallium-detected or sesti-MIBI–detected reperfusion defect, a decline in ejection fraction with exercise, or new LV wall motion occurring with stress (Table 4-2). Predicting the amount of ischemia (i.e., the amount of myocardium in jeopardy) is difficult. It appears to be inversely related to the double product at the onset of signs or symptoms of ischemia. ST-segment elevation over diagnositc Q waves is the only ECG response specifically associated with LV dysfunction (see Table 4-2). This indicates depressed LV function and possibly large aneurysms. Clinical markers include a history of congestive heart failure (CHF) or MIs, large Q waves, bundle-branch block, LV hypertrophy, gallops, and cardiomegaly. Test markers of decreased LV function all relate to estimates of ejection fraction. The exercise responses due to both ischemia and LV dysfunction include chronotropic incompetence or heart rate impairment, systolic BP drops, and a poor exercise capacity. Their association with both ischemia and dysfunction explains why these exercise responses are so important in predicting prognosis.

The pathophysiology of vavular dysfunction, the third key feature, can be due to sclerosis (aortic stenosis), congenital abnormalities (bicuspid aortic valve), autoimmune reactions (rheumatic disease leading to mitral stenosis), histocompatibility abnormalities (ankylosing spondylitis), infection (tricuspid endocarditis associated with intravenous drug use), or myxomatous degeneration (mitral valve prolapse, aortic root dissection). The resultant heart failure or susceptibility to endocarditis explains the morbidity and mortality. It can be secondary to LV dilation resulting in enlargement of the atrioventricular rings with resultant insufficiency of the mitral or tricuspid valve.

It remains uncertain specifically why exercise capacity, the fourth key feature, is an independent predictor of mortality, though this is most likely because of the combination of factors that are part of the integrated response to exercise (i.e., lungs, heart, and other organs). In many different classifications of patients with heart disease, poor exercise capacity has been identified as an independent predictor of subsequent cardiac events, including myocardial infarction and death. However, exercise capacity poorly correlates with LV function in patients without signs or symptoms of right-sided heart failure. Exercise testing is not very helpful in identifying patients with

Table 4-2.   Clinical Exercise Testing Variables Associated with Cardiac Disease

Ischemia	Left Ventricular Function	Both
Angina	ST-segment elevation over Q waves	Low heart rate response
ST-segment depression (≥ 0.1-mV flat or downsloping)	Q waves on resting ECG and exercise-induced elevation in the leads with the Q wave	Flat or drop in systolic BP during exercise
ST-segment elevation without Q waves		Low METs for age
Reperfusion defect with thallium 201 or sesti-MIBI		
Failure of ejection fraction to rise with exercise		
New left ventricular wall motion with stress		

moderate LV dysfunction, a group known to have improved survival after coronary bypass surgery. Moderate LV dysfunction is better recognized by a history of CHF, physical examination, resting ECG, echocardiography, or radionuclide ventriculography.

The fifth key feature, arrhythmia status, does not appear to be independently predictive of coronary artery disease because the prognosis of arrhythmias is closely related to LV abnormalities except in rare circumstances (e.g., the several thousand individuals in the world with prolonged QT-interval syndrome, a genetic abnormality). Exercise-induced dysrhythmias indicate electrical instability most often due to LV dysfunction rather than to ischemia (except for exercise-induced ST-segment elevation in a normal ECG, which is very arrhythmogenic) and do not appear to have independent predictive power.

Statistical Methods for Prognostication

To determine the prognostic implications of clinical and test variables, follow-up studies must be performed and survival analysis (special statistical methods) applied. Survival analysis consists of a group of univariate and multivariate mathematical techniques that consider person-time of exposure and use it to calculate hazard or risk.

Censoring is done at the time of "lost to follow-up," removal from risk (e.g., coronary artery bypass surgery, percutaneous transluminal coronary angioplasty, cardiac transplantation, valve replacement), or study termination. Comparisons are made between person-time units of survival or exposure. The following explains why this is necessary. Consider two groups of 100 patients, both with 10 deaths in a year of follow-up (a 10% mortality). However, in this example, all 10 in one group die at the beginning of the year, while in the other group they all die at the end of the year. The former situation certainly would have a worse significance than the latter but only would be detected by appropriate survival analysis and not by simple proportion testing (i.e., both had a 10% death rate).

The two most commonly used survival techniques are Kaplan-Meier survival curves for univariate analysis and the Cox hazard model for analysis. Multivariate analysis is necessary because many of the variables interact. Univariately, variables can be associated with death, but the association may be through other variables. For instance, digoxin use associates with death through CHF, and exercise-induced ST-segment elevation associates with death most often through the underlying Q waves.

The study of prognosis is further complicated by the fact that cardiac death occurs in a spectrum; there are patients with myocardial damage who die of CHF (or pump failure) and those with normal ventricles in whom ischemia precipitates death. The clinical and test markers would be expected to be quite different for patients who die at the extremes of this spectrum. While markers of myocardial damage (history of CHF, Q waves) track the former, markers of ischemia (angina, ST-segment depression) better predict the latter. Still other markers, such as arrhythmias, poor exercise capacity, and exertional hypotension, are associated with both. Further complicating prediction algorithms, "damage" markers predict short-term deaths, while "ischemic" markers predict deaths occurring 2 years or later. Given this etiologic milieu, associating clinical and test markers with death as an outcome becomes quite difficult. Differences in populations may favor one or the other type of mortality (pump failure versus ischemia). This may explain why ischemic variables are more predictive in some populations and myocardial damage variables more predictive in others. Table 4-3 lists the prognoses for different conditions associated with the five key features.

Table 4-3. The Specific Prognoses for Different Types of Conditions Associated with the Five Key Features of Heart Disease

Key Features	Type	Prognosis
Myocardial dysfunction	Systolic (dilated cardiomyopathy)	10 to 25% annual mortality
	Diastolic (hypertrophic cardiomyopathy)	Depends on cause; lower mortality than dilated cardiomyopathy
Myocardial ischemia	Angina	2 to 4% annual mortality
	Post MI	2 to 30% mortality in first year depending on clinical features
	Variant angina	Uncertain mortality; low prevalence
Valvular disorders	Original	Poor when valvular or myocardial dysfunction occurs
	Prosthetic	Depends on type and specific characteristics
Exercise intolerance	Cardiac cause	Prognostic equation scores include METs
	Noncardiac cause	Underlying disease determines the prognosis
Arrhythmias	Atrial fibrillation	Expected mortality doubles and 5% annual risk for cerebrovascular accident
	Complete heart block	If syncope occurs, mortality high
	Ventricular tachycardia	Depends on characteristics and associated conditions

MI = myocardial infarction.

SPECIALIZED TESTS
Echocardiography
Indications
The indications for echocardiography are as follows:

Diagnosis of cardiac murmurs, rubs, or enlargement suggested by physical examination or ECG; or diagnosis of specific chamber enlargement or pericardial effusion after cardiomegaly is noted on a chest x-ray

Evaluation of cardiac function and morphology (i.e., as part of work-up for CHF, MI, dyspnea on exertion [DOE], and hypertension)

Identification of intercardiac thrombus associated with syncope, stroke, transient ischemic attacks (TIAs), or high risk for thrombus (particularly in patients with an MI, dilated cardiomyopathy, or atrial fibrillation)

Estimation of severity and serial follow-up for valvular disease

Confirmation and follow-up of subacute bacterial endocarditis (SBE)

Contraindications, Risks, and Dangers
Although the test may be technically difficult and the results less reliable in smokers, the obese, patients with chronic obstructive pulmonary disease (COPD), or patients who are tachypneic, there are no contraindications, risks, or dangers.

Description
Sound waves are both broadcast on a plane (in two dimensions) and received by a probe held by hand on the chest wall. The waves reflected off structures are imaged on a screen representing a plane cut through the heart at various angles. This allows for accurate measurements of wall and chamber size. With Doppler techniques, the direction and velocity of blood flow can be estimated. The color Doppler makes it possible to recognize diastolic dysfunction and to estimate valvular gradient and area. Red usually signifies forward flow and blue backward flow, enabling recognition of stenosis and regurgitation. Due to the attenuation of ultrasound signals by the chest wall and lungs (particularly of smokers), passing an ultrasound transducer down the throat (transesophageal echocardiography) allows for better visualization of thrombus, vegetations, and wall motion abnormalities.

Preparation of Patient
The patient is instructed to lie down on the table, turned on the left side, in a darkened room. The probe is pressed to the chest and will be moved and twisted. The patient will be asked to breathe in and out on command and to hold the breath out. The patient should not have smoked or overeaten in the 2 hours prior to the test.

Interpretation
An example of an echocardiogram report is given below (Fig. 4-5). The interpreter must develop considerable skill so that the appropriate views can be recognized in order to make the various measurements. Artifacts make the measurements more difficult than anticipated, but experience can usually prevent major errors. Fractional shortening is merely the percent shortening along a single axis and is only valid as an indicator of LV function if there are no major localized wall motion abnormalities. Equations can be used to estimate ejection fraction but not all echocardiography laboratories provide this measurement. Thrombus is not always easy to detect but pedunculated clots can be mobile and very easy to image.

```
SMITH,DAVID W    ID#: 999-68-8731    Room/Clinic        DOB: 03/16/47
              PROCEDURE DATE/TIME: 11/01/95 11:01
- - - - - - - - - - - - - - - - - - - - - - - - - - - - - - - - - - - - -
WARD/CLINIC: MCCU

REFERRING PHYSICIAN: NEEDY, JANE MD

   AGE: 48                    SEX: MALE

   HT IN: 75       WT LBS: 145     BSA:  1.9

RESTING SYSTOLIC BP: 144     DIASTOLIC BP:  78    HEART RATE: 76

INDICATIONS: EVALUATE MYOCARDIAL AND VALVULAR FUNCTION

STUDY TYPE: TRANSTHORACIC OR TRANSESOPHAGEAL

QUALITY OF STUDY:

TEST RESULTS:

            M-MODE MEASUREMENTS (CHAMBER SIZES AND WALL THICKNESS)

LEFT ATRIUM:           (25-45mm)        LV IN DIASTOLE:      (37-57mm)
AORTIC ROOT:           (20-40mm)        LV IN SYSTOLE:
RV IN DIASTOLE:        (10-25mm)
% FRACTIONAL SHORTENING (LVS/LVD X 100):        (25-45)
ANTERIOR RV WALL:        (2-4mm)
INTRAVENTRICULAR SEPTUM IN DIASTOLE:            (6-14mm)
E POINT SEPTAL SEPARATION:                      (0-5mm)
INTRAVENTRICULAR SEPTUM IN SYSTOLE:             (8-20mm)
LV POSTERIOR WALL THICKNESS IN DIASTOLE:        (5-13mm)
LV POSTERIOR WALL THICKNESS IN SYSTOLE:         (9-21mm)


                  TWO DIMENSIONAL/DOPPLER FINDINGS

REGURGITATION:    AVR        MVR        TVR        PVR

OUTFLOW OBSTRUCTION/VALVE AREA:        AVA        MVA

VALVE MORPHOLOGIES/VEGETATIONS/FLOWS:

ESTIMATED LV FUNCTION:

WALL MOTION ABNORMALITIES/LV THROMBUS:

PERICARDIAL EFFUSION:

ESTIMATED PA PRESSURE:

   CONCLUSION:
```

Fig. 4-5. Example of an echocardiogram report.

Radionuclide Tests

Cardiac Imaging of Technetium Pyrophosphate Injection
INDICATIONS. Imaging with the radionuclide technetium pyrophosphate is used for diagnosing MI when other tests are not valid (e.g., ECG shows LBBB, enzyme levels already returned to normal).

CONTRAINDICATIONS, RISKS, AND DANGERS. There are virtually no contraindications, risks, or dangers. The cancer risk is very low.

DESCRIPTION. Pyrophosphate binds to calcium released by cell death, and the tagged technetium creates a "hot spot" on the image proportionate to the infarct size.

PREPARATION OF PATIENT. After intravenous injection, the patient is imaged with a standard gamma scintillation camera for about ½ hour.

INTERPRETATION. A hot spot proportionate to the infarct size is seen in planar or single-photon emission computed tomography (SPECT) images. Bone or other calcium deposits can cause hot spots that are artifacts or that interfere with interpretation. This test has been used to recognize MIs as a complication of cardiac surgery but currently is used only rarely.

Radionuclide Ventriculography
(Multi-ECG-Gated Acquisition or MUGA)
INDICATIONS. This test is used to estimate ejection fraction and ventricular wall motion.

CONTRAINDICATIONS, RISKS, AND DANGERS. There are no contraindications. However, because imaging is dependent on the ECG dividing the cardiac cycle into equal windows for count accumulation, atrial fibrillation or frequent premature ventricular contractions lessen the accuracy.

Although it is necessary for the patient to lie stationary for at least 5 minutes, the risk or danger posed by the radiation is minimal. Technetium has a 6-hour half-life, which exposes patients to less than 5 mrem of radiation (roughly equivalent to the radiation exposure of many standard clinical x-ray studies).

DESCRIPTION. After intravenous injection of technetium tagged to RBCs by tin, a scintillation camera is placed over the heart and imaging is begun. The usual single-crystal camera only produces images by processing the imaging counts into a computer. The ECG is used to divide the cardiac cycle into a series of timed windows in which the counts are gathered for imaging. The images created in these windows are then visualized sequentially like an endless loop cine film. This provides an image similar to a left ventricular angiogram. Although no geometric assumptions are necessary, as for radiographic imaging, the measurement of ejection fraction is affected by the background settings and other artifacts.

PREPARATION OF PATIENT.   An intravenous line must be placed and secured; electrodes are necessary to obtain an ECG signal for gating the images. The patient must be able to lie still for at least 5 minutes.

INTERPRETATION.   Wall motion programs usually automate the process of identifying wall motion and estimating ejection fraction. Normal sinus rhythm is essential for gating the images, and mitral regurgitation makes the ejection fraction appear to be associated with a better-than-expected ventricular function because of the unloading of the ventricle due to backward flow of blood expelled with each contraction through the mitral valve.

Thallium or Isonitrile (sesti-MIBI) Perfusion Scanning

INDICATIONS.   Imaging after administration of thallium or an isonitrile is used to recognize viable, perfused myocardium. Resting studies have been used to determine whether there is viable myocardium that might benefit from reperfusion. Higher doses of radionuclide must be used with resting studies than with exercise studies because of the lower coronary blood flow, but viable myocardium is present if the area in question is visualized (i.e., lights up).

CONTRAINDICATIONS, RISKS, AND DANGERS.   The half-life, normal-dose, and radiation exposure for thallium and technetium are considered here because either can be used (technetium is tagged to the perfusion agent sesti-MIBI). Technetium 99m decays by photon emission with a peak energy component at 140 keV and a half-life of 6 hours. The risk of developing cancer from the normal dose is 1 in 2,000, an increase of 0.05% over the expected risk of cancer, which is 0.25%. Thallium 201 has a half-life of 3 days and decays giving off x-rays with a peak energy component at 80 keV. Because thallium has a longer half-life than technetium, the amount of thallium given to the patient must be reduced so that the radiation exposure is the same. The lower half-life of technetium allows for a higher dose to be given. Because of this and the higher emission energy that results in less scattered radiation, technetium results in better images than does thallium.

There are no contraindications.

DESCRIPTION.   At peak exercise, either thallium 201 or technetium tagged to an isonitrile is injected into a peripheral arm vein, and imaging with a scintillation crystal is begun. Thallium 201 is a radioactive agent that behaves like potassium and is taken up by viable, perfused myocardial and other muscle cells. It gives off low-energy x-rays that are subject to scatter. When injected at peak exercise, it is taken up more avidly by myocardium than when injected at rest, due to the higher coronary flow during exercise. The presence of a cold spot on the image during exercise could result from ischemia or scar. Imaging is then repeated 4 hours later; if the cold spot fills in, the spot was caused by ischemia. However, in 25% of cases of severe ischemia, the cold spots do not fill in within 4 hours. For patients without history or ECG evidence of MI in whom the cold spot does not fill in, most laboratories repeat the imaging procedure. For convenience, this is usually performed 24 hours later, and a higher dose of radionuclide must be used because there is less avid takeup by the myocardium at rest.

Sesti-MIBI is an isonitrile chemical that also accumulates in viable muscle cells in the heart and other muscles. It is tagged with technetium, which gives off gamma rays that have imaging characteristics superior to those of thallium. A cold spot noted after injection at peak exercise still signifies ischemia or scar, but technetium does not redistribute like thallium. Instead, a second injection is required. This is actually helpful because the time from injection to imaging is not as critical an issue for recognizing ischemia as it is when thallium is used, which requires immediate postexercise imaging in order not to miss exercise-induced ischemia.

PREPARATION OF PATIENT.   An intravenous line must be placed and secured; electrodes are necessary to obtain an ECG signal for gating the images. The patient must be able to lie still for at least 15 minutes; the prone position is preferred, to lessen artifacts in the inferior wall due to diaphragmatic uptake.

INTERPRETATION.   These agents can be imaged using planar or SPECT techniques. The latter creates three-dimensional images that are more subject to artifact, resulting in a lower specificity. A cold spot or defect is a scar or relative ischemia. If the patient is imaged again and filling in or redistribution of the cold spots occurs, ischemia is present.

Exercise Testing

Standard ECG Exercise Testing

INDICATIONS.   The four major indications for exercise testing [6] are as follows:

1. Diagnosing coronary artery lesions significant enough to cause myocardial ischemia
2. Establishing the severity of coronary artery disease and estimating cardiovascular mortality
3. Evaluating exercise capacity
4. Evaluating interventions such as medications, surgery, and exercise training

CONTRAINDICATIONS, RISKS, AND DANGERS.   Before an exercise test is started, contraindications to exercise testing must be addressed. If any contraindications are present, the patient should either be rescheduled for testing or considered for another method for evaluation. Risk-increasing contraindications can be identified from the history, physical examination, or ECG findings.

Specific questions from the history would include the following:

1. Is the patient's disease stable? Are the symptoms stable or unstable (new or increasing symptoms)?
2. Does the patient have true angina pectoris? Question the patient regarding any chest pain characteristics and make a determination as to whether the pain is noncardiac, typical, or atypical?
3. Does the patient have CHF? Check the patient's history and tests documenting CHF.
4. What is the patient's neurologic status? Is there a history of stroke or syncope?
5. What is the arrhythmia status? Is there a history of palpitations, arrhythmias, syncope, sudden death, or cardioversion?
6. Is there a history of uncontrolled hypertension?
7. Is there a change in activity status?

A brief physical examination should always be performed to rule out significant obstructive aortic valvular disease, obstructive or nonobstructive cardiomyopathy, and dilated cardiomyopathy. If a patient is diagnosed with dilated cardiomyopathy, signs of CHF and LV dysfunction should be noted. If a patient has recently had an exacerbation of heart failure or CHF with a recent MI, the test should *not* be performed. If the patient has aortic stenosis as shown by history and examination, usually an echo-cardiogram including a Doppler assessment of the aortic gradient should be obtained before the exercise test is performed.

A baseline supine ECG should be compared to previous ECGs to determine significant changes and baseline abnormalities.

The MI status (new or old) and its severity should be determined and whether a maximal or submaximal proto-col should be used must be decided.

Possible contraindications to exercise testing include

- Recent MI
- Unstable angina
- Variant angina
- Previous problems with testing
- Episode of sudden death/ventricular tachycardia requiring treatment
- Exercise-induced syncope or arrhythmia
- CHF or evidence for LV dysfunction, complicated MI
- Obstructive aortic outflow disorder (asymmetric septal hypertrophy, aortic stenosis)
- Uncontrolled hypertension
- Pericardial tumors or cysts
- Cardiac vegetations or endocarditis
- Acute pericarditis

Due to the publication of strict guidelines, the danger of testing level is very low. Approximately four events (including CPR, MI, or death) can be expected per 10,000 tests.

DESCRIPTION.   The patient walks on a motor-driven treadmill with controlled speed and grade, or pedals a cycle with controlled resistance, until signs or symptoms occur or until exhaustion. A submaximal target is usually used if the test is performed within 3 weeks of an MI. A 12-lead ECG is recorded throughout exercise and recovery. Various continuous, progressive protocols have been uti-lized. BP must always be monitored during exercise test-ing; manual sphygmomanometry is the best way to do this (the automated systems are not reliable during exercise). Exercise capacity (in METs or VO_2 max) can be estimated from the treadmill speed and grade or by the bike work-load. Scores from the Borg scale of perceived exertion (Fig. 4-6) should be recorded every 2 minutes. Angina should not be allowed to exceed the usual level that occurs with everyday activities. Hyperventilation should not be per-

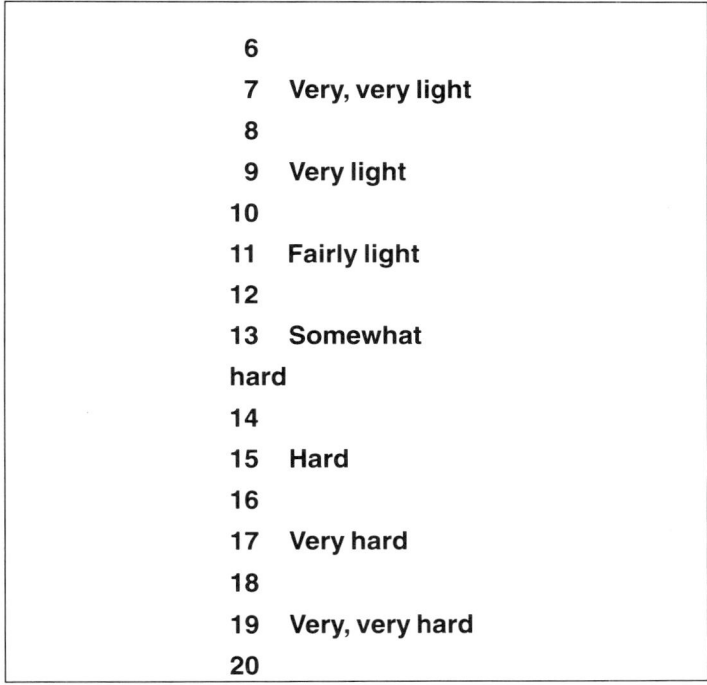

6

7 Very, very light

8

9 Very light

10

11 Fairly light

12

13 Somewhat hard

14

15 Hard

16

17 Very hard

18

19 Very, very hard

20

Fig. 4-6. The linear Borg scale of perceived exertion.

formed prior to testing. The patient should lie down as soon as possible after the test. The 3-minute recovery period ECG is critical for ST-segment analysis, and ECG strips should be recorded immediately after exercise and at each minute thereafter for 5 minutes or longer until changes have stabilized.

PREPARATION OF PATIENT. Preparations for exercise testing include the following:

1. The patient should be instructed not to eat or smoke at least 2 to 3 hours prior to the test, and to come dressed to exercise.
2. A brief history should be obtained and physical examination performed to rule out any contraindications to testing and to determine the patient's activity level.
3. Specific questioning should determine which drugs are being taken, and potential electrolyte abnormalities should be considered. The labeled medication bottles should be requested of the patient so that the drugs can

be identified and recorded. Because of the life-threatening rebound phenomena associated with beta-blockers, they should not be stopped routinely prior to testing. However, if testing is performed for diagnostic purposes, they can be gradually stopped if a physician or nurse carefully supervises the tapering process.

4. If the reason for the exercise test is not apparent, the referring physician should be contacted.

5. A 12-lead ECG should be obtained for both the supine and the standing position. The supine ECG should be compared to previous supine ECGs. This is an important rule, particularly in patients with known heart disease, as an abnormality or a change may prohibit testing. On occasion, a patient referred for an exercise test will instead be admitted to the coronary care unit.

A worksheet is provided in Appendix C.

INTERPRETATION. **ST-Segment Analysis.** The interpretation of the exercise test requires an understanding of physiology and pathophysiology gained through training and experience. The American College of Physicians has guidelines on clinical competence for physicians performing exercise testing [7]. The criteria of 1 mm of horizontal or downsloping ST-segment depression measured at the J-junction continues to provide optimal test characteristics. ST-segment depression is a representation of global subendocardial ischemia, with direction determined largely by the placement of the heart in the chest; thus, the most important ST-segment depression occurs in lead V_5. ST-segment depression does not localize coronary artery lesions. The degree of ST depression should be measured at the end of the QRS complex (also known as the J-junction or ST0) (Fig. 4-7). ST depression in the inferior leads (II, aVF) is most often due to the atrial repolarization wave, which begins in the PR segment and can extend to the beginning of the ST segment. Severe transmural ischemia, resulting in wall motion abnormalities, causes a shift of the vector in the direction of the wall motion abnormality. However, preexisting areas of wall motion abnormality (e.g., scar), usually indicated by a Q wave, also cause such a shift resulting in ST-segment elevation without ischemia being present. When the resting ECG shows Q waves of an old MI, ST-segment elevation is due to ischemia or wall motion abnormalities or both. When the resting ECG is normal, however, exercise-induced ST-segment elevation is due to severe ischemia (spasm or a criti-

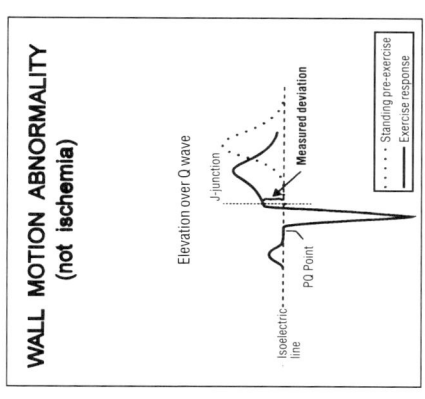

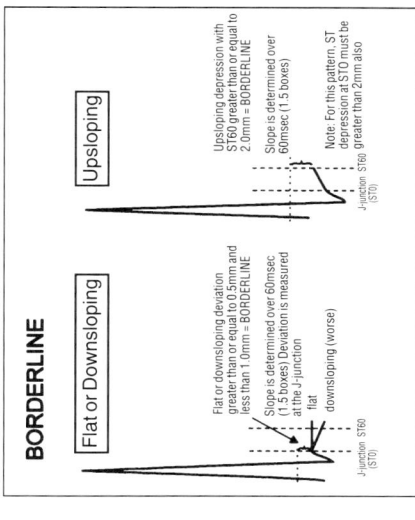

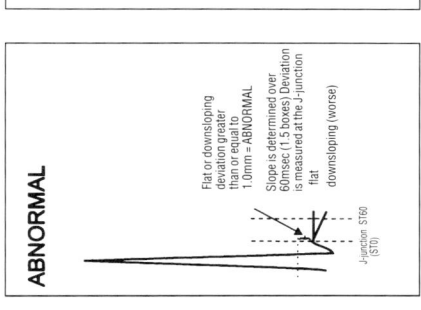

Fig. 4-7. Examples of ST-segment responses to exercise.

cal lesion). ST-segment depression limited to the recovery period does not generally represent a false-positive response. Avoidance of a cool-down walk and inclusion of ST-segment analysis during this time period increases the diagnostic yield of the exercise test. Figure 4-7 provides examples of ST-segment responses to exercise. Figure 4-8 illustrates how to account for the ST level during standing before exercise.

Arrhythmias. As with resting ventricular arrhythmias, the significance of exercise-induced ventricular arrhythmias is related to the disease processes they are associated with (syncope, sudden death, a large heart, murmurs, ECG showing prolonged QT interval, preexcitation, Q waves). If there are no signs or symptoms of associated diseases, then the clinician can usually ignore exercise-induced ventricular arrhythmias (do not behave as if in a coronary care unit). In most patients with coronary disease, ventricular arrhythmias occurring during exercise testing most likely do not have an independent association with death; that is, other variables can provide a better prediction. Most likely, there are a small percentage of patients in whom exercise-induced ventricular arrhythmias are independently predictive of death. Nonsustained ventricular tachycardia is uncommon during routine clinical treadmill testing, is well tolerated, and is associated with a relatively good prognosis. Outcome is primarily determined by concomitant clinical features such as ventricular function, ischemia, and symptoms.

Hemodynamic Responses. Rather than relying on functional classifications, physicians frequently use exercise testing for disability evaluation because it can objectively demonstrate exercise capacity. No questionnaire, submaximal test, or nonexercise stress test can give the same results as a symptom-limited exercise test. Exercise capacity should be reported in METs rather than in minutes of exercise. METs are multiples of basal ventilatory oxygen consumption. They can be estimated from different activities or calculated from treadmill speed and grade using the following equation:

METs = (mph × 26.8 [0.1 + {% grade × 1.8}] + 3.5)/3.5

Age-predicted maximal heart rate targets are relatively useless for clinical purposes. It is surprising how much steeper the age-related decline in maximal heart rate is in referred populations as compared to age-matched normal

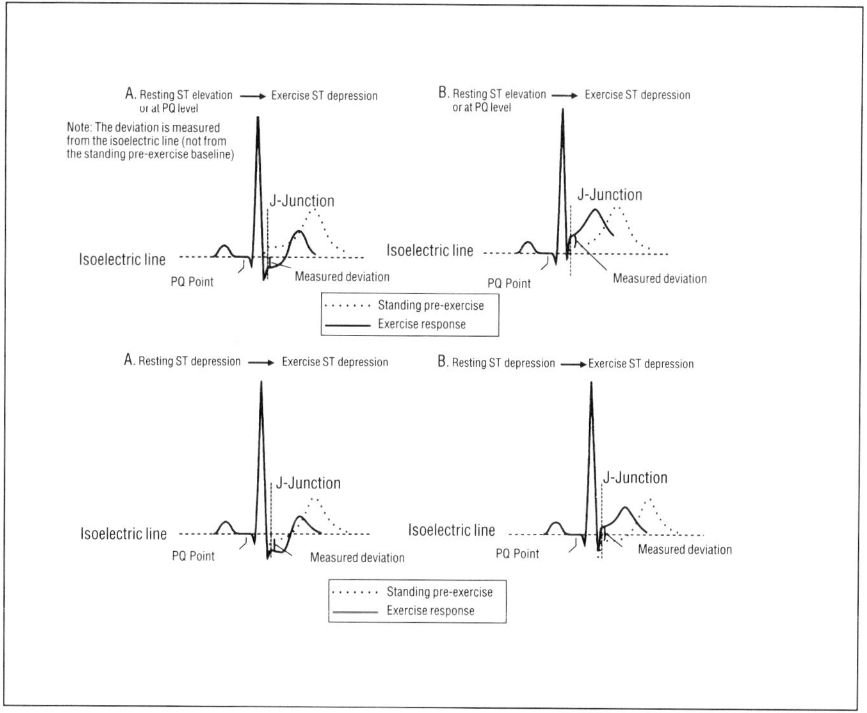

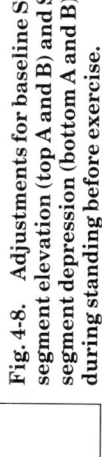

Fig. 4-8. Adjustments for baseline ST-segment elevation (top A and B) and ST-segment depression (bottom A and B) during standing before exercise.

subjects or volunteers. A relatively poor relationship of maximal heart rate to age has been a consistent finding in population studies. Correlation coefficients of -0.4 are usually found with a standard error of the estimate of 10 to 25 bpm. In general, this wide range has not been narrowed by considering activity status, weight, cardiac size, maximal respiratory quotient, or perceived exertion. One should not consider a test "inadequate" if 85% of the age-predicted maximum is not reached. More than 25% of normal individuals giving maximal effort will still fall short of the 85 percent. Effort is actually best judged by using the Borg scale of perceived exertion (see Fig. 4-6).

Exertional hypotension, best defined as a drop in systolic BP below standing resting systolic BP, is very predictive of severe angiographic coronary artery disease and a poor prognosis. It is also associated with cardiac arrests in the exercise laboratory; therefore, considerable care should be taken to monitor BP. A failure of systolic BP to rise is particularly worrisome after an MI.

Nomograms.   Nomograms greatly facilitate the description of exercise capacity relative to age and enable comparison between patients [8]. There are many benefits to reporting exercise capacity as a percentage, with 100% as normal for age. Figure 4-9 is a nomogram based on METs from expired gas analysis in normal volunteers. Figure 4-10 is based on estimated METs in "normal" patients referred for evaluation.

Symptoms.   Because anginal histories can often be vague or patients can use denial or limit themselves to avoid the occurrence of angina, the exercise test provides an excellent opportunity to evaluate a patient's exercise-induced symptoms. Pains with an ectopic location or sensations other than pain (discomfort, pressure) can be evaluated as presenting angina. The angina should be clearly separated from noncardiac pain (such as sharp or nonprogressive pains) and be classified according to the Duke angina index as 1 for present and 2 if it is the reason for stopping the test. A score of 2 is more likely to be associated with severe coronary artery disease and adversely affects prognosis. Other symptoms such as shortness of breath are difficult to equate as an anginal equivalent, but palpitations can be recognized as resulting from arrhythmias. Dyspnea and fatigue are common reasons for termination. The medical history and examination can determine whether these symptoms are due to pulmonary disease.

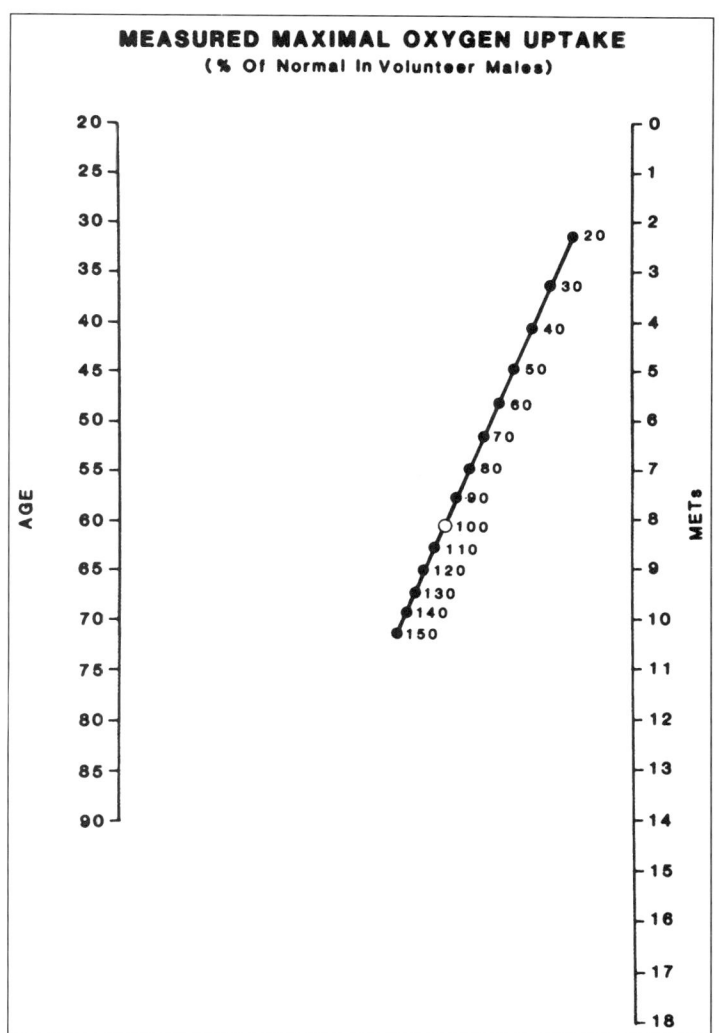

Fig. 4-9. Nomogram of METs for age in healthy normal volunteers, with 100% being as expected for age.

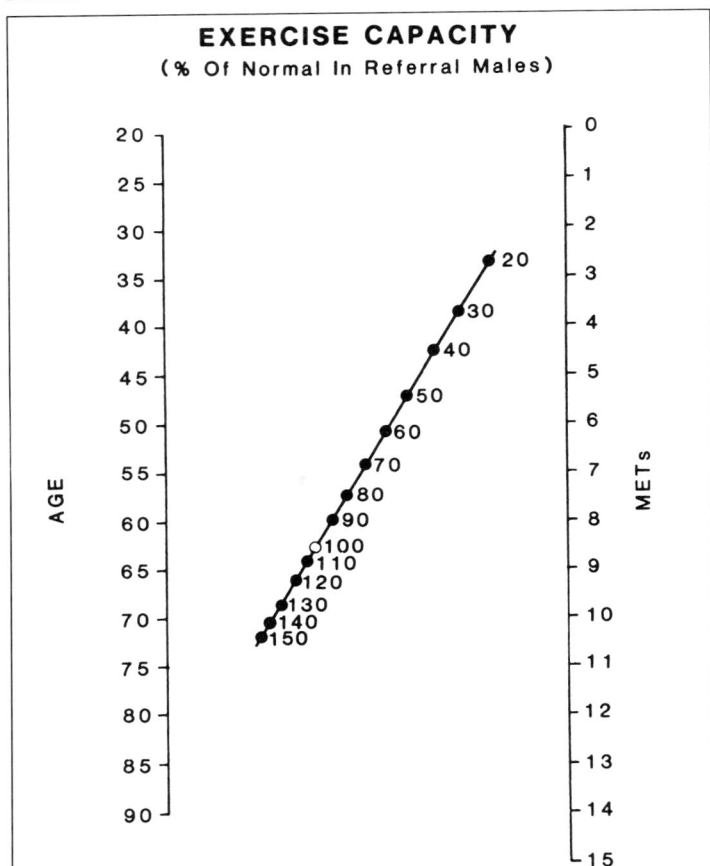

Fig. 4-10.   Nomogram of METs for age in men referred for evaluation of possible heart disease, with 100% being as expected for age.

Diagnosis and Prognosis.   One millimeter of horizontal or downsloping ST-segment depression measured at the J-junction (the junction of the QRS complex and the ST segment), usually occurring in lead V_5 during exercise or at 3 minutes of recovery, has the optimal test characteristics for diagnosing atherosclerotic coronary artery disease severe enough to cause ischemia. The ST-segment measurement must take into consideration the ST level while standing prior to testing. The most common situation is the normally seen ST-segment elevation called early repolarization. When this is present, the exercise ST-segment measurement is made relative to the PQ isoelectric line. When there is ST-segment depression during standing, the exercise ST measurement is made from the point (see Fig. 4-8). With these criteria the exercise test has approximately 65% sensitivity and 85% specificity for any coronary artery disease. The sensitivity is higher for more serious forms, such as left main coronary artery or triple-vessel disease. More ST-segment depression, downsloping depression, more leads involved, occurrence at lower double products, and greater persistence of depression are more diagnostic. The characterization of angina (not nonspecific chest pain) and how it impacts the test (is it the reason for stopping or not?) also adds to the diagnostic characteristics of the test.

The Duke nomogram permits a reproducible and accurate estimate of annual cardiovascular mortality using simple exercise test responses (Fig. 4-11) [9].

Exercise Testing with Expired Gases
INDICATIONS.   Ventilatory gas exchange techniques have generally been used in human performance laboratories, but applications in clinical settings have increased due to technologic advances [10]. Measurements of VO_2 max permit a more accurate and reproducible assessment of cardiopulmonary function as compared to estimating work from treadmill speed and grade. In addition to some inherent variability in predicting oxygen uptake from external work, factors such as treadmill experience, exercise protocol, and presence of heart disease contribute to these errors. Various methods of expressing efficiency of ventilation, breathing patterns, physiologic dead space, and oxygen kinetics can be useful in characterizing the presence of and gauging responses to therapy in certain heart and lung diseases. It can also help distinguish whether shortness of breath is due to lung or heart disease, but actually the resting pulmonary function tests are most informative. These methods are most important for assessing the fitness of athletes, prescribing exercise training, identifying patients for cardiac transplantation, and performing drug studies (i.e., assessing antianginal medications or vasodilators for CHF).

CONTRAINDICATIONS, RISKS, AND DANGERS.   Contraindications, risks, and dangers are the same as for standard ECG exercise testing.

DESCRIPTION.   While performing a standard exercise test, the patient breathes through a mouthpiece like a

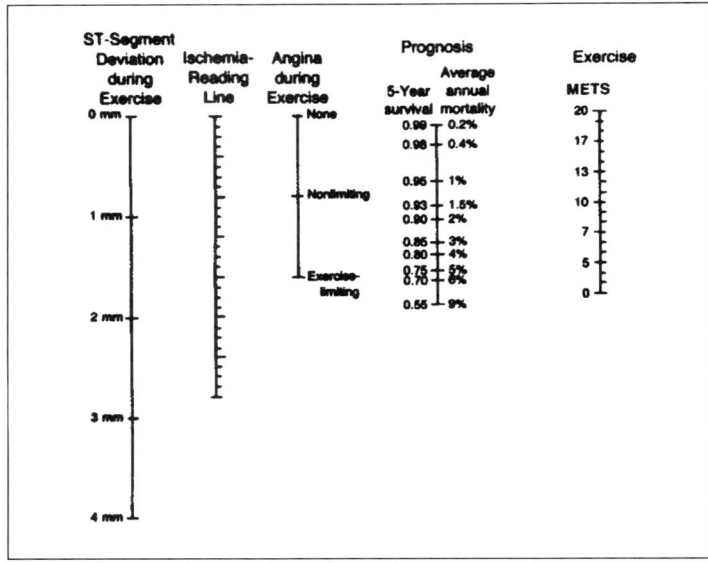

Fig. 4-11.   The Duke nomogram estimates prognosis from the parameters of the Duke score in five steps. First, the observed amount of ST-segment depression is marked on the ST-segment deviation line. Second, the observed degree of angina is marked on the line for angina, and these two points are connected with a straight edge. Third, the point where this line intersects the ischemia-reading line is noted. Fourth, the observed exercise capacity in METs is marked on the line. Finally, the mark on the ischemia-reading line is connected to the mark on the MET line, and the estimated 5-year survival or average annual mortality rate is read from the point at which this line intersects the prognosis scale. For instance, even patients with 2 mm of ST-segment depression and angina occurring during the test will still have less than a 3% annual cardiovascular mortality rate if their exercise capacity is 7 METs or greater. (Modified from Mark D, et al. Exercise treatmill score for predicting prognosis. *N Engl J Med* 1991;325:849–853.)

snorkel with the nose closed using a clip, or through a face mask. The volume of expired air is measured, and the contents of inspired and expired oxygen and carbon dioxide are determined.

PREPARATION OF THE PATIENT.   In addition to the instructions for standard exercise testing, the patient must be instructed in hand signs to communicate the presence of symptoms. False teeth are usually required to be in place during testing, but a loose fit or loose teeth can be problematic. Use of a face mask can avoid these problems; the new versions allow for an adequately tight fit.

INTERPRETATION. The measurement of METs (VO_2) is more accurate than estimates and should be unaffected by serial testing. Gas exchange anaerobic threshold and oxygen kinetics can be measured; however, their clinical utility in routine practice is uncertain. There is a higher VO_2 with treadmill than cycle testing but the maximal heart rates obtained are similar.

Exercise Testing with Radionuclides

LEFT VENTRICULAR RESPONSE (MUGA) TO SUPINE OR SITTING CYCLE EXERCISE. Indications. This test is used to diagnose ischemia due to coronary artery disease or to evaluate LV and valvular functions during exercise [11].

Contraindications, Risks, and Dangers. The dangers are the same as those for resting technetium 99m imaging and standard exercise testing. The contraindications are the same as for the standard exercise test.

Description. The LV is visualized so that wall motion abnormalities and ejection fraction can be determined during and after exercise. Exercise-induced ischemia can produce decreased motion or bulges (e.g., hypokinesia or dyskinesia) associated with fixed coronary lesions. Ejection fraction normally increases with exercise, and a drop in ejection fraction has been associated with ischemia, hypertension, aging, and valvular disease.

Preparation of Patient. The preparation is the same as for standard testing, except that an intravenous line is needed.

Interpretation. Abnormalities in wall motion, end-systolic volume, and ejection fraction should be noted. Unfortunately, the specificity of these abnormalities for coronary disease has been poor (60%). Some investigators use the ejection fraction response in valvular disease to time the need for valve replacement, but there is no consensus on the validity of this practice.

PERFUSION SCINTIGRAPHY WITH THALLIUM OR ISONITRILES TAGGED WITH TECHNETIUM. Indications. This test is used to diagnose ischemia and to determine its severity and location. Due to test characteristics thought to exceed the standard exercise ECG, it has been recommended as the best secondary noninvasive test for coronary artery disease. However, it is usually indicated when the resting ECG makes ST-segment analysis uncertain (e.g., left bundle-branch block, Wolff-Parkinson-White syndrome, LV hypertrophy with strain) or when the ST response is thought to represent a false positive or a false negative. Because it can localize ischemia, it has been used to determine the "culprit" lesion by comparison with the coronary angiogram. Negative perfusion study results identify a low-risk group of patients with an excellent prognosis.

Contraindications, Risks, and Dangers. The contraindications, risks, and dangers are the same as for the standard exercise test.

Description. The description is the same as for the standard exercise test except that an intravenous line must be placed before the test begins so isotope can be injected at the point of maximal exercise.

Preparation of Patient. The patient must be informed of the need for intravenous placement and must have a suitable venous access site. Otherwise, the preparation is the same as for the standard exercise test.

Interpretation. Images in multiple views are gathered immediately following exercise. A cold spot present in an area where there should be cardiac muscle could represent scar or ischemia. If the area fills in when imaging is repeated later, ischemia is the cause of the defect. If the defect persists, it is due to scar. The septal area is the most reproducible and is highly associated with proximal left anterior descending (LAD) coronary artery disease. The inferior area is most confused by artifact, but this problem can be lessened by positioning the patient prone for imaging. Increases in LV size and lung uptake are less specific abnormalities that can be interpreted by experts, but carry a poor prognosis.

Echocardiographic Exercise Testing

INDICATIONS. Echocardiographic exercise testing is used for diagnosing coronary artery disease and ischemia and localizing the site and extent of the ischemia [12]. It is particularly helpful and cost-effective when resting ECG abnormalities confound ST-segment analysis or in women or when digoxin is being administered. The impression from inadequate studies comparing exercise echocardiography to coronary angiograms is that echocardiography has better test characteristics than does standard exercise ECG testing. The exercise images are actually taken after a standard treadmill test, as imaging during exercise is not essential.

CONTRAINDICATIONS, RISKS, AND DANGERS. These are the same as for standard exercise testing. Some patients, particularly those with lung disease, those currently smoking, and those who are obese, are very difficult to image. If resting images are not suitable (the endocardial surface cannot be distinguished) then the exercise echocardiogram will be futile.

DESCRIPTION.   After the patient is connected to the ECG machine, he or she is instructed to lie down in the left lateral decubitus position so that resting images can be obtained. This includes the four standard views: parasternal long axis, parasternal short axis, apical four chamber, and apical two chamber. All views must be stored in the four-screen format for later comparison.

Immediately after exercise, the patient is again instructed to lie down, and imaging should begin within 1 minute. These images are captured in the four-screen format, with four cardiac cycles (one for rest) of each view. The images must be captured within the first minute after exercise and must be during expiration.

PREPARATION OF PATIENT.   The preparation is the same as for standard exercise testing and rest echocardiography.

INTERPRETATION.   After exercise image acquisition, the best cardiac cycle for each of the four views is chosen. These four poststress images are then displayed next to the corresponding resting images. This display facilitates the comparison of wall motion before and after stress. With the four views, each of the 16 areas defined by the American Echocardiographic Society are scored as follows: 1 = normal, 2 = hypokinetic, 3 = akinetic, 4 = dyskinetic, 5 = aneurysmal, 6 = aneurysmal with scar, and 7 = dyskinetic with scar. A wall motion score index and the percentage of normal muscle are calculated. These preexercise and postexercise scores are compared as are visual findings.

Nonexercise Stress Techniques

DIPYRIDAMOLE AND ADENOSINE PERFUSION IMAGING.   Indications.   The test is used to diagnose ischemia in patients who are unable to exercise on a treadmill or in those who give an inadequate effort. Inability to exercise can be due to strokes, orthopedic problems, handicaps, claudication, instability, and so on. Use of thallium or sesti-MIBI also makes it possible to localize ischemia and significant lesions. This test has been advocated as part of the preoperative work-up of patients with peripheral vascular disease, but patients should be selected for testing according to their symptoms and history. Asymptomatic patients are unlikely to benefit from such testing.

Contraindications, Risks, and Dangers.   Contraindications for dipyridamole include unstable angina, recent MI, severe bronchospastic lung disease, and hypotension. Not all patients with lung disease need to be excluded, only those with a bronchospastic component. For adenosine, contraindications also include heart block and sick sinus. Adenosine causes more GI (nausea and epigastric pain) and CNS (flushing, headache, and dizziness) symptoms and hypotension than does dipyridamole. It is usually contraindicated in patients with COPD or asthma. Aminophylline must be available to reverse bronchospasm or hypotension by blocking the adenosine receptors (60–240 mg IV). There has only been one serious side effect per 1,000 studies reported. Adenosine is more likely to interfere with cardiac conduction. The extremely short intravenous half-life of adenosine allows for a rapid normalization of rhythm as soon as adenosine infusion is stopped.

Description.   Dipyridamole given intravenously or in an oral bolus causes an increase in the plasma level of endogenous adenosine. This results in vasodilation of nondiseased coronary vessels, "stealing" blood from diseased vessels and causing reduced tracer uptake. Intravenously administered adenosine directly causes the same effect.

Preparation of Patient.   The patient should be told to avoid methylxanthine medications and foods containing caffeine for at least a day prior to the test.

Interpretation.   Fixed defects found on scanning with a scintillating camera are due to scar, and defects that later fill in are due to ischemia.

DOBUTAMINE ECHOCARDIOGRAPHY. **Indications.**   This test is used to diagnose ischemia in patients who are unable to exercise on a treadmill or who give an inadequate effort.

Contraindications, Risks, and Dangers.   Contraindications include hypertrophic cardiomyopathy and severe hypertension. Arrhythmias, hypertension, hypotension, and severe ischemia are all rare possibilities that are more probable if the drug is not properly titrated. Dobutamine echocardiography does not pose any threat of bronchospasm, which can be secondary to adenosine or dipyridamole administration. Its side effects can be reversed by a beta-blocker.

Description.   Dobutamine is a synthetic catecholamine that acts directly on beta-1 and beta-2 receptors. It increases the force of myocardial contractility more than it increases heart rate. It is titrated intravenously from low to higher doses while the four views described above for exercise echocardiography are observed. Wall motion abnormalities are caused by the associated increased demand for myocardial oxygen and shortening of coronary artery filling time resulting from the increase in heart rate.

Preparation of Patient.   An intravenous line is necessary for the dobutamine infusion. The patient should be made aware of this and an appropriate venous access must be available.

Interpretation.   If ischemia is induced, a wall motion abnormality appears at a specific heart rate.

Ambulatory Monitoring (Holter Monitor / Event Recorder)
INDICATIONS.   There are two techniques for ambulatory monitoring: the continuous recording of selected ECG leads over a period of time (Holter monitoring) and the patient-triggered recording of symptomatic events (event recording) [13].

Holter monitors provide a quantitative assessment of all events, including cyclic and periodic arrhythmias, silent and activity-related ischemia, and variant angina. These devices stratify the risk of evaluating patients with conditions that increase the possibility of dangerous arrhythmias, such as post-MI LV damage, cardiomyopathy, and severe valvular disease. Holter monitors can also be used in serial studies for the evaluation of treatments. Duration of the continuous ECG recording can be up to 48 hours and a new device enables recording of all 12 leads.

Event recording enables the assessment of relatively infrequent outpatient cardiac events such as palpitations, syncope, and dizziness. Such events can result from arrhythmias or from electronic pacemaker malfunction in pacemaker-dependent patients. They can be kept on the patient indefinitely.

CONTRAINDICATIONS, RISKS, AND DANGERS.   There are none; however, given the cost of the recorders, it is advisable to exclude patients likely to lose, damage, or fail to return the units.

DESCRIPTION.   **Holter Monitor.**   Electrodes are applied to skin that has been mildly abraded to improve recording quality, and then connected to a portable recording device. If ischemia is an issue, lead V_5 should be included. Before the device is connected, leads are reviewed to ensure good signal qualities, including P-wave amplitude (usually lead II or aVF) for rhythm analysis. Although the most common recording device had been analog recording tape, newer units use a digitized system for storing ECG signals on digital magnetic media. Recordings are made continuously for 24 or 48 hours and then analyzed by a computer. This quantitates heart rate and detects, identifies, and quantitates arrhythmias and ischemia on an hourly basis. Patients are given diaries to record symptoms or significant daily activities. They can also mark symptomatic events by activating a marker on the recorder.

Event Recorder.   Applied to the skin or fastened as wristbands, electrodes provide a signal to a small recording device with a continuous-loop recording of the ECG [14]. When a symptomatic event occurs, the patient activates the recording device, which stores the event. The unit can be programmed to also record a fixed interval before and after activation by the patient. The stored event is then transmitted telephonically and reported as a rhythm strip to the physician. This system is most cost-effective in patients with infrequent symptoms that are likely to be missed by only a day or two of monitoring.

It is important that the recorder and the playback unit meet the American Heart Association specifications for ECG devices.

PREPARATION OF PATIENT.   Electrode placements are as defined above. Optimal utilization of the information requires the patient to record symptoms or symptomatic events; therefore, the patient needs to be adequately trained in the use of equipment and in diary recording.

INTERPRETATION.   The Holter monitor provides quantitative information about heart rate, arrhythmias, and ST-segment changes over 1 to 2 days. Standard ECG analysis is employed. Keep in mind that early repolarization, which is a normal ST-segment elevation, sinks to the baseline with increasing heart rate. If the reverse occurs when going from a fast to a slow heart rate, the resulting normal ST-segment elevation should not be misinterpreted as a result of ischemia. Correlation of the ECG information with patient symptoms is an important component of complete interpretation.

Event recorders provide rhythm strips at times of symptomatic events, which also enable correlation of events with symptoms. Tracings should be reviewed to confirm the computer identification of ectopic beats or pauses and to prevent recording artifact being interpreted as arrhythmia.

Cardiac Catheterization

Coronary Angiography

INDICATIONS.   Coronary angiography is the "road map" for any invasive revascularization procedure [15]. It is used for diagnosing coronary artery disease when symptoms are out of proportion to the findings of noninvasive testing or when a false result is suspected (false negative or positive). The combination of triple-vessel or left main artery disease along with depressed myocardial function (ejection fraction < 50%) is a pattern that identifies patients who will have a better chance of survival with surgical revascularization than with medical management.

CONTRAINDICATIONS, RISKS, AND DANGERS.   In an emergency setting, this procedure can be lifesaving, so contraindications can be waived. In the nonacute outpatient setting, contraindications include recent stroke, progressive renal insufficiency, GI bleeding, fever due to infection, short life expectancy due to complicating illness, severe anemia, history of anaphylaxis to contrast material, digoxin toxicity, electrolyte problems, and uncontrolled high BP. Embolic strokes, arterial complications, hematomas, MI, and death are all rare but possible complications. The risk to life should be less than 0.2% and that for major adverse effects (stroke, MI, or bleeding) less than 0.5%. However, certain circumstances, such as the presence of left main artery disease or recent thrombolysis for MI, can raise the odds. Concern must always be given to the danger of inducing irreversible renal damage in patients with chronic renal insufficiency.

DESCRIPTION.   A preformed catheter is inserted over a guide wire that has been inserted percutaneously into the femoral artery in the groin. The catheter is advanced up to the aorta and twisted until it pops into a coronary ostium. Two catheters must be used because a different shape is needed for the right and left coronary ostia. Care must be taken not to traumatize the artery or to wedge the catheter too tightly. Once the catheter is aligned, several milliliters or contrast material is injected to fill the coronary lumen. The patient is positioned in several alignments to best illustrate certain parts of the vessels. Caudad tilts are helpful for visualizing the left main coronary artery.

PREPARATION OF PATIENT.   The patient must sign an informed consent form for this invasive procedure and should be instructed not to eat for at least 6 hours prior to the procedure. Mild sedation is often used, but the patient must be alert enough to cooperate with breathing instructions during the procedure. Today, cardiac catheterization is frequently performed as an outpatient procedure.

INTERPRETATION. The multiple views, variations in anatomy, and effects of disease can make reading a coronary angiogram difficult. The left-hand model shown in Figures 4-12 and 4-13 and the recognition of particular anatomic landmarks facilitate interpretation.

To teach coronary artery anatomy and distribution for interpreting coronary arteriography, the left hand can serve as a three-dimensional model of the coronary arterial system. If the thumb, index, and second fingers are formed into a curved position similar to a left-handed baseball pitcher's grip, the relationship of the three main coronary vessels can be readily visualized. The right coronary artery (RCA) is represented by the thumb, while the index and second fingers assume the roles of the LAD and left circumflex artery (LCX), respectively (see Figs. 4-12, 4-13). The hand may then be turned into various degrees of rotation, simulating the commonly used arteriographic viewing positions. Thus, one can demonstrate changes in the cineradiographic relationships of arteries brought about by rotation of the patient during catheterization. This facilitates recognition of confusing arterial patterns, and demonstrates the three-dimensional concept that must be kept in mind when viewing arteriograms; problems such as superimposition of vessels, double shadows, and foreshortening effects of viewing vessels "end on" can be readily demonstrated.

Remember that the LCX (second finger) and RCA (thumb) form one plane (the mitral-tricuspid plane), while the LAD (index finger) lies on a perpendicular plane (septal plane) that has its posterior edge formed by the posterior descending artery. A helpful mnemonic is the *d*iagonals come off of the LA*D* (both have D's) while *m*arginals come off of the circu*m*flex (both have M's).

Fortunately, the skilled angiographer often provides the practitioner with labeled snapshots, with arrows pointing to the pertinent lesions. Because the contrast material fills the lumen of the artery, lesions are estimated by comparison to nearby areas assumed to be nondiseased. Although two-dimensional imaging allows for the calculation of luminal area, this is rarely done. Thus, for clinical purposes, a percent lumen lessening of 75% is considered meaningful. Recognizing the two planes of the heart (the atrioventricular [AV] valve plane highlighted by the late filling of the coronary sinus and the septum highlighted by

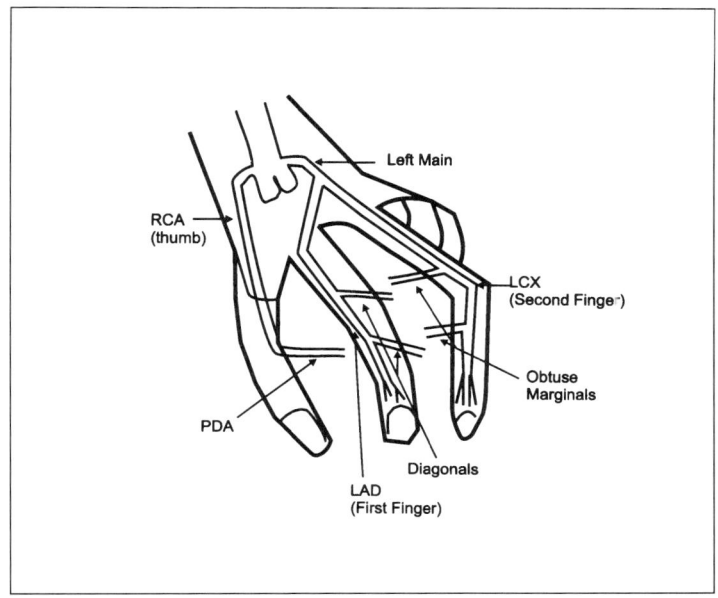

Fig. 4-12.   Left-hand model for interpreting the coronary angiogram: the left anterior oblique projection. RCA = right coronary artery; PDA = posterior descending artery; LAD = left anterior descending artery; LCX = left circumflex artery.

the septal blush and the perforating branches) is critical. Dominance is actually determined by whether the right or left coronary artery provides the main supply to the posterior surface of the heart.

Ventriculography

INDICATIONS.   As part of all coronary angiography, ventriculography is routinely performed to demonstrate the ejection fraction, valvular insufficiency, and any wall motion abnormalities.

CONTRAINDICATIONS, RISKS, AND DANGERS.   When the 15- to 20-ml contrast load may damage chronically insufficient kidneys or may push a weakened heart into CHF, this procedure is often postponed or replaced by MUGA or echocardiography. The risks and dangers are similar to those of coronary angiography.

DESCRIPTION.   Contrast medium is injected into the LV and x-ray cine films of the heart are exposed simultaneously. Cine film is gradually being replaced with digital imaging techniques.

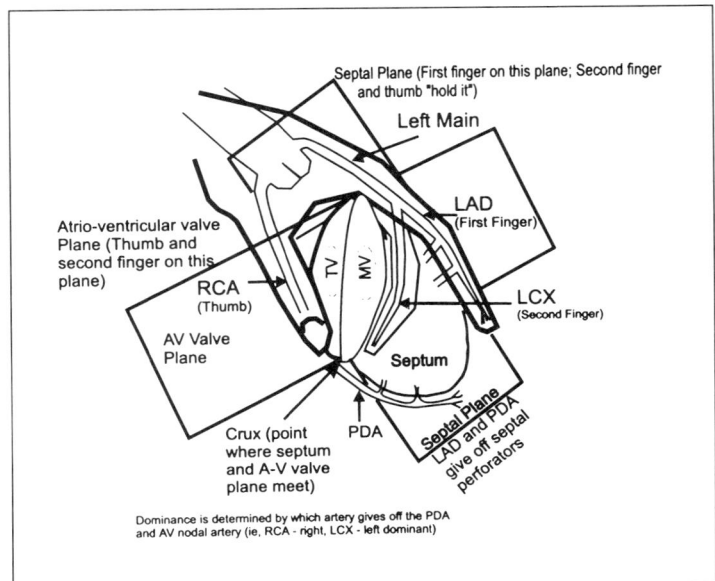

Fig. 4-13.   Left-hand model for interpreting the coronary angiogram: the right anterior oblique projection. RCA = right coronary artery; LAD = left anterior descending artery; LCX = left circumflex artery; TV = tricuspid valve; MV = mitral valve; PDA = posterior descending artery.

PREPARATION OF PATIENT.   Patient preparation is the same as for coronary angiography.

INTERPRETATION.   Wall motion is classified as normal, hypokinetic, akinetic, or dyskinetic. Ejection fraction is measured by tracing the endocardium, estimating the volume at end diastole and at end systole using the proloid ellipse equation, and dividing stroke volume by end-diastolic volume. A normal ejection fraction should be over 55%. The ventricular volumes are normalized for body size, and LV mass is estimated from the thickness of the left ventricle. Normal values for each laboratory are provided with the report.

Electrophysiologic Studies
INDICATIONS.   Electrophysiologic studies are used to evaluate the origin of arrhythmias in patients with documented or suspected arrhythmias, to evaluate arrhythmias or conduction abnormalities as the etiology of syncope, and to assess the efficacy of antiarrhythmic drugs or implanted cardioverter or defibrillators [16]. Some

arrhythmias, particularly supraventricular tachycardia due to reentrant circuits involving accessory pathways (Wolff-Parkinson-White) or the AV node, can be eliminated by the application of radiofrequency current to the tachycardia circuit [17]. Modification or elimination of AV node conduction by radiofrequency current can modify ventricular response during atrial fibrillation.

CONTRAINDICATIONS, RISKS, AND DANGERS. This procedure often involves induction of life-threatening arrhythmias in order to demonstrate their presence and to try a drug therapy. Normal rhythm must be restored electrically during the procedure if chemical cardioversion fails. In addition, placement of multiple venous catheters can lead to thrombosis and clot with embolization.

DESCRIPTION. Multiple multielectrode catheters are placed via venous access (usually from the femoral veins) and positioned fluoroscopically in various positions in the heart. These catheters are used for both pacing and recording intracardiac electrical activity. Multiple surface ECG leads are also placed, and defibrillator electrodes are placed on the back and chest. An intravenous line is maintained for the administration of antiarrhythmic agents and emergency drugs. During the study, the electrode catheters are paced in sequential fashion (programmed stimulation) to assess the conduction system and attempt to induce or terminate tachycardias. Multiple episodes may be induced to fully characterize the arrhythmia. Drugs such as isoproterenol, adenosine, or procainamide may be administered to assess the response.

PREPARATION OF PATIENT. The patient must sign an informed consent form for the placement of multiple catheters with the risk of clot or hemorrhage, the risk of life-threatening arrhythmias, and the need for electrical cardioversion. Often the consent for radiofrequency ablation is also obtained prior to the study so that the patient can be sedated or treated with analgesia for the discomfort of lying supine for a protracted period of time. The patient must be alert enough to cooperate during the procedure.

INTERPRETATION. Unfortunately, the response to many antiarrhythmic agents is different when given acutely (i.e., during the procedure) as compared to chronically. One of the most important antiarrhythmic agents, amiodarone, has no immediate effect. Also, the strength and timing of stimuli associated with the induction of ominous ventricular tachycardias are uncertain. If they are sufficiently strong or timed inappropriately, even the normal heart will fibrillate. Holter monitoring is often a better option to assess the response to drug therapy in patients with a high degree of spontaneous ventricular ectopy. Comparisons of the use of Holter monitoring and exercise testing to electrophysiologic studies to evaluate ventricular arrhythmias suggest that the noninvasive approach may be more cost-effective [18]. Electrophysiologic studies are often indicated to diagnose tachyarrhythmias of uncertain etiology.

**APPLICATION OF TESTS
FOR THE FIVE KEY FEATURES**
The following sections highlight the appropriate use of these tests to assess each of the key features (see also Appendix Tables F-3, F-4, F-6, F-7, F-9, F-10, F-12, F-13, F-15, and F-16).

Myocardial Dysfunction
Exercise Test
Exercise capacity is not directly related to myocardial dysfunction. This is probably due to the fact that exercise capacity is only strongly affected by LV dysfunction when pulmonary artery and right ventricular pressures are elevated. The correlation between resting ejection fraction and measured or estimated maximal oxygen consumption (i.e., METs) is poor. However, in some circumstances, a drop in systolic BP, a low maximal heart rate (chronotropic incompetence), or poor exercise capacity can be due to myocardial dysfunction more than ischemia. In fact, this should be suggested when there are no signs of ischemia in a patient who has these hemodynamic responses. The exercise capacity is important to estimate for prognosis, and measured gas analysis is frequently used as a criteria for cardiac transplantation.

Echocardiography
Echocardiography is the best noninvasive way of evaluating myocardial function. The M-mode was limited because it only gives an ice pick view and can cut across good or bad areas of myocardial function. This is particularly the case in a regional disease such as coronary disease. However, when there is diffuse disease, an accurate estimate of ventricular function can be obtained even with the M-mode. Two-dimensional echocardiography cuts across a single plane at a time, but segmental wall motion analysis can be interpreted with reasonable accuracy because four views

are imaged. The equations and formula for estimating ejection fraction from two-dimensional echocardiography have been well validated. Doppler imaging adds a noninvasive means to estimate hemodynamic measurements including gradients and cardiac output. The main advantage of echocardiography with Doppler over other techniques of ejection fraction measurement is that it detects mitral regurgitation (i.e., one can tell when the ventricle is unloading backward, allowing myocardial function to appear better than it would be if mitral regurgitation was not present). The most common cause of pericardial effusion seen on the echocardiogram is CHF due to myocardial dysfunction. As mentioned before, echocardiography can be performed after exercise. Wall motion abnormalities brought out by the exercise as compared to rest are due to ischemia rather than LV damage. Echocardiography can identify the confounders and rarities that simulate myocardial dysfunction including a right ventricular infarct, cardiac tamponade, constrictive pericarditis, and isolated diastolic dysfunction.

Nuclear Cardiology
Radionuclide ventriculography provides a means of viewing the LV and estimating ejection fraction. It is not totally noninvasive like echocardiography because an intravenous line must be established. Both the first-pass technique and the multigated acquisition (MUGA) technique enable measurements of ejection fraction. The use of the MUGA technique yields better resolution, enabling the formulation of ventricular wall motion estimates and rough ventricular volume estimates. Also, sequential interventions can be applied to see how ejection fraction responds. The argument has been made that this should be the best way of measuring ejection fraction because it depends on total counts and geometric assumptions are unnecessary, but that is only theoretical. Technical problems that affect the results obtained include chamber separation, choice of a background area, and proper edge detection. In addition, atrial fibrillation and frequent premature beats make it less accurate. These limitations vary from laboratory to laboratory, making quality assessment critical to clinical utility of these techniques.

Nonexercise Stress Tests
This class of tests addresses a high-risk group of patients, those unable to exercise. Every study that has considered

patients with coronary artery disease has identified those unable to exercise as at higher risk of death and cardiovascular events. These tests are for the evaluation of ischemia, not of LV function or damage.

Holter Ambulatory Monitoring
Holter monitoring cannot be used to estimate myocardial function. However, patients with myocardial damage and dysfunction frequently are monitored because they often have atrial and ventricular arrhythmias and are in danger of arrhythmic systemic embolization and sudden death.

Cardiac Catheterization
This is the gold standard for evaluating ventricular function, as well as for coronary anatomy. The measurement of ejection fraction during LV angiography is the gold standard for EF, and it is most accurately performed biplane. When the ventricle loses its ellipsoid shape due to dilation, measurements are less accurate. Hemodynamic measurements including pressure data (LV end-diastolic pressure and other chamber and vessel pressures), cardiac output, isovolumic change in pressure over time (DP/DT), and ejection phase indices give estimates of myocardial function. The response of the ventricle and of cardiovascular hemodynamics to exercise can demonstrate the function of the heart.

Myocardial Ischemia
Exercise Test
The standard exercise ECG test is the key method for non-invasively confirming the diagnosis of myocardial ischemia, estimating the severity of disease, and estimating prognosis. It should be the first test used for diagnosis of CAD in both adult men and women with non-acute chest pain, including patients receiving digoxin, with less than one millimeter of resting ST depression or with right bundle branch block. The markedly positive response on the exercise test (including signs or symptoms of ischemia at a low double product, a low exercise capacity, multiple lead involvement, and prolonged ST-segment depression into recovery) and exertional hypotension increase the probability for having triple-vessel or left main coronary artery disease.

Myocardial oxygen demand and ventilatory oxygen consumption (or uptake) are two important estimates to be made during exercise testing. Although they are directly related statistically, they represent different physiologic processes. Myocardial oxygen demand depends on the work demands on the heart itself. Though altered by LV volume and contractility, it is most easily estimated by the heart rate–systolic BP product. Usually, patients with fixed lesions develop angina or ST-segment depression, or both, at the same product (called rate pressure product or double product). The higher product achieved during exercise (normal > 25,000, depending on age), the less the amount of ischemic myocardium. Ventilatory oxygen consumption is the amount of oxygen taken from the air breathed to perform the work of the body and is presented in METs rather than minutes. Maximal ventilatory oxygen uptake is the amount consumed during maximal work. It can be estimated from the workload performed.

Exercise-induced ST-segment depression is the most sensitive and specific ECG marker of myocardial ischemia, which is most often due to coronary artery disease. Flat or downsloping depression in lateral leads (V_4, V_5, V_6) is the most predictive. The leads in which it occurs do not localize the site of ischemia nor the artery involved. One millimeter at J-junction is considered abnormal, but more depression and a downward slope are more predictive. False abnormal depression can occur during digoxin treatment, in women, and with left bundle-branch block, LV hypertrophy, and mitral valve prolapse. Elevation over Q waves diagnostic of infarction does not necessarily mean ischemia, but elevation occurring with a normal ECG usually means severe ischemia due to coronary spasm or a tight proximal lesion in the myocardial area over which the leads are located.

If after testing, the clinical impression is that the exercise ECG result is a false positive or a false negative, then one should apply the best-performed exercise add-on that is available. This could be coronary angiography but usually will be a nuclear perfusion test. If the patient was unable to give an adequate effort to exercise, then nonexercise stress test should be considered.

Echocardiography
Left main coronary artery occlusion has been visualized using two-dimensional echocardiography, but this is not a reliable tool for this diagnosis. Segmental wall motion abnormalities at rest imply an old MI but can be due to other causes of myocardial scarring. If spontaneous or induced ischemia occurs (i.e., after treadmill exercise), wall motion abnormalities can be detected by echocardiog-

raphy. Echocardiography will recognize the confounders causing chest pain, including pericarditis, aortic aneurysm, and aortic stenosis.

Nuclear Cardiology

Thallium exercise scintigraphy is an accurate means of diagnosing myocardial ischemia. It should be the first test used for diagnosis of CAD in patients with more than one millimeter of resting ST depression, left bundle branch block, or WPW. It is complicated by the fact that in some patients with severe ischemia, the cold spots do not fill in at 4 hours after exercise, giving the appearance of a scar. Also, in patients with prior myocardial infarction, the scar complicates the recognition of additional defects. Computer programs to analyze thallium scintigraphy appear to increase sensitivity but decrease specificity. SPECT imaging that provides three-dimensional cuts of the ventricle is now widely used, but it has a lower specificity than planar imaging. Radionuclide ventriculography performed in conjunction with exercise can detect ischemic wall motion abnormalities and drops in global ejection fraction, but this test response has a poor specificity.

Nonexercise Stress Tests

Two tests now enable diagnosis of coronary disease and quantification of the ischemic risk in patients unable to exercise: scintigraphy with dipyridamole or adenosine as the stressor and thallium or a technetium 99m–labeled isonitrile as the perfusion agent and echocardiography with dobutamine. Dipyridamole and adenosine cause myocardial "steal" with relative hypoperfusion, and dobutamine increases myocardial oxygen demand in a manner similar to exercise. These tests are essential for diagnosing ischemia in patients unable to exercise or who give an inadequate exercise response. Dipyridamole must be avoided in patients with active bronchospastic disease; otherwise, the best-performed method available locally should be used.

Holter Monitoring

The frequency response of many of the recorders and playback units now permits accurate assessment of ST-segment changes. However, appropriate lead systems must be used in order for Holter monitoring to be used to evaluate myocardial ischemia. For typical ST depression, V_5 is optimal to monitor. If one is trying to diagnose coronary artery spasm or variant angina, the leads should be placed appropriately to the artery that may undergo spasm. If the

circumflex or right coronary arteries are involved, an inferior lead should be monitored, and if the LAD artery is
involved, lateral or anterior leads should be monitored.
Due to the cyclic nature of variant angina, and to the fact
that only 50% of patients with this diagnosis will have
abnormal exercise tests, Holter monitor results can be
helpful in recognizing them. Often in addition to ST-segment elevation, ECG findings such as complete heart
block, ventricular tachycardia, and even ventricular fibrillation can be noted. Another use for Holter monitoring is to
evaluate patients, particularly those who cannot exercise,
for ischemia during everyday activities.

Cardiac Catheterization
This is the gold standard for evaluating myocardial ischemia. It should be noted, however, that it represents an
anatomic evaluation and not a functional one. The lesions
that can create myocardial ischemia during exercise are
accepted to be those with 50% narrowing of the diameter
or 75% reduction in cross-sectional area. Angiographic
measurement of atherosclerotic lesions usually underestimates the actual size. The severity of ischemia can be estimated by the diameter narrowing and the number of vessels involved. Categorizing ischemia as single-, double-,
and triple-vessel disease is a simplistic approach, and
other coronary artery scores are more accurate but have
found little clinical utilization. Angiographic scores considering lesion location actually provide a more accurate
estimation of myocardium in jeopardy. The prognosis in
patients with coronary artery disease is directly related to
the number of vessels: Single-vessel disease has a 3%
annual mortality; two-vessel disease, an 8% annual mortality; triple-vessel disease, a 12% annual mortality; and
left main coronary artery disease, a 16% annual mortality.
Prognosis is greatly altered by the associated ejection fraction, with values over 50% being protective. Ten-year
follow-up of the consolidated coronary artery bypass grafting randomized trials demonstrated that triple-vessel and
left main coronary artery disease with an abnormal ejection fraction (<50%) are the only anatomic patterns associated with improved survival after bypass surgery compared to medical therapy [19].
   Assessment of coronary artery reserve is a method of
evaluating the response of coronary flow to vasodilator
drugs. One study suggested that this was a better marker
of ischemia than quantification of coronary lesions. Mea-

suring coronary reserve is a technically difficult procedure and currently is limited to assessment of patients with single-vessel coronary disease for research purposes [20].

In addition, pressure measurements may identify pulmonary artery hypertension as a cause of chest pain.

Valvular Function
The key issue is to weigh the risk of surgery for valve replacement or repair and the subsequent limitations of an artificial valve (inherent outflow obstruction, risk of SBE and valve degeneration, and need for anticoagulation) against the symptoms and risks of the diseased valve. This is usually a very difficult decision, best made by a cardiac surgeon and an experienced cardiologist together after appropriate tests have been performed and in conjunction with an informed patient. Relative quality-of-life issues must be carefully weighed.

Exercise Test
The exercise test is the only means of truly demonstrating a patient's exercise capacity and of documenting disability secondary to valvular disease. Exercise testing can even be performed in patients who have aortic stenosis, but it should be done with careful recording of the systolic BP. Echocardiography and catheterization are often indicated prior to use of the exercise test if the history or physical findings suggest tight aortic stenosis. Exercise responses can help one to decide whether surgery or medical management of valvular abnormalities is best. Measurement or estimation of changes in intracardiac pressures, ejection fraction, and cardiac output through the use of catheters in the cardiac chambers, of MUGA, or of echocardiography has been used as a means of determining the need for valve replacement surgery.

Echocardiography
Echocardiography is the optimal noninvasive means of evaluating valvular function. The addition of Doppler studies has made it possible to assess regurgitation and estimate pressure gradients and cardiac output. Valve size and pressure can be estimated with considerable accuracy. Coexistent regurgitation can confound these estimates.

Nuclear Cardiology
Perfusion imaging has been recommended as a means to identify ischemia in patients with valvular disorders, and exercise MUGA has been used to determine which patients with aortic insufficiency need surgery, but these uses are

unsubstantiated at this point. The nonexercise stress tests have no indication for evaluation of valvular disease but can help to determine if chest pain or ST-segment depression is due to ischemia. However, the ischemia could be due to low cardiac output instead of coronary disease.

Holter Monitoring

Holter monitoring is not helpful in evaluating valvular function, but it may detect paroxysmal arrhythmias that cause myocardial decompensation leading to symptoms. Recognition of a propensity for atrial fibrillation and other arrhythmias is important and can also explain symptomatic episodes.

Cardiac Catheterization

This is the gold standard for evaluating valvular function. Pressure measurement, visualization with contrast media, and hemodynamic measurements make it possible to grade stenosis and insufficiency of all valves. Multiple valvular defects combining stenosis and insufficiency or defects in more than one valve can make the measurements less accurate. Along with coronary angiography it is always indicated prior to valve surgery. Even if atherosclerosis is unlikely, coronary emboli are always a possibility in patients with valvular disease.

Exercise Capacity

Exercise Test

The exercise test is the gold standard for determining exercise capacity. It demonstrates maximal dynamic exercise capacity. Maximal exercise capacity can be estimated from the treadmill workload and grade, which have equivalent oxygen costs. Oxygen cost can be calculated in milliliters of oxygen per kilogram per minute, or in multiples of 3.5 ml of oxygen per kilogram per minute. One MET is 3.5 ml of oxygen per kilogram per minute and is the oxygen cost of maintaining life at rest. For instance, a satisfactory or "normal" exercise capacity would be 35 ml of oxygen per kilogram per minute, or 10 METs in a middle-aged individual. In general, exercise capacities below 5 METs are associated with a poor survival, whether an individual is treated medically or surgically. Treadmill time should not be used because it is specific to a protocol. Rather, the MET or oxygen consumption level reached is the value to be given for exercise capacity. The test can also suggest when deconditioning or pulmonary disease is the cause of a poor exercise capacity.

Echocardiography, Nuclear Techniques, Holter Monitoring, Nonexercise Stress Techniques, and Cardiac Catheterization

These procedures have little utility for determining exercise capacity. However, they may provide evidence for myocardial or valvular dysfunction, which can limit exercise performance.

Arrhythmias

Exercise Test

The exercise test is particularly valuable for evaluating exercise-induced ventricular arrhythmias or symptoms that could result from them. The nonexercise stress tests have no indication for evaluation of arrhythmias.

Echocardiography

Echocardiography can be used to evaluate the underlying cause of ventricular arrhythmias. Myocardial trabeculations, right ventricular dysplasia, ventricular aneurysms, mitral valve prolapse, asymmetric septal hypertrophy, LV dysfunction, and other cardiac findings have been associated with an increased prevalence of ventricular dysrhythmias.

Nuclear Cardiology

Frequent dysrhythmias can distort data gathered using the MUGA technique. The associated cardiac diseases can be delineated with these tests if clinically indicated.

Holter Monitoring

Holter monitoring is the gold standard for evaluating arrhythmias. It enables beat counts, classification, and determination of whether the arrhythmias are related to symptoms. Although computerized methods of counting arrhythmias are fraught with problems, particularly artifact recognition, the technology is always improving. Event recorders often have advantages, particularly for symptoms that occur infrequently.

Cardiac Catheterization

Electrophysiologic studies are the definitive means of diagnosing cardiac dysrhythmias and evaluating their response to medications. However, the voltage and number of stimulations needed to cause sustained ventricular tachycardia or fibrillation are still under investigation. In addition, the reproducibility of responses to drugs has been poor. Holter monitoring and exercise testing may be more cost-effective.

REFERENCES

1. Philbrick JT, Horwitz RI, Feinstein AR. Methcd-ologic problems of exercise testing for coronary artery disease: groups, analysis and bias. *Am J Ccr-diol* 1980;46:807.

2. Detrano R, et al. Bayesian probability analysis: a prospective demonstration of its clinical utility in diagnosing coronary disease. *Circulation* 1984;69:541–550.

3. Reid MC, Lachs MS, Feinstein AR. Methodologic standards in diagnostic test research. *JAMA* 1995;274:645–651.

4. Rosanski A, et al. The declining specificity of exercise radionuclide ventriculography. *N Engl J Med* 1983;309:518–522.

5. Guyatt GH. Readers' guide for articles evaluating diagnostic tests: What ACP Journal Club does for you and what you must do yourself. *ACP J Ciub* 1991;115:A-16.

6. Froelicher VF. *Handbook of Exercise Testing*. Boston: Little, Brown, 1996. P. 17.

7. Schlant RC, Friesinger GC, Leonard JL. Clinical competence in exercise testing. *Circulation* 1990;5:1884–1888.

8. Morris CK, et al. Nomogram based on metabolic equivalents and age. *J Am Coll Cardiol* 1993;22(1):175–182.

9. Mark DB, et al. Exercise treadmill score for predicting prognosis in coronary artery disease. *Ann Intern Med* 1987;106:793–800.

10. Myers J. *Essentials of Cardiopulmonary Testing*. Ontario: Human Kinetics, 1996. P. 20.

11. Ritchie JI, et al. Guidelines for clinical use of cardiac radionuclide imaging. A report of the American Heart Association/American College of Cardiology Task Force. *Circulation* 1995;91(4):1278–1303.

12. Froelicher VF, Myers J, Follansbee W, Labovitz A. *Exercise and the Heart* (3rd ed.). St. Louis: Mosby Yr Bk, 1993. P. 220.

13. Knoebel S, et al. Clinical competence in ambulatory electrocardiography. A statement for physicians from the AHA/ACC/ACP Task Force on Clinical Privileges in Cardiology. *Circulation* 1993;88(1):337–341.

14. Kinlay S, et al. Cardiac event recorders yield more diagnoses and are more cost-effective than 48-hour

Holter monitoring in patients with palpitations. A controlled clinical trial. *Ann Intern Med* 1996;124(1): 16–20.

15. Kirklin JW, et al. ACC/AHA Guidelines and Indications for Coronary Artery Bypass Graft Surgery. *JACC* 1991;17:543–589.

16. Guidelines for Clinical Intracardiac Electrophysiological and Catheter Ablation Procedures. ACC/AHA Task Force Report. *Circulation* 1995;92(3):673–691.

17. Radio frequency ablation for treatment of cardiac arrhythmias. *Med News Let* 1996;38:40–41.

18. Mason JW. A comparison of electrophysiologic testing with Holter monitoring to predict antiarrhythmic-drug efficacy for ventricular tachyarrhythmias. *N Engl J Med* 1993;329:445–451.

19. Yusuf S, et al. Effect of coronary artery bypass graft surgery on survival: overview of 10-year results from randomised trials by the Coronary Artery Bypass Graft Surgery Trialists. *Lancet* 1994;344(8922):563–570.

20. Wilson RF, et al. Accuracy of exercise electrocardiography in detecting physiologically significant coronary arterial lesions. *Circulation* 1991;83(2):412–421.

Treatment According to the Diagnoses Within the Key Features

Table 5-1 provides an overview of the specific treatments and goals for the most common disease presentations associated with the five key features.

DYSFUNCTION: KEY FEATURE 1— MYOCARDIAL DYSFUNCTION

Treatment for Acute Myocardial Dysfunction

Treatment for acute myocardial dysfunction manifested as pulmonary edema consists of oxygen, intravenous (IV) administration of furosemide (Lasix) and morphine sulfate, and at times administration of aminophylline and use of rotating tourniquets. The doses are 5 mg of morphine sulfate over 3 minutes, 40 to 60 mg of furosemide over 2 minutes (which causes vasodilation first, diuresis later), and 5 mg/kg of aminophylline in 10 minutes followed by a constant infusion of 0.9 mg/kg/hr. Vasodilators can be used, particularly if the arterial pressure is elevated. Nitroglycerin (NTG) in sublingual or topical form can be tried, but absorption is erratic and some patients become hypotensive. IV NTG can be titrated better. The dose is 20 mg/min and can be increased another 5 mg every 4 minutes until a response is obtained. The primary cause of the pulmonary edema should be identified and treated once the above-described therapy is effective. If chronic myocardial dysfunction is not due to systolic dysfunction and a dilated heart, consider diastolic dysfunction. If congestive heart failure (CHF) is semiacute and persisting due to ischemia, beta-blockers can be considered. Calcium antagonists are not helpful even if the CHF is due to diastolic dysfunction. IV furosemide is indicated for its immediate vasodilatory effect and because it causes a much-needed diuresis. Digoxin's many effects may be helpful in the acute treatment of CHF due to dilated cardiomyopathy, but it should be avoided in CHF of other causes. If atrial fibrillation is implicated as the precipitator of CHF, digoxin or diltiazem can be used to slow the ventricular response.

Table 5-1. A Summary of Specific Treatments and Goals for the Most Common Disease Presentations Within the Five Key Features

Key Features	Type	Prognosis	Treatment for Symptoms	Treatment for Prognosis
Myocardial dysfunction	Systolic (dilated cardiomyopathy)	10 to 25% annual mortality	Fluid and salt restrictions, diuretics, digoxin	ACE inhibitor, vasodilation, transplantation
	Diastolic (hypertrophic cardiomyopathy)	Varies; lower mortality than systolic	Control high BP; type-specific treatment	Control high BP; ?
Myocardial ischemia	Angina	2 to 4% annual mortality	Nitrates, beta-blockers, calcium antagonist, PTCA	CABS (for >3 vessel CAD and EF<50)
	Post MI	2 to 30% mortality in first year	Treat for dysfunction and/or ischemia	Aspirin, beta-blockers, risk factor modification
	Variant angina	Uncertain; rare	Nitroglycerin, nifedipine	?
Valvular disorders	Original	Poor when valvular or myocardial dysfunction occurs	Fluid and salt restrictions, diuretics, and digoxin for CHF	Yearly follow-up, timely surgery
	Prosthetic			Anticoagulation for CVA
Exercise intolerance	Cardiac cause	<5 METs from prognostic equations	Treatments for ischemia or dysfunction above	Exercise training program
	Noncardiac cause	For underlying disease	Treat underlying disease	Treat underlying disease
Arrhythmias	Atrial fibrillation	Mortality doubles; 5% annual CVA risk	Diltiazem, digoxin, ECT	Anticoagulation, ECT
	Complete heart block	If syncope occurs, mortality increases	Pacemaker	Pacemaker
	Ventricular tachycardia		Antiarrhythmic	AICD, beta-blockers

CVA = cerebrovascular accident; PTCA = percutaneous transluminal coronary angioplasty; CHF = congestive heart failure; ECT = electrocardioversion; CABS = coronary artery bypass surgery; CAD = coronary artery disease; EF = ejection fraction; AICD = automatic implantable cardio-defibrillator.

Treatment for Chronic Myocardial Dysfunction

Important Causes of Cardiomyopathy

The possible causes of myocardial damage or dysfunction listed below should be considered so that treatment can be directed to the etiology. Within the list, the four most common causes of systolic dysfunction resulting in a dilated cardiomy-opathy have been emphasized by italics. These four *(alcohol, HPB, ischemic, idiopathic)* account for 95% of the patients with chronic CHF seen in the ambulatory care clinic.

1. Inflammatory: infective and collagen
2. Metabolic
   a. Nutritional: vitamin deficiency, obesity
   b. Endocrine: pheochromocytoma, diabetes mellitus, hypothyroidism or hyperthyroidism
   c. Altered metabolism: gout, porphyria
3. Cellular damage: *alcohol,* venoms, heavy metals, toxins, antitumor drugs, cobalt
4. Infiltrative: amyloid, sarcoid, hemochromatosis
5. Fibroplastic
6. Hematologic: sickle cell anemia, leukemia
7. Hypersensitivity: drugs, rejection
8. Genetic: hypertrophic cardiomyopathy, neuromuscular
9. Miscellaneous acquired: *hypertensive, ischemic*, postpartum, valvular
10. *Idiopathic*
11. Physical agents: heat stroke, hypothermia, radiation

Overview of Therapy

The treatment of CHF includes relieving symptoms and improving prognosis with afterload reducers and angiotensin-converting enzyme (ACE) inhibitors [1]. The inotropic agents do not prolong life, but the vasodilators and ACE inhibitors clearly do. The side effects of the ACE inhibitors include a cough and renal dysfunction. A general guideline is to titrate the ACE inhibitor to the highest tolerated dose but not to allow the patient to become symptomatic from orthostatic hypotension or to become hyperkalemic. The clinician should not overlook the "standard therapy" of digoxin and diuretics. Changes in diuretic doses, even admissions for IV administration, can be very effective. Addition of potassium-sparing diuretics or metolazone can also yield the desired result. However, potassium-sparing diuretics and ACE inhibitors must be used together carefully, because they may precipitate hyperkalemia. Beta-blockers have been used in selected patients with obvious hypercatecholamine states (propranolol, 10 mg qid), but they can cause some patients to go into CHF. Recent emphasis on the hormonal dysfunction in CHF (i.e., recognition that catecholamine levels are directly related to mortality) has led to new beta-blocking agents that hold great promise in CHF. Also, agents that work at other points in the angiotensin cascade without affecting bradykinin levels may have the same results as the ACE inhibitors without the side effects (irritating cough and renal dysfunction).

Antiarrhythmic therapy for ventricular arrhythmias is controversial, especially since amiodarone did not reduce mortality in a randomized trial of patients with chronic CHF [2]. However, amiodarone is often used in these patients and can certainly complicate their management. The possible associated hyperthyroidism or hypothyroidism can exacerbate CHF while the former can increase arrhythmias [3]. Also, the pulmonary effects of amiodarone (lipid lesions, decreased diffusion capacity) can be confused with CHF.

Nonpharmacologic Therapy
Serial measurements of weight are the key to managing patients with CHF. This can be confounded by other illnesses, true caloric changes, changes in thyroid status, and problems with appetite due to digoxin toxicity. Increases in weight and swelling should indicate to the informed patient to increase his or her diuretics and to decrease salt and water intake. While a patient can make these changes, the physician should be sure that the patient does not increase the warfarin (Coumadin) or digoxin dose with the rationale that more may be better. It is important to remind the patient that he or she has a more narrow window of tolerance for other illnesses because of the heart muscle disease. Even the most informed patient can forget medications, catch a cold, consume extraneous added salt, or drink too much fluid.

Reduction of fluid and salt intake is critical to the management of CHF. Patient education regarding foods high in sodium is imperative for compliance. Sodium intake should be restricted to 2 g/day or less. Fluid intake should be reduced to 1,500 ml/day or less. Limitations on fluids should be guided by symptoms. Diuretic therapy is most effective and can be minimized when patients adhere to limitations of sodium and water intake. Patients should be educated regarding potassium-rich foods because most diuretics waste potassium, which can lead to arrhythmias and generalized weakness. Avoidance of alcohol is critical.

Digoxin

It has been suggested that digoxin is ineffective in CHF patients in sinus rhythm. This is primarily based on the finding that in selected patients, stopping chronic digoxin has no adverse effects. Also, the beneficial hemodynamic changes due to chronically administered digoxin are relatively modest and do not apply to every patient. For instance, one should not expect a systematic increase in ejection fraction. Perhaps it has its greatest effect when pulsed like many other drugs or when the right ventricle is involved [4]. Digoxin *should not* be used in patients only with diastolic dysfunction or with hypertrophic cardiomyopathy.

DIGOXIN TOXICITY.   The prevalence of digoxin toxicity has greatly decreased for many reasons, including the following:

1. Preparations other than digoxin are no longer used, and digoxin is now produced with a very consistent bioavailability.
2. Loading doses are rarely used.
3. The dangers of electrolyte abnormalities are now appreciated and they are treated or avoided.
4. Clinical situations for which 0.125 mg qd or less than the usual of 0.25 mg qd is now used include renal failure, age older than 65, and chronic obstructive pulmonary disease (COPD).
5. That loss of appetite can be the first symptom of digoxin toxicity and that any arrhythmia may be precipitated are now appreciated.
6. Patients with atrial fibrillation who need high doses of digoxin may become toxic if they revert to sinus rhythm.

Appreciation of these points makes measurement of digoxin levels rarely necessary. The problem of increased blood levels due to quinidine is greatly exaggerated. Although some experts recommend regular measurements of digoxin levels, we have not found this to be cost-effective. It is better to measure levels if the symptoms of digoxin toxicity—nausea, color perception changes, or arrhythmias—occur. Titration of the digoxin dose according to the level measurement is not indicated.

Vasodilators

Hydralazine (Apresoline) and long-acting nitrates are vasodilators that can improve survival in patients with CHF who cannot tolerate ACE inhibitors. The rationale for using an arteriolar dilator such as hydralazine is to break the cycle in which low cardiac output (mediated by potent neurohumoral mechanisms) leads to increased systemic resistance, which further increases the resistance to ejection and further reduces cardiac output (Fig. 5-1). Filling pressure is not changed much after vasodilators are given, but stroke volume and stroke work can be increased by 50%.

Venodilation increases the capacitance of the peripheral veins, thereby reducing volume in the heart and lungs, with a consequent reduction in right and left atrial filling pressures and relief of dyspnea. Nitrates, the most potent venodilators, have these effects. Nitrates reduce filling pressure without having much effect on stroke volume. Tolerance to nitrates must be considered, however. For the best balance between efficacy and tolerance, a drug such as isosorbide dinitrate should be given three or four times a day (40–120 mg). Oral nitrates have to be used in higher doses than other forms, to compensate for their first-pass metabolism by the liver.

The acute response to nitrates does not necessarily predict chronic effect; a poor acute response can be followed by a good chronic response, and vice versa. This finding has put less emphasis on acute hemodynamic monitoring to determine efficacy and dosage, but sometimes monitoring is indicated for safety reasons. In reducing the resistance to forward ejection, nitrates also have a beneficial effect on mitral regurgitation, a very common dysfunction among CHF patients. Using a venodilator to reduce heart size appears to improve the competency of the mitral valve apparatus. Nitroprusside in acute and chronic mitral regurgitation shows a striking reduction in the V wave on wedge pressure tracings, a marker for regurgitation.

Vasodilators can also confer dramatic clinical improvement and hemodynamic benefit while producing very little change in ejection fraction, in echocardiographic or chest x-ray appearance, or in any of the other parameters used to objectively measure left ventricular (LV) function.

Angiotensin-Converting Enzyme Inhibitors

Angiotensin II has three effects that can be deleterious in heart failure and can be inhibited by the relatively new class of drugs called ACE inhibitors:

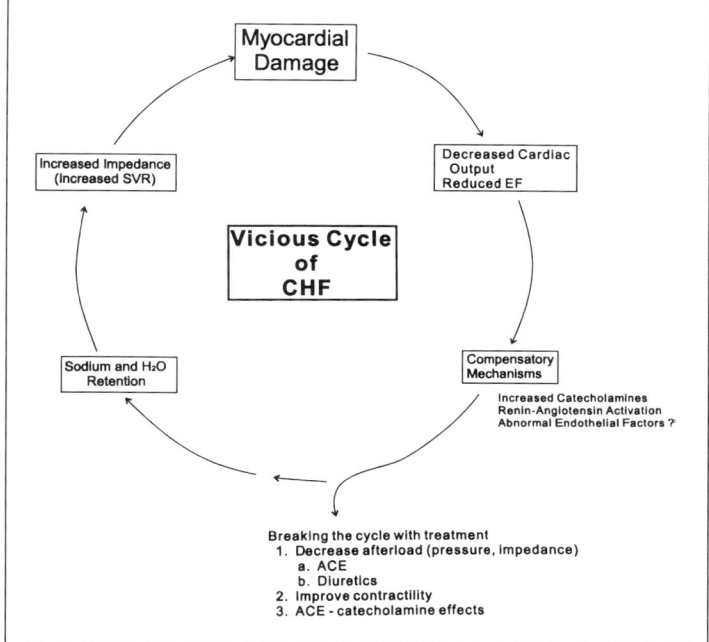

Fig. 5-1. The cycle of congestive heart failure, showing the points where the cycle can be broken by treatment. CHF = congestive heart failure; SVR = systemic vascular resistance.

1. It is a potent vasoconstrictor and therefore may contribute directly to increased systemic resistance.
2. It facilitates sympathetic outflow and thus tends to increase catecholamines.
3. Feedback of angiotensin II to the adrenals causes the release of aldosterone and the consequent retention of salt and water.

Captopril (Capoten) acutely produces a reduction in systemic resistance, and even with a single dose there is a moderate increase in cardiac output and a reduction in wedge pressure. Chronic administration is associated with a sustained decrease in systemic resistance; moderate increase in cardiac output; sustained reduction in arterial, left atrial, and wedge pressures; and not much change in heart rate. Improvement in clinical class, including an increase in exercise duration, can occur. The current emphasis on the neurohumoral aspects rather than the hemodynamic aspects of CHF has been strengthened by the success of the ACE inhibitors. Besides being vasodilators, they decrease catecholamine levels.

ACE inhibitors reduce mortality over a year by about 15%, compared to placebo, in patients with moderate to severe LV dysfunction. They are also associated with an improvement in the quality of life, less hospitalizations, and fewer exacerbations of CHF. During the acute and immediate infarction phase, ACE inhibitors lessen infarction expansion and facilitate healing.

A particular advantage of ACE inhibitors is their ease of titration. Once the converting enzyme has been blocked, the inhibitor is effective. In more than 90% of patients, the optimal dose of captopril is 25 mg tid. For initial administration, 6.25 mg tid is recommended, working up to 25 mg tid. A disturbing side effect that occurs in about 15% of patients is a histamine- or bradykinin-induced cough. Even though captopril can delay the need for dialysis in patients with diabetic nephropathy, it can also cause renal dysfunction, requiring that the dose be reduced when hyperkalemia occurs. Enalapril can be given twice a day (2.5–20.0 mg) and lisinopril once a day (10–40 mg).

ACE inhibitors including enalapril (Vasotec) and lisinopril (Prinivil, Zestril) improve survival and quality of life and lessen hospitalizations of patients with chronic CHF, even when only mild LV dysfunction is present. They also improve survival and lessen infarction expansion at the time of a myocardial infarction (MI). These agents are a *must* therapy in patients with chronic CHF [5], just as beta-blockers are a *must* in the first year after an MI has occurred.

Angiotensin Reception Blockers
A new class of antihypertensive drugs that are similar to ACE inhibitors but are angiotensin II receptor blockers has just been approved. They appear to have fewer side effects (kidney dysfunction or cough) than ACE inhibitors but there are no data demonstrating an improved survival rate in hypertensive or CHF patients.

Diuretics
Despite more than 60 years of empiric diuretic use for heart failure, the actual database regarding the long-term efficacy, adverse effects, and altered mortality outcome in heart failure is relatively small [6]. In addition to altered electrolyte transport and total-body electrolyte depletion, diuretics may be associated with adverse neurohormonal activation. Thus, guidelines for acute and long-term ther-

apy with diuretics in heart failure remain somewhat empirical. Diuretics will remain a mainstay for the treatment of edema in CHF patients but must be accompanied by moderate sodium restriction. However, large clinical trials of diuretics will be necessary to demonstrate that improved clinical efficacy with edema reduction is not offset by adverse effects, which include electrolyte depletion, ventricular arrhythmias, and subsequent increased mortality.

It is important to emphasize that the clinical effectiveness of diuretics depends on adherence to a restricted-sodium diet. Patients should be instructed to limit their daily intake of sodium to 2,000 mg or less, although this amount can be reduced further depending on the severity of edema. The sites of diuretic actions are shown in Figure 5-2.

LOOP DIURETICS.   Loop diuretics are compounds that exert their primary action on the thick ascending loop of Henle. To reach the intraluminal site of action, these organic acids must first be secreted into the proximal tubule via the organic acid pathway. Once the drug is in the lumen, active resorption of chloride is inhibited in both the medullary and the cortical portions of the loop of Henle. Decreased sodium resorption also occurs, since the chloride ion is cotransported with sodium and potassium. Loop diuretics decrease renal vasculature resistance and increase total and coronary renal blood flow. Sodium depletion and diuretic therapy tend to increase renin and aldosterone levels.

The three loop diuretics used to treat the edema of CHF are ethacrynic acid, furosemide, and bumetanide. Despite equal efficacy, clinicians often substitute one for another, with the hope of improved efficacy, but this strategy is typically not effective.

THIAZIDES.   Thiazide diuretics (hydrochlorothiazide and metolazone) are also organic acids that are highly bound to protein. Since they cannot be filtered, they gain access to the tubular lumen via the organic acid secretory pathway of the proximal tubule. The additive response observed with metolazone used in combination with a loop diuretic results from its sodium blockade at the distal portion of the nephron. Differences among pharmacokinetic characteristics of thiazide-type agents are minimal. The addition of IV chlorothiazide to IV loop diuretic therapy results in a more predictable blockade of both the thick ascending limb of the Henle and the distal tubule. This is important because absorption is impaired in CHF.

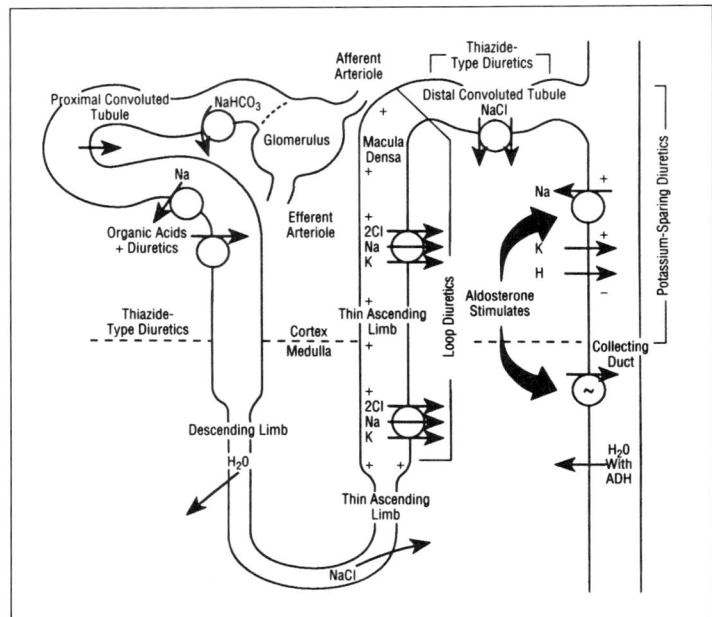

Fig. 5-2.   Sites of diuretic actions. ADH = antidiuretic hormone. (Reproduced with permission from RJ Cody. Diuretic treatment for the sodium retention of congestive heart failure. *Arch Intern Med* **1994;154:1905–1914. Copyright 1994 by American Heart Association.)**

POTASSIUM-SPARING DIURETICS. Although potassium-sparing diuretics act at the distal nephron and collecting duct, their effect is achieved by two different mechanisms. Active sodium resorption in the distal tubule and the collecting duct occurs in exchange for potassium and hydrogen. One mechanism is mediated by aldosterone and may be antagonized by spironolactone, which is a competitive receptor antagonist. The effects of triamterene and amiloride are independent of mineralocorticoids, and they act by direct inhibition of sodium transport. Differing from spironolactone, these two drugs must first reach their site of action by means of glomerular filtration and the organic base secretory pathway of the proximal tubule. Overall, these agents decrease sodium resorption, reduce potassium excretion, and theoretically potentiate hyperkalemia.

ADVERSE EFFECTS OF DIURETICS. The majority of the adverse effects of the diuretics are the result of altered renal tubular electrolyte transport and therefore may be related to the intensity and duration of therapy. Some adverse effects are specific for certain classes. For instance, hyperkalemia with potassium-sparing agents occurs in 2 to 10% of patients. Spironolactone produces gynecomastia in 10% of men and is dose dependent.

Electrolyte and metabolic disorders are the most common adverse effects of all diuretics. Long-term diuretic use may produce hypokalemia, hyponatremia, hypocalcemia, hypomagnesemia, hyperuricemia, and metabolic alkalosis. The reported incidence of these electrolyte and metabolic disorders is anywhere from 14 to 60%. The most common of these is hypokalemia, mediated by both direct transport into the tubular lumen and hypersecretion of aldosterone, which blocks distal resorption. Most patients with heart failure require the concomitant use of potassium supplements to correct hypokalemia. Hypokalemia and hypomagnesemia may be associated with myalgias, leg cramps, and an increase in ventricular arrhythmias. As high-grade ventricular arrhythmias and sudden death are frequently observed in patients with heart failure, the adverse effects of diuretics on electrolyte balance are of particular concern. Additional adverse effects, including a rash, may be seen with loop diuretics. Hyperuricemia occurs in 18 to 40% of patients and may precipitate an acute episode of gout, but this typically occurs in patients with a history of gout. GI tract disturbances are more frequent with ethacrynic acid than with furosemide or bumetanide, but occur in less than 10% of patients. Ototoxic effects also can occur with the use of ethacrynic acid more than with furosemide, but in less than 5% of patients.

ACUTE INTRAVENOUS DIURETIC THERAPY. IV diuretic therapy can be used acutely in several clinical situations. In pulmonary edema, the obvious benefit of acute IV diuretic therapy is the rapid clearance of pulmonary congestion, likely mediated by natriuresis and diuresis, a reduction of intravascular volume, and vasodilation. Acute IV diuretic therapy can also be used to supplement long-term oral therapy for sodium retention, to augment diuresis in the outpatient setting. For acute reversal of sodium retention and fluid overload, therapy with a loop diuretic is indicated. It should be given IV, to a high dose that is twice the normal oral dose (e.g., furosemide, 80 mg; bumetanide, 2 mg), and increased as necessary, in combination with other agents. A thiazide-type diuretic in combination with a loop diuretic is often effective. However, an oral thiazide-type diuretic, particularly metolazone, may require several days to achieve its maximum favorable response, because of delayed absorption. IV chlorothiazide (Diuril) is not considered as often as it should be. Unlike hydrochlorothiazide, chlorothiazide can be given IV in a dose of 250 to 500 mg, which is equivalent to an oral hydrochlorothiazide dose of 25 to 50 mg; when combined with a loop diuretic, chlorothiazide will produce greater diuresis than the loop diuretic alone.

DIURETIC RESISTANCE.   Patients should be considered to have diuretic resistance when they demonstrate progressive edema despite increasing doses of oral or IV diuretic therapy in combination with appropriate sodium and fluid limitations. Renal insufficiency can reduce tubular secretion of the diuretic as well as the filtered load of sodium. Therefore, patients with decreased renal function caused by heart failure or due to age frequently have reduced responses to diuretics. Indomethacin and other nonsteroidal anti-inflammatory drugs (NSAIDs) reduce the maximal response to furosemide. Mesenteric congestion may limit the absorption and bioavailability of orally administered medications.

Several therapeutic interventions can be used to augment diuretic responses in patients with refractory edema. An increasing dosage of IV loop diuretics is the most common approach, and the dosage should be rapidly doubled until the desired effect is produced. An ultrahigh dose of loop diuretic may be effective; however, the overall response to ultrahigh doses is often unimpressive. Alternatively, and perhaps more physiologically oriented, is the combination of a thiazide and a loop-type diuretic, in view of the structural hypertrophy of the distal nephron. Although precise dose limits are difficult to define, when a patient achieves a requirement of, for instance, 240 mg of furosemide daily, addition of an IV (chlorothiazide) or oral thiazide-type diuretic will be more effective than further increases of the loop diuretic. The combination of a loop and a thiazide diuretic will be more effective than high doses of a loop diuretic alone. Using supplement thiazide-type diuretics only on a temporary basis tends to reduce the cumulative long-term diuretic exposure.

Other Agents

IV infusions of dobutamine can be effective in increasing cardiac output in severe cardiomyopathies. The action can persist for days after the infusion is discontinued. Levodopa has been given orally.

Anticoagulation

The incidence of arterial thromboembolism in patients with CHF ranges from 0.9 to 5.5 events/100 patient-yr, with the largest studies reporting incidences of 2.0% and 2.4%. Findings regarding the relationship between ventricular function and thromboembolic events are contradictory. No controlled trial has assessed the efficacy or risks of anticoagulation for patients with heart failure and sinus rhythm, and reported efficacy rates in case series range from 0 to 100%. Until adequate studies are performed, anticoagulation should be discouraged for patients with heart failure who are in sinus rhythm and free of LV clot.

Coronary Artery Bypass Surgery

Coronary artery bypass grafting (CABG) improves 3-year survival rates by approximately 30 to 50% and exercise capacity in patients with moderate to severe LV dysfunction (EF of 30 to 50%), limiting angina, and three-vessel or left main coronary artery disease [7]. However, the operative mortality ranges from 5 to 30%, depending on ejection fraction and comorbidity. It is not clear whether patients whose predominant symptom is heart failure rather than angina benefit from bypass surgery or how much ischemia is required to justify surgical intervention. Clinical outcomes after angioplasty have not been adequately studied to determine the relative risks and benefits compared with bypass grafting in CHF patients [8].

Cardiac Transplantation

The nonspecialist should understand selected aspects of the treatment of patients being evaluated for and undergoing cardiac transplantation [9]. Cardiac transplantation is a potential therapeutic option for a variety of irreversible cardiac disorders when the symptomatic status and anticipated survival after transplantation exceed that of the patient's condition. The timing of cardiac transplantation with respect to prognosis is aided by the measurement of baseline hemodynamics and maximal aerobic capacity and must be made by an experienced cardiologist. Major cardiac problems that occur after transplantation include an increased early risk of acute allograft rejection and, later, the occurrence of allograft coronary artery disease. Furthermore, cardiac transplant recipients have unique "normal" physiologic alterations with respect to intracardiac hemodynamics, exercise capacity, the effects of denervation, and expected ECG and echocardiographic findings.

Cardiac transplantation should be a therapeutic consideration to improve the survival or symptoms of irreversible heart disease. Since 1986 when it was approved by Medicare, this operation has been accepted as the best therapy for end-stage heart failure, with over 20,000 cardiac transplantations performed. The most common heart diseases in patients undergoing transplantation are dilated cardiomyopathy and ischemic heart disease. Other diagnoses include valvular or congenital heart disease, hypertrophic cardiomyopathy, angina (unresponsive to drugs and not amenable to CABG), myocarditis, sarcoidosis, and amyloidosis. Indications include maximal ventilatory oxygen consumption of less than 14 ml of oxygen/kg/min (or <40% of age predicted) measured during a maximal exercise test as well as uncontrolled ischemia, arrhythmias, or CHF. A low ejection fraction alone is not an indication. Absolute contraindications include emotional or psychiatric impairment, fixed pulmonary high BP, cerebrovascular disease, and coexistent life-limiting disorders.

EVALUATION AND LISTING.   In addition to exercise testing with expired gas analysis, evaluation should include complete cardiac catheterization with coronary angiography and measurement of right-sided heart pressure, which must be less than 50 mm Hg. Reversibility of the high BP should be tested with vasodilators. Once approved for transplantation, the patient is placed on the transplant list ("listed") and can anticipate a 3- to 6-month wait. Some of the 10,000 patients listed every year can be removed from the list because they improve or respond to new therapies. Remember that 50% of patients with recent onset of a nonischemic cardiomyopathy will spontaneously improve and avoidance of alcohol can also lead to improvement. Half of the listed patients receive heart transplants from donors matched to recipients by blood type and body size. Consideration of genetic markers (HLA) improves the match, however. Patients in common blood groups such as type O vie for more donors and thus tend to have a longer wait. The severity of the symptoms and of the condition also impacts the wait, with the sicker patients having a higher priority. Currently only 2,000 appropriate donor matches are found each year and this number is declining with the increased use of airbags in cars. This limitation may be removed if a new strain of allogenic pigs can be used to harvest hearts that will not be rejected by human recipients.

AFTER TRANSPLANTATION—GENERAL FACTS. The operative mortality is 14% for the sickest patients and 6% for the remainder. Most early deaths are due to infections or graft failure. Follow-up by a transplant team is required weekly for several months with increasingly frequent laboratory tests, then monthly for the rest of the first year, and then every 3 months thereafter. The early follow-up targets the tolerance and dosage of medications and monitoring for rejection. Quality of life should approximate normal and some recipients can overcome prejudices and return to work. While only 30 to 40% return to work, more than 80% report leading an active lifestyle. The major problems recipients encounter are infections and other immunosuppression side effects including osteoporosis, cataracts, and accelerated coronary disease. It is important to realize that even though coronary artery disease and MIs are usually late complications and rejection is an early complication, they can occur at any time.

IMMUNOSUPPRESSION. The commonly used triple therapy includes azathioprine, corticosteroids, and cyclosporine. Lympholytic agents can induce immunosuppression and lessen the doses of the triple-therapy drugs. Cyclosporine is the key drug but its side effects include neurotoxicity (tremors), high BP, and renal dysfunction. The levels of cyclosporine must be followed because it is affected by many drugs including diltiazem and antibiotics. Azathioprine is an antifolate drug that affects DNA synthesis. It can cause anemia, pancreatitis, and abnormal liver function. Allopurinol can potentiate leukopenia and so should not be given with azathioprine. *When cyclosporine and lovastatin are given together, there is a 30% incidence of myositis.*

REJECTION. Rejection is characterized by CHF and fatigue, with ECG findings of bradyarrhythmias and atrial arrhythmias, but most frequently rejection is asymptomatic at first. When rejection is suspected, a biopsy is indicated. Echocardiography appears to be the most helpful noninvasive tool, with changes in LV size and function as well as increased pericardial effusions being indicative of rejection. Echocardiography should be performed and the results interpreted by the same experienced individuals. Accelerated coronary atherosclerosis is the major limiter of long-term survival.

GENERAL FINDINGS. Right bundle-branch block and tachycardia are frequently present. Though exercise capacity improves, it is not normal but can be further

improved by an exercise program. Sympathetic denervation results in a higher resting heart rate ($\geq$100 bpm) and
lower than predicted maximal exercise heart rate. Hypertension is frequently encountered and should be tested.
Antibiotic prophylaxis is indicated for dental and surgical
procedures. Consultation with the transplantation team is
indicated for noncompliance, abnormal laboratory results,
CHF, arrhythmias, and medication problems.

Practical Considerations and
Summary of Therapy for CHF

Patients should be encouraged to participate in their management. Counseling and education can improve patients'
adjustment to their illness and decrease unnecessary hospitalizations. Because of alcohol's direct depressive action
on cardiac function, it should be avoided. Daily measurement of weight on an accurate scale is essential. Salt intake
should be limited to 2 g or less a day and fluid restriction to
1.5 liters, particularly when weight is increasing. BP
should be measured daily and kept at or below 110/80 mm
Hg. Patients who can follow these guidelines and understand the volume overload that occurs with CHF can even
be expected to adjust their diuretic doses with weight
changes. They certainly should know to call their physician
when they note increases in abdominal girth, pedal edema,
shortness of breath, and weight. Exercise, particularly
walking, is safe and can improve exercise duration and
symptoms. Adherence to the treatment plan should be
stressed along with daily weight measurement, and monitored at each visit. Clinicians should inform patients of the
seriousness of their disease and their prognosis, but they
should emphasize that patients can continue to remain
active and enjoy a reasonable quality of life (see also
Appendix A for sodium and potassium content in foods).

A careful history can help to explain an exacerbation
of CHF; failure to follow dietary restrictions and medical
prescriptions, alcohol ingestion, and symptoms of hypokalemia are all to be considered. Recent interesting
patients include a cook who drank pickle brine not realizing
it contained salt, and a patient on amiodarone who had a
tachycardia and gallop even though his weight was down—
hyperthyroidism had developed due to the amiodarone.
Hypokalemia can develop, particularly after a large diuresis, requiring that potassium levels be maintained by
ingestion of fresh vegetables and fruits, supplemented during times of increased fluid loss, and measured along with
renal function at least quarterly or with symptoms.

It is necessary to take care in coprescribing drugs. NSAIDs, calcium channel– or beta-blocking agents, steroids, terfenadine (Seldane), and lithium should be used with great caution, if at all, in patients with CHF.

ACE inhibitors should be given to all patients unless specific contraindications exist. Diuretics should be used judiciously early in treatment to prevent excessive diuresis that could prevent titration of ACE inhibitors to target doses. Digoxin has not been shown to affect the natural history of heart failure but it is often helpful in those with right-sided symptoms. Isosorbide dinitrate and hydralazine hydrochloride should be tried in patients who cannot tolerate ACE inhibitors, as these vasodilators can prolong life.

Diagnosis and Treatment of Venous Thromboembolism: A Confounder of CHF
Venous thromboembolism is being seen with increasing frequency in outpatients; because it can be a complication of CHF and the pedal edema can confound the diagnosis of CHF, it is presented in this section. Venous thromboembolism involves venous thrombosis and its two major complications—pulmonary embolism (discussed later) and the postthrombotic syndrome [10]. The increased incidence of venous thromboembolism in outpatients is due to the early hospital discharge of postsurgical patients, the performance of outpatient surgery, and the use of the femoral vein for outpatient angiography. It is more frequently identified because of the availability of reliable noninvasive diagnostic tests.

Risk Factors
Most patients with venous thromboembolism have one or more well-recognized clinical risk factors. The most common risk factors are recent surgery, trauma, and immobility, as well as serious illness, including CHF, stroke, malignancy, and inflammatory bowel disease. *The common risk factors in outpatients include hospital admission within the past 6 months, malignancy, presence of antiphospholipid antibody, and familial thrombophilia.* Less common associations are paroxysmal nocturnal hemoglobinuria, nephrotic syndrome, and polycythemia vera.

Pathophysiology of Venous Thrombosis
Venous thrombi are composed predominantly of fibrin and red blood cells. They usually arise at sites of vessel damage or in the large venous sinuses of the calves or the valve

cusp pockets in the deep veins of the calves. Thrombosis occurs when blood coagulation exceeds the natural anticoagulant mechanisms and the fibrinolytic system. Coagulation is usually triggered when blood is exposed to tissue factor on the surface of monocytes or endothelial cells activated in response to tissue damage or vascular trauma. Clinical risk factors that activate blood coagulation include extensive surgery, trauma, burns, malignant disease, MI, cancer chemotherapy, and local hypoxia produced by venous stasis. Malignant cells contain a cysteine proteinase that activates factor X and thus leads to coagulation. Venous stasis and damage to the vessel wall increase the thrombogenic effect of blood coagulation. Venous stasis is produced by immobility, by obstruction or dilation of veins, by increased venous pressure, and by increased blood viscosity. Tissue damage, by stimulating the release of inflammatory cytokines, also results in impaired fibrinolysis.

Increased central venous pressure, which produces venous stasis in the extremities, explains why venous thrombosis is common in patients with CHF. Stasis resulting from venous dilation occurs in elderly patients, in patients with varicose veins, and in women who are pregnant. Venous obstruction contributes to the risk of venous thrombosis in patients with pelvic tumors and to the risk of recurrent venous thrombosis in patients with persistent obstruction resulting from proximal vein thrombosis. Increased blood viscosity, which also causes stasis, may explain the risk of thrombosis in patients with polycythemia vera, hypergammaglobulinemia, or chronic inflammatory disorders. Direct venous damage can lead to venous thrombosis in patients undergoing hip surgery, knee surgery, or varicose vein stripping and in patients with severe burns or trauma to the lower extremities.

Most venous thrombi produce no symptoms and are confined to the intramuscular veins of the calf. Many calf vein thrombi undergo spontaneous lysis, but some extend into the popliteal and more proximal veins. Complete lysis of proximal vein thrombosis is rare. Most symptomatic pulmonary emboli and all fatal emboli arise from thrombi in the *proximal veins of the legs*. Extensive venous thrombosis causes venous valvular damage, which leads to the postthrombotic syndrome. Patients with previous venous thrombosis are more likely to experience additional episodes, particularly when exposed to high-risk situations.

Untreated or inadequately treated venous thrombosis is associated with a high rate of complications, which can be decreased considerably by adequate anticoagulant therapy. About 25% of untreated calf vein thrombi extend into the popliteal vein, and about 50% of untreated proximal vein thrombi cause pulmonary embolism. Patients with proximal vein thrombosis who are inadequately treated have a recurrence rate of about 40% and patients with symptomatic calf vein thrombosis who are treated with a 5-day course of intermittent IV heparin without continuation of oral anticoagulant therapy have a recurrence rate higher than 20% over the next 3 months.

In contrast, fewer than 5% of patients with proximal vein thrombosis experience a clinically detectable recurrence during the initial period of heparin therapy if an adequate anticoagulant response is achieved, and fewer than 4% of patients experience recurrence during the subsequent 3 months of treatment with moderate-intensity oral anticoagulant therapy or moderate-dose subcutaneous heparin therapy. After 3 months of anticoagulant therapy, patients have an annual recurrence rate of about 3% if the thrombosis developed after a reversible provocation, such as surgery, or as high as 15% if the thrombosis was idiopathic or associated with ongoing conditions, such as prolonged immobilization or cancer. In patients with more than one documented episode of deep venous thrombosis or pulmonary embolism, the recurrence rate in the first year after a 3-month course of anticoagulant therapy is approximately 25%, and the mortality is approximately 5%.

SUPERFICIAL VENOUS THROMBOSIS. Venous thrombosis usually occurs in superficial or deep veins of the legs. Generally benign and self-limiting, thrombosis in a superficial vein of the leg can be serious if it extends from the long saphenous vein into the common femoral vein or if it is associated with deep venous thrombosis that is clinically silent. Superficial thrombophlebitis is easily recognized by the presence of a tender vein surrounded by an area of erythema, heat, and edema. A thrombus can often be palpated in the affected vein. Superficial thrombophlebitis may be associated with deep venous thrombosis. In most cases, superficial disease can be treated conservatively by elevating the affected limb, applying local heat, and administering anti-inflammatory drugs and antibiotics for suspected infections.

DEEP VENOUS THROMBOSIS. Thrombosis involving the deep veins of the leg may be confined to calf veins or may extend into the popliteal or more proximal veins. Thrombi confined to calf veins are usually small and are rarely associated with pulmonary embolism. About 20% of calf vein thrombi, however, extend into the popliteal vein and beyond, where they can cause serious complications. About 50% of patients with symptomatic proximal vein thrombosis also have silent pulmonary embolism, and about 70% of patients with symptomatic pulmonary embolism have deep venous thrombosis, which is usually clinically silent.

The clinical features of venous thrombosis, such as localized swelling, redness, tenderness, and distal edema, are nonspecific and should always be confirmed by objective tests. About 70% of ambulatory patients with clinically suspected venous thrombosis have another cause for their symptoms. Confounders that are most likely to simulate venous thrombosis are ruptured Baker's cyst, cellulitis, muscle tear, muscle cramp, muscle hematoma, external venous compression, superficial thrombophlebitis, and postthrombotic syndrome. Of the 30% of patients who have venous thrombosis, about 85% have proximal vein thrombosis and the rest have thrombosis confined to the calf. *CHF results in edema in both legs while peripheral venous thrombosis usually only involves one leg.*

Although clinical features cannot be used to confirm or exclude a diagnosis of venous thrombosis, careful history taking and documentation of the signs and symptoms at presentation can be useful in diagnosis. Evidence suggests that patients can be classified as having a high, intermediate, or low probability of having venous thrombosis according to the presence or absence of risk factors such as recent immobilization, hospitalization within the past 6 months, and malignancy, as well as the clinical manifestations at presentation. Patients with classic signs and symptoms of deep venous thrombosis (e.g., localized pain, tenderness, swelling, and discoloration) who have at least one risk factor have an 85% probability of having venous thrombosis; those with atypical symptoms and no risk factors have only a 5% probability. Patients in the intermediate probability group have a 35% chance of having venous thrombosis.

The pretest classification of patients by the probability of their having venous thrombosis can be used in combination with the results of objective noninvasive tests to determine the diagnosis in approximately 60% of symptomatic patients. Thus, a diagnosis of venous thrombosis can be excluded in patients with a low pretest probability of venous thrombosis and negative findings on noninvasive testing, obviating further testing. A high pretest clinical probability and an abnormal noninvasive test provide a definitive diagnosis of venous thrombosis. Patients with low pretest probabilities and an abnormal noninvasive test and those with high pretest probabilities and a normal noninvasive test should undergo venography. For the one-third of patients in the intermediate-probability group, an abnormal noninvasive test indicates a diagnosis of venous thrombosis; repeat testing is often indicated if clinical suspicion is high.

Diagnostic Tests
Three objective tests—venography, impedance plethysmography (IPG), and venous ultrasonography—are available for diagnosing venous thrombosis [11]. Venography detects both proximal vein and calf vein thrombosis; IPG is moderately sensitive and specific for proximal vein thrombosis in symptomatic patients but is insensitive to calf vein thrombosis; and venous ultrasonography is more sensitive and specific for symptomatic proximal vein thrombosis than is IPG and detects about 50% of calf vein thrombi.

Venography, which involves the injection of a radiocontrast agent into a distal vein, is the standard for the diagnosis of venous thrombosis. However, this test has been replaced clinically by the noninvasive tests.

IMPEDANCE PLETHYSMOGRAPHY.   IPG is a noninvasive test that uses electrical resistance, or impedance, to reflect blood volume changes in the calf produced by inflation and deflation of a pneumatic thigh cuff [12]. The changes in blood volume are reduced if the popliteal or more proximal veins are obstructed. Because IPG does not distinguish between thrombotic and nonthrombotic obstruction to venous outflow, it can give false-positive results if the vein is compressed by an extravascular mass or if venous outflow is impaired by elevated central venous pressure.

VENOUS ULTRASONOGRAPHY.   Venous ultrasonography (duplex, which includes color flow, or gray scale) has greater sensitivity and specificity than IPG and is *the preferred noninvasive method of diagnosis for venous thrombosis*. The common femoral vein, superficial femoral vein, popliteal vein, and proximal deep calf veins are compressed with the transducer probe and flow characteristics recorded.

Treatment of Thromboembolism

The objectives of treating patients with venous thromboembolism are to prevent fatal pulmonary embolism, the postthrombotic syndrome, and thromboembolic pulmonary hypertension and to alleviate the discomfort of the acute event. Anticoagulants can effectively reduce morbidity and mortality caused by pulmonary embolism. Vena caval interruption, which is usually achieved with an inferior vena caval filter, is also effective but is more complicated, expensive, and invasive. For these reasons, it is used only if anticoagulant therapy has failed or is contraindicated because of the risk of serious hemorrhage.

ANTICOAGULANT THERAPY.   Anticoagulants are the major treatment for venous thromboembolism. Superficial disease can usually be treated conservatively by elevating the affected limb, applying local heat, and administering anti-inflammatory drugs and antibiotics for suspected infections. Most patients with proximal vein thrombosis, calf vein thrombosis, and pulmonary embolism should be treated first with high-dose heparin and then with moderate-intensity oral anticoagulant therapy (international normalized ratio [INR], 2.0–3.0) for 3 months. The acute episode of thromboembolism should be treated with heparin, which can be administered by continuous IV infusion or subcutaneous injection. The anticoagulant effect of IV heparin is immediate. With subcutaneous injection, the anticoagulant effect is delayed for about an hour; peak levels occur at 2 to 3 hours and are maintained for about 12 hours with therapeutic doses. Heparin therapy is usually monitored by the activated partial thromboplastin time (APTT) and less frequently by heparin assays. For IV heparin therapy, a bolus of 5,000 units should be followed by a continuous IV infusion at a dosage of 1,300 units/hr. The initial dosage of subcutaneous heparin should be 35,000 units/day, given in two divided doses. Heparin should be administered for a total of 5 to 7 days, and warfarin should be commenced 24 to 48 hours after heparin treatment begins. The dose of heparin should be adjusted to maintain the APTT at 1.8 to 2.5 times the control value. The APTT should be measured 6 hours after the bolus dose was given, so that it reflects the anticoagulant effects of the infusion, and the dose should be adjusted according to

a dose-adjustment nomogram. If twice-daily subcutaneous heparin is given, the APTT should be measured 6
hours after injection. The INR is used to monitor oral anticoagulant therapy, and the dose of warfarin is adjusted to
achieve an INR of 2.0 to 3.0.

Long-term anticoagulant therapy should be considered
for patients with recurrent venous thromboembolism and
for those with continuing risk factors, such as hereditary
thrombophilia, malignancy, and the antiphospholipid
antibody syndrome.

Postthrombotic Syndrome
Pulmonary embolism (discussed later) is the most serious
complication of venous thrombosis, but the postthrombotic syndrome, which occurs as a long-term complication
in 30 to 60% of patients with symptomatic proximal vein
thrombosis, is responsible for much greater morbidity
[13]. Over a 2-year follow-up, 20% of patients with a first
episode of symptomatic deep venous thrombosis will experience a reoccurrence. Cancer or impaired coagulation
raises the risk of reoccurrence. Nearly 33% of patients
with these complications will develop the postthrombotic
syndrome after 8 years. Clinically, the postthrombotic syndrome can mimic acute venous thrombosis or CHF, or it
can manifest as chronic leg pain that is associated with
edema and that worsens at the end of the day. Some
patients also have stasis pigmentation, induration, and
skin ulceration; a smaller number of patients have venous
claudication on walking.

The postthrombotic syndrome is caused by venous
hypertension that usually results from valvular destruction and leads to increased ambulatory pressure in the
deep calf veins. This increased pressure, in turn, produces
edema with chronic pain and swelling. In patients with
extensive thrombosis involving the iliofemoral veins, the
swelling and pain may never disappear. Typically, however, the symptoms subside after a period of weeks to
months but return years later. The early manifestations
include pain in the calf and swelling after prolonged
standing or exercise, which subsides with rest and elevation of the leg. In more severe cases, progressive skin pigmentation and induration of the subcutaneous tissues
around the ankle and the distal part of the calf occur.
These conditions can lead to cellulitis and venous ulceration.

Treatment and Work-up for High Blood Pressure

Work-up

Since high BP is a cause of myocardial hypertrophy and damage, its work-up is presented here [14]. While high BP is highly prevalent, most of the time it does not have a specific known cause, so the work-up must be simple and inexpensive.

MEDICAL HISTORY.   The patient should be questioned regarding personal or family history of hypertension, symptoms or previous diagnoses or complications of hypertension, and previous therapy. Important historical features include duration and severity of hypertension and the presence of factors known to ease or worsen hypertension such as salt and alcohol ingestion, exercise, and the use of medications such as diet, decongestants, and birth control pills. Evidence of organ damage such as CHF, stroke, and renal dysfunction should be sought. Symptoms of secondary causes of hypertension including palpitations, diaphoresis, feelings of impending doom (pheochromocytoma) or weakness, muscle cramps, and polyuria (hypokalemia and primary hyperaldosteronism) should be included in the history.

PHYSICAL EXAMINATION.   Critical to diagnosing and managing hypertension is accurate measurement of the BP. Guidelines for standardized measurement of the BP by the American Heart Association (AHA) and the American Society of Hypertension should be followed. Proper equipment should be used, with a mercury manometer being preferred to an aneroid one. Manometers should be calibrated on a regular basis to the nearest 2 mm Hg. The cuff must be free of air leaks and be the proper size. The bladder length should be at least 80% of the arm circumference and the bladder width should cover at least two-thirds of the upper arm. The recorded BP should be the average of two or more readings taken minutes apart and should be obtained with the patient sitting and standing. The bell of the stethoscope should be used for auscultation. The cuff should be inflated at least 30 mm Hg above the patient's palpated systolic pressure to avoid underestimating the BP due to the presence of an auscultatory gap (disappearance and reappearance of the Korotkoff sounds between systole and diastole). Funduscopy should be performed to evaluate the degree of retinopathy and the abdomen auscultated to detect bruits suggestive of renal artery stenosis.

LABORATORY TESTS.   Urinalysis for active parenchymal renal disease, serum BUN, creatinine, and potassium measurements, and an ECG should be obtained. A chest x-ray study may assist in a diagnosis of an aortic coarctation and CHF. Hypokalemia suggests possible primary hyperaldosteronism. The place of echocardiography is being resolved, with the possibility that a "quick look" could document LV hypertrophy (associated with increased morbidity and mortality) at a lower cost than a complete echocardiographic study. Currently, ambulatory BP monitoring is not recommended for initial or routine use in the evaluation and treatment of hypertension.

EVALUATION OF SECONDARY HYPERTENSION. The secondary causes of hypertension are so rare and the expense and risk of the studies necessary to rule them out are so high that routine testing for secondary hypertension is not recommended. Signs and symptoms suggestive of secondary causes of hypertension include an abdominal bruit (possibly due to renal artery stenosis); a history of anxiety, tremor, or rapid pulse (pheochromocytoma or hyperthyroidism); diaphoresis (pheochromocytoma); and muscle weakness or cramps (due to primary hyperaldosteronism). Physical findings of Cushing's syndrome and diminished or delayed femoral pulses due to aortic coarctation should be considered. Patients at high risk for having secondary causes would be those who have the above signs or symptoms, who are less than 30 years old, in whom medical therapy fails to control BP, and in whom BP control suddenly worsens.

Treatment

The fifth Joint National Committee on Detection, Evaluation, and Treatment of High Blood Pressure (JNC V) recommended a new algorithm for treating hypertension that emphasizes the use of drugs shown in randomized clinical trials to reduce cardiovascular morbidity and mortality—namely, diuretics and beta-blockers [15]. The report contains several new sections, including new data from the National Health and Nutrition Examination Survey (NHANES III) on the prevalence, awareness, treatment, and control of hypertension; a new classification schema that includes systolic and diastolic criteria; and sections on the effects of cocaine, lithotripsy, cyclosporine, and erythropoietin to induce or aggravate hypertension. Other topics have been greatly expanded, including special populations and situations, primary prevention of hypertension, and lifestyle modifications. The JNC V report also added alpha-1-adrenergic blocking agents and the alpha-beta-blocker labetalol to the list of drugs suitable for initial monotherapy in managing hypertension. The data suggesting that calcium antagonists are associated with increased morbidity and mortality, particularly at higher doses, make them less attractive for the treatment of high BP.

The report highlighted the importance of systolic hypertension and recommended that hypertension should be diagnosed, regardless of age, when systolic BP readings are consistently 140 mm Hg or higher. JNC V reflected the opinion in JNC IV that several drug classes, including diuretics, beta-blockers, ACE inhibitors, calcium antagonists, and alpha-blockers, are suitable for initiating antihypertensive therapy. However, *JNC V gave preference to diuretics and beta-blockers because these drug classes reduced the incidence of stroke and cardiovascular events in clinical trials; similar studies with the newer drug classes have not been completed yet*. This recommendation is highly controversial because the benefits of diuretic and beta-blocker use are most evident in the elderly, and the beneficial effects of these drugs on the incidence of coronary events are relatively modest [16]. Further, growing experience with ACE inhibitors and calcium antagonists shows that these agents lack the metabolic disadvantages of older agents and can exhibit antiatherosclerotic and antihypertrophic vasoactivity. Although to date the clinical benefits of the newer agents have been documented in conditions other than hypertension, the data are persuasive and indicate a probability that these drugs will improve prognosis in hypertensive patients. JNC V also emphasized lifestyle modifications; however, even when they decrease BP, dietary and other nonpharmacologic strategies have not been shown to lower the incidence of clinical events.

Results of trials of the primary prevention of coronary heart disease suggest that treating hypertension with high doses of thiazide diuretic drugs might increase the risk of sudden death from cardiac causes. In contrast, treatment with low doses of thiazide reduces the risk of coronary heart disease. To examine the association between thiazide treatment for hypertension and the occurrence of primary cardiac arrest, a population-based case-control study of enrollees of a health maintenance organization was conducted [17]. The case patients were 114 persons with hypertension who had a primary cardiac arrest between 1977 and 1990. The control patients were a stratified random sample of 535 persons with hypertension. The risk of primary cardiac arrest among patients receiving combined thiazide and potassium-sparing diuretic therapy was lower than that among patients treated with a thiazide without potassium-sparing therapy (odds ratio, 0.3). As compared with low-dose thiazide therapy (25 mg daily), moderate-dose therapy (50 mg daily) was associated with a moderate increase in risk (odds ratio, 2) and high-dose therapy (100 mg daily) was associated with a larger increase in risk (odds ratio, 3.6). The addition of a potassium-sparing drug to low-dose thiazide therapy was associated with a reduced risk of cardiac arrest (odds ratio, 0.4). Both the dose of thiazide drugs and the addition of potassium-sparing drugs influence the risk of primary cardiac arrest. *Must-use* drugs for initial treatment of high BP are a low-dose thiazide along with a potassium-sparing diuretic (Maxzide [triamterene and hydrochlorothiazide] is a good combination, 1 tablet/day) and then a beta-blocker (atenolol is cardiospecific and does not cross the blood-brain barrier, 50 mg once a day).

LIFESTYLE MODIFICATIONS.   There appears to be considerable impact of small reductions of diastolic BP, such as those achievable by lifestyle modification, on the incidence of coronary heart disease and stroke [18]. Published data from the Framingham Heart Study, a longitudinal cohort study, and from the NHANES II, a national population survey, were used to examine the impact of a population-wide strategy aimed at reducing diastolic BP by an average of 2 mm Hg in a population including normotensive subjects. A reduction of 2 mm Hg in diastolic BP results in a 17% decrease in the prevalence of hypertension as well as a 6% reduction in the risk of coronary heart disease and a 15% reduction in risk of stroke and transient ischemic attacks (TIAs). From an application of these results to U.S. white men and women aged 35 to 64 years, it is estimated that a successful population intervention alone could reduce coronary heart disease incidence more than could medical treatment for all those with a diastolic BP of 95 mm Hg or higher. It could prevent 84% of the events prevented by medical treatment for all those with a diastolic BP of 90 mm Hg or higher. For stroke (including TIAs), a populationwide 2 mm Hg reduction could prevent 93% of the events prevented by medical treatment for those with a diastolic BP of 95 mm Hg or higher and 69% of the events for those with a diastolic BP of 90 mm Hg or higher. A combination strategy of both a population reduction in diastolic BP and targeted medical intervention is most effective and could double or triple the impact of medical treatment alone. Adding a population-based intervention to existing levels of hypertension treatment could prevent an estimated additional 67,000 coronary heart disease events (6%) and 34,000 stroke and TIA events (13%) annually among all those aged 35 to 64 years in the United States. The small reduction of 2 mm Hg in diastolic BP in the mean of the population distribution, in addition to medical treatment, could have a great public health impact on the number of coronary heart disease and stroke events prevented. Such diastolic BP reductions can be achieved through lifestyle interventions, particularly through sodium reduction, only with the cooperation of the food industry, government agencies, and practitioners.

Treatment of Hypertrophic Cardiomyopathy:
A Confounder of CHF

Hypertrophic (obstructive, nonobstructive) cardiomyopathies are familial, occurring in less than 1% of the population and with varying degrees of penetrance. The hypertrophy leads to diastolic dysfunction; the obstructive form leads to pressure differential across the aortic outflow because of septal asymmetry and mitral valve involvement. The hypertrophy can be localized (i.e., septal or apical). Septal hypertrophy is known by numerous names—asymmetric septal hypertrophy (ASH), hypertrophic obstructive cardiomyopathy (HOCM), and idiopathic hypertrophic subaortic stenosis (IHSS). Apical hypertrophy appears to be benign but causes deeply inverted lateral T waves simulating an MI. Anginal-type chest pains occur with hypertrophic cardiomyopathy, even though normal coronary arteries are usually demonstrated by cardiac catheterization. There can be a family history of sudden death or CHF. Hypertrophic cardiomyopathy is the most common cause of sudden disease in young athletes [19]. On physical examination, patients with ASH have a characteristic brisk carotid pulse and harsh systolic ejection murmur that increases with Valsalva's maneuver. The ECG shows LV hypertrophy with strain, left bundle-branch block, and sometimes pseudoinfarction Q waves due to the septal hypertrophy. Deeply inverted anterolateral T waves are seen with apical hypertrophy. Echocardiography is more diagnostic than the chest x-ray since valves, function, and chamber and wall dimensions can be determined. In ASH, the septum to posterior wall ratio exceeds 1.3.

There can be systolic anterior motion of the anterior mitral leaflet, which causes the outflow obstruction.

ASH is best treated with beta-blockers or calcium antagonists but recently flecainide has been used despite its anticholinergic side effects. The danger of using verapamil in patients with ASH or IHSS has been made apparent by 5 deaths reported to the National Institutes of Health (NIH). Although this agent can be very effective for the symptoms of hypertrophic cardiomyopathy, much care must be taken in prescribing it, particularly in patients with conduction disorders. In addition, the calcium antagonists can cause constipation, which could lead to straining during bowel movements. The associated Valsalva maneuver in these patients could be dangerous. Their chest pains are often treated with NTG but nitrates can worsen obstruction by decreasing LV volume. This is also the case for many of the standard therapies of CHF which can mistakenly be directed to treat congestive symptoms. *Digoxin, nitrates, and diuretics should be avoided because they can worsen outflow obstruction.* Digoxin increases contractility and nitrates and diuretics decrease ventricular volume. *Patients with obstructive hypertrophic cardiomyopathy should always be followed by a cardiologist* because they are so difficult to manage. While they are at increased risk of sudden death, the features that predict this are still uncertain. Therapies that have been attempted are septal surgery, mitral valve replacement, and sequential chamber pacing. Young patients with ASH often must be counseled not to participate in competitive athletics [20].

ISCHEMIA: KEY FEATURE 2— MYOCARDIAL ISCHEMIA
Treatment for Myocardial Ischemia
Unstable Angina
Unstable angina is conventionally treated with hospitalization and bed rest, nitrates, aspirin, and beta-blockade [21]. If the patient is already on these medications, then their doses can be increased and other abnormalities treated. It is imperative to continue treatment with beta-blockers because hemodynamic rebound or hyperactivity after these agents are stopped is an established phenomenon that can cause infarction or death. Since calcium antagonists can sometimes worsen angina and do not cause rebound, their withdrawal should be considered. Calcium antagonists can be added if new ST-segment ele-

vation is present in non-Q-wave areas, IV NTG can be used if systemic BP is elevated, and diuretics can be added to treat volume overload associated with CHF. If the pain and ECG changes cannot be controlled, cardiac catheterization to consider surgical intervention or percutaneous transluminal coronary angioplasty (PTCA) is indicated. In general, this can be delayed if the symptoms and signs can be controlled. Thrombosis appears to play some role in this process, which has led some investigators to try acetylsalicylic acid (ASA), dipyridamole, heparin, and thrombolytic agents, but only ASA and heparin are recommended for use. ASA is a *must*-use drug for ischemic pain [22]. One 5-grain ASA (300 mg) should be given immediately to all patients with unstable angina.

PRACTICAL CONSIDERATIONS. The risk of unstable angina is not as great as it once was because nearly all patients can be stabilized using bed rest, nitrates, aspirin, and beta-blockers. Some patients appear to have chronic unstable angina because of failure to comply with their medical regimen, exercise prescription, or substance use recommendations. All patients with angina should take their medications as prescribed, have nitrate-free periods so they do not develop tolerance, walk or perform another aerobic exercise for 30 minutes every day, avoid cigarette smoking, and follow an appropriate diet. A statin-type drug for lowering cholesterol is usually indicated because statin-type drugs affect the progression of atherosclerosis and decrease the number of cardiac events, including the need for CABG and hospitalization.

Variant Angina
Variant angina is best treated with nitrates and a calcium antagonist, nifedipine being the preferred agent. Although theoretically beta-blockers could exacerbate the spasm, they are frequently helpful, particularly when ventricular arrhythmias occur. This rare condition requires cardiac catheterization. While in half the patients, coronary spasm is all that is found, in the others atherosclerosis is that cause, and occasionally a tight proximal lesion is found that responds to PTCA.

Typical Angina Pectoris
Typical angina pectoris is treated medically in stepwise fashion with nitrates, beta-blockers, and calcium antagonists. Rarely occurring angina is often better treated by sublingual NTG as needed rather than by increasing regular doses.

PRACTICAL CONSIDERATIONS. Patients with angina should learn about the characteristics of angina, what causes and what exacerbates it, and when to seek treatment. They are often more concerned with the sharp stabbing pains, which are rarely due to ischemia, until instructed not to take NTG for them. Also pains that last all day are not of cardiac origin. Since angina is exacerbated by cold, overeating, and isometric exercise, these should be avoided. Progressive increases in exercise are to be recommended over sudden exertion, and a cooldown walk is often helpful in avoiding symptoms in the postexercise period. All patients with angina should take their medications as prescribed, have nitrate-free periods so that they do not develop tolerance, perform aerobic exercise (e.g., walking, biking, swimming, etc.) every day, avoid cigarette smoking, and follow an appropriate diet. A statin-type drug for lowering cholesterol is usually suggested. Antianginal medications can be dosed according to the timing of symptoms; night pain can be targeted with a dose of long-acting nitrates taken at bedtime, and NTG can be taken before sexual activity or exercise.

NITRATES. The placebo effect in anginal therapy has never been more apparent than with physician and patient acceptance of transdermal Band-Aid preparations of NTG [23]. These preparations won immediate acceptance as a clinically effective treatment for angina and chronic CHF. However, after their introduction, most studies found them to be ineffective in objectively increasing exercise capacity or in lessening objective signs of ischemia. Although tolerance may be a problem, most likely these preparations do not achieve high enough blood levels because of their limited surface area. Tolerance has always been a problem with evaluating long-acting nitrates. If given acutely, these preparations show an extended hemodynamic effect but their effect lessens if administered chronically. Hemodynamic effects (i.e., a drop in resting and exercise systolic BP) are most likely markers of a satisfactory response to nitrate therapy for angina or chronic CHF. Our recommendation for such therapy with long-acting nitrates is titration with isosorbide dinitrate (Isordil), 10 to 80 mg qid, or 0.5 to 1.5 inches of NTG paste three times a day under an occlusive cover until a hemodynamic response occurs (i.e., a drop of 10–20 mm Hg in resting systolic BP ½ hour after the usual dose). Isosorbide is also useful.

Nitrate action occurs in many areas: It causes coronary artery dilation (which could result in "steal" away from areas supplied by fixed lesions but is very important in treating spasm), venodilation with a decrease in LV filling pressure and diastolic volume, and a drop in systolic BP.

BETA-BLOCKERS.   Many different beta-blockers are now available. Their most important clinical features are beta-1 selectivity, lipophilicity, intrinsic sympathetic activity, and length of action. Beta-1 receptors are mainly in the heart and when blocked, result in decreased heart rate and contractility, thus decreasing myocardial oxygen demand. These receptors are also involved in anginal pain, explaining why the beta-blockers lessen this pain even if ST-segment depression is not reduced. Beta-2 receptors are largely in the lungs and peripheral vessels, and when they are blocked, bronchospasm and arterial constriction occur. Beta-1 selectivity in the beta-blockers is dose related, but when beta-2 effects are avoided, most of the side effects of beta-blockers are avoided. Lipophilicity leads to passage through the blood-brain barrier with resultant CNS side effects such as fatigue, nightmares, and sexual problems. Intrinsic sympathetic activity in a beta-blocker is to be avoided because it overcomes the ability of the beta-blockers to increase the fibrillatory threshold and to decrease premature ventricular contractions (PVCs).

Beta-blockers are the major drug for treating angina. They should always be used except:

- In patients with bronchospastic lung disease or with peripheral vascular disease, if their symptoms are exacerbated by beta-blockers.
- In patients with unstable diabetes, if the hypoglycemic symptoms can be masked by beta-blockade.
- In patients whose systolic dysfunction is worsened by beta-blockers, resulting in symptoms of CHF.
- In patients who develop symptomatic bradycardias.
- In patients who otherwise do not tolerate beta-blockade.

Propranolol (Inderal, 40 mg qid) is the prototypic beta-blocker that requires multiple daily doses. For the patients who require higher doses and have the side effects or require once-a-day dosing, atenolol (Tenormin, 50–100 mg/day) and metoprolol (Lopressor) are both beta-1 selective, have little lipophilicity or intrinsic sympathetic activity, and are relatively long-acting.

A computerized literature search was performed to consider the problem of sudden death from heart disease and the role of beta-blockers and other agents in preventing sudden death and to review perceived problems with beta-blocker therapy, such as effects on blood lipids, complications in diabetes, and adverse effects on heart failure and quality of life [24]. More than 400 original and review articles were evaluated, of which the most relevant were selected. Of all of the therapies currently available for the prevention of sudden cardiac death, none is more established or more effective than beta-blockers. The evidence that beta-blockers have a cardioprotective effect is compelling. They probably reduce the rate of atheroma formation; they reduced the risk for ventricular fibrillation in animal models of myocardial ischemia; they reduced cardiac mortality in primary prevention trials; and they reduced mortality, particularly from sudden death, in patients who had infarction. Withholding beta-blockers because of problems perceived to be associated with them is usually not warranted and may frequently prevent their use in those who will benefit the most. Clinicians should reappraise the evidence for the significant effect of beta-blockers on morbidity and mortality, and they should recognize the importance of initiating and maintaining beta-blocker therapy.

CALCIUM ANTAGONISTS.   This class of agents has a broad range of effects due to their action on calcium metabolism. In addition to a cardiac depressant action and a vasodilatory action on all blood vessels (i.e., they lower BP, decreasing afterload, and lessen coronary artery tone), they also are effective for exercise-induced bronchospasm. They are the agents of choice for ischemic syndromes due to coronary artery spasm, but also are effective in stable angina due to fixed lesions. They should be the third choice in treating angina (except for variant or vasospastic angina) except in patients with concurrent bronchospastic lung disease, in patients with insulin-dependent diabetes who are prone to hypoglycemic attacks, or and in patients with claudication exacerbated by beta-blockers. Calcium antagonists are currently overprescribed because of an enormous amount of advertising. This advertising has overemphasized the effects of beta-blockers and diuretics on lipids and played heavily on their hypothetical impact on stopping calcium from being deposited in atherosclerotic lesions. It is important to realize that the only antihypertensive agents to lessen the morbidity and mortality associated with high BP are beta-blockers and diuretics, and the only anti-ischemic agents known to lessen mortality are the beta-blockers (in patients in the first year after MI). In most randomized trials of patients with heart disease, calcium antagonists had a tendency toward worsening mortality. However, calcium antagonists have been incredibly successful in treating patients with the rare condition of vasospastic variant angina.

Verapamil has the greatest effect on atrioventricular (AV) conduction and can be effective in some patients with exercise-induced ventricular tachycardia. The myocardial depression it causes is a problem when treating patients with LV dysfunction. This has made analogues like felodipine and amlodipine popular because they do not have an effect on the conduction system nor do they depress the myocardium. Nifedipine has the greatest effect on coronary artery spasm and the least on conduction but has the most side effects (constipation and pedal edema). Diltiazem lies between nifedipine and verapamil in terms of its action and side effects. Approximately 10% of patients treated with nifedipine experience worsening of angina rather than an improvement and must be switched to another agent. Beta-blockers and calcium antagonists that affect the conduction system probably should not be used together in any patient with a history or ECG suggestive of conduction system disease. Recent concern with increased morbidity and mortality, particularly with high doses of calcium antagonists, makes them less attractive agents for treating high BP or angina, but they are still specific and clearly indicated for variant angina. Side effects include nausea; pedal edema, particularly for nifedipine; and constipation with verapamil.

Screening for Hyperlipidemia
The American College of Physicians published a controversial change in their clinical guidelines for screening for preventing coronary disease in adults [25]. The new guidelines are as follows:

1. Patients in whom screening for lipoprotein abnormalities is appropriate should have total cholesterol levels measured.
2. In patients who are screened for the primary prevention of heart disease, the total cholesterol level should be measured once.
3. Screening for total cholesterol levels is not recommended for young men (<35 years old) or women (<45

years old) unless the family history or physical examination suggests a familial lipoprotein disorder or at least two other risk factors for heart disease are present.

4. Screening for total cholesterol levels in the primary prevention of coronary heart disease is appropriate, but not mandatory, for men 35 to 65 years old and for women 45 to 65 years old.

5. Evidence is insufficient to recommend or discourage screening for the primary prevention of coronary heart disease in men and women 65 to 75 years old.

6. Screening is not recommended for men and women 75 years or older.

7. All patients with known coronary heart disease or those with vascular disease that places them at high risk for coronary heart disease should have lipid analysis, including but not limited to measurement of total cholesterol levels.

These guidelines conclude that screening with total cholesterol levels is most likely useful when done in populations at high short-term risk for dying of coronary heart disease such as middle-age men surviving MI with multiple cardiac risk factors. In these populations, cholesterol reduction appears to be both effective and cost-effective. In other populations, the benefits of reduction are much smaller or are uncertain. The AHA Task Force on Risk Reduction [26] and the National Cholesterol Education Program (NCEP) [27] objected to these guidelines and *recommended that all adults over 20 years old have serum cholesterol levels measured.*

Treatment of Hyperlipidemia

LIPID ABNORMALITIES AND CORONARY ARTERY DISEASE. An elevated level of low-density-lipoprotein (LDL) cholesterol is a common disorder that increases the risk of cardiovascular disease. Many patients can be managed with dietary fat restriction, particularly saturated fat. In patients requiring drugs, 3-hydroxy-3-xymethylglutaryl coenzyme A (HMG CoA) reductase inhibitors (statins) and bile acid–binding resins are the first- and second-line drugs; niacin is third, but often should be added in low dosage to a statin.

Two common mixed hyperlipidemias are polygenic hypercholesterolemia and obesity-induced hypertriglyceridemia. They are often associated with hypertension and low high-density-lipoprotein (HDL) levels and most probably an increased risk of coronary artery disease. Exercise and weight loss are the mainstays of management. When indicated, niacin, HMG CoA reductase inhibitors, and gemfibrozil are the main drugs.

Isolated hypertriglyceridemia is less common and its association with cardiovascular risk uncertain. Exercise and weight loss are the management strategies. If there is a history of pancreatitis, a positive family history of coronary disease, or very low HDL levels, then drug management can be indicated. Niacin and gemfibrozil are the first- and second-line drugs.

LIPID-LOWERING DRUGS.   Bile Acid–Binding Resins: Cholestyramine (Questran) and colestipol (Colestid).

Indications: Elevated LDL levels (with normal triglyceride levels).

Actions: Dose related; 15 to 30% decrease in LDL level. Maximum response is evident within 2 to 4 weeks. HDL levels may increase up to 5% and there may be a rise in triglycerides of 5 to 20%, which may or may not persist.

Mechanism: Bind to bile acids in the intestine, interrupting enterohepatic circulation and increasing fecal excretion of the acids. This increases the synthesis of bile acids from hepatic cholesterol stores. This in turn leads to an increase in the number of hepatic LDL receptors and an increase in the activity of HMG CoA reductase, both of which are compensatory changes to increase cholesterol stores in the liver to allow for increased bile acid synthesis. The increased extraction of LDL from the bloodstream via LDL receptors lowers LDL concentration in the plasma.

Contraindications: Severe diverticulosis with recent diverticulitis; troublesome hemorrhoids.

Side effects: Constipation, unpalatability, elevation in triglyceride levels; rarely elevation of liver function, or abdominal pain.

Drug interactions: Decreased absorption of certain other drugs, including thiazides, warfarin, digitalis, thyroxine, and beta-blockers.

Available from pharmacy:
   Cholestyramine (Questran)—box of 60 4-g packets or 378-g cans.
   Colestipol (Colestid)—box of 30 5-g packets or 500-g bottle.

Administration: Usually start with 1 packet or scoop twice daily. Must be mixed with fluids (usually juice) before ingestion. Increase over 1 to 2 weeks to desired dose. If constipation develops, add 1 teaspoon of psyllium seed (Metamucil) to mixture. Prescribe other drugs to be taken 1 hour before or 4 hours after the resin. Cholestyramine has an orange flavor; colestipol is gritty and must be mixed with applesauce or juice.

Dosage:
> Cholestyramine—maximum dose is 24 g/day up to three times a day.
>
> Colestipol—maximum dose is 30 g/day up to three times a day.

Bile acid–binding resins may be combined with nicotinic acid, lovastatin, gemfibrozil, or probucol. Simultaneous administration with nicotinic acid does not impair the absorption of nicotinic acid.

Nicotinic Acid (Niacin).
Indications: Elevated LDL, elevated triglycerides, or both [28].

Actions: 15 to 30% decrease in LDL, 20 to 50% decrease in triglycerides, 20 to 30% increase in HDL.

Mechanism: Inhibits very-low-density lipoprotein (VLDL) synthesis in the liver by unclear mechanism; inhibits the release of free fatty acids from adipose tissue and increases the activity of lipoprotein lipase.

Contraindications: Active liver disease, active peptic ulcer disease.

Side effects: Cutaneous flushing, pruritus, abdominal discomfort; nausea; vomiting; diarrhea; elevations in glucose, uric acid, liver enzymes; malaise; rarely, peptic ulceration, hyperpigmentation, acanthosis nigricans, postural hypotension, arrhythmia, maculopathy. Severe hepatotoxicity has been reported, more commonly with the time-release form of the medication. Niacin can cause diabetes to go out of control by interacting with oral hypoglycemic agents.

Drug interactions: Associated with an increased risk of myopathy when taken with lovastatin (the risk of myopathy is 0.15% with lovastatin, and this risk increases over 10 times when niacin is added to lovastatin).

Available from pharmacy (nicotinic acid, which is a B vitamin, is an over-the-counter medication): Crystalline nicotinic acid tablets: 50, 100, 250, and 500 mg; time-release nicotinic acid capsules and tablets not recommended because of association with hepatic failure.

Nicotinic acid (niacin) is not the same as nicotin-amide (niacinamide). Nicotinamide does not lower lipid levels.

Approach to use: Use crystalline nicotinic acid because the time-release form is associated with more GI complaints and liver toxicity. Start with a low dose three times a day, and gradually work up to at least 1.5 g/day. Less than 1.5 g/day usually does not produce a therapeutic response. Increase the dose as needed for lipid response. The usual dose is 1.5 to 3.0 g/day. The maximum dose is usually 6 g/day, although higher doses may occasionally be appropriate. An asymptomatic increase in liver transaminase levels as high as twice the upper limit of normal does not require discontinuation. If the patient develops side effects at a dose higher than 1.5 g/day, consider reducing the dose and adding another lipid-lowering medication rather than discontinuing niacin altogether.

Strategies to minimize flushing: (1) The patient should always take the dose after meals, (2) the dose should be increased gradually, and (3) the patient should take 80 to 325 mg of aspirin up to 30 minutes before taking nicotinic acid. Glucose, uric acid, and liver enzyme levels should be checked once the 1.5-g/day dose is reached, and then peri-odically (i.e., about three times a year) when a stable dose of nicotinic acid is reached. Niacin can be combined with other lipid-lowering drugs.

Instructions for Taking Nicotinic Acid (Niacin).   Nicotinic acid can be accelerated to higher doses more quickly, with larger increments at shorter intervals. Some may have to increase the dose more slowly. One should start with 50 to 100 mg tid, and increase the dose every week until the desired dose is reached. In most cases, one can increase to a total dose of 1,500 mg/day before lipids, glucose, uric acid, and liver enzyme levels are rechecked. The patient should begin with the 100-mg tablets of unmodified nico-tinic acid, and then take 100 mg tid after meals for 1 week, 200 mg tid after meals for 1 week, 300 mg tid after meals for 1 week, 400 mg tid after meals for 1 week, and then switch to 500-mg tablets of nicotinic acid and take 500 mg tid after meals.

HMG CoA Reductase Inhibitors ("Statins").

Indications: Elevated LDL; may be useful when triglyc-eride levels are mildly elevated in addition.

Actions: Dose related; 20 to 40% decrease in LDL, 5 to 10% rise in HDL, and 10 to 20% decrease in triglycerides.

The maximum lowering of LDL cholesterol will be seen 4 weeks after starting therapy.

Mechanism: Inhibit HMG CoA reductase, the rate-limiting enzyme in cholesterol synthesis. Reduced production of cholesterol within hepatocytes stimulates the synthesis of new LDL receptors. Increased numbers of LDL receptors lead to enhanced clearance of VLDL remnants (the precursor particles to LDL) and LDL from the bloodstream.

Contraindications: Active liver disease, pregnancy and lactation, unexplained persistent elevations in serum transaminases.

Side effects: 2% incidence of marked persistent increases of transaminases (more than three times the upper limit of normal), which resolves on discontinuation. For lovastatin there is a 0.5% incidence of myopathy associated with a rise in creatine kinase; incidence is uncertain for other statins. The rise in creatine kinase and symptoms resolves promptly on discontinuation of the drug. The myopathy risk is about 30% when taking cyclosporine. Myopathy can lead to rhabdomyolysis and acute renal failure. There has been a 5% incidence of myopathy in patients taking lovastatin with gemfibrozil, and a 2% incidence in those taking lovastatin with nicotinic acid. In patients taking none of these drugs, the incidence of myopathy is 0.15%. Rhabdomyolysis has also occurred in patients taking lovastatin concomitant with erythromycin. Fluvastatin has a different structure from the other statins and may have less skeletal muscle complications. Other complications include rash, GI symptoms, headache, and insomnia.

Drug interactions: There is increased myopathy prevalence with cyclosporine, nicotinic acid, and gemfibrozil. Adding lovastatin to warfarin can increase the prothrombin time or bleeding or both.

Available from pharmacy: Lovastatin comes in 10-, 20-, and 40-mg tablets; pravastatin comes as 10- and 20-mg tablets; simvastatin comes as 5-, 10-, 20-, and 40-mg tablets; fluvastatin comes in 20- and 40-mg capsules.

Approach to use:

Lovastatin: The usual starting dose is 1 tablet (20 mg) with dinner. For people with very elevated cholesterol levels (i.e., >300 mg/dl), the starting dose may be 40 mg in a single or divided dose. The maximum dose is 80 mg/day in a single or divided dose. Twice-daily dosing may be slightly more effective.

Pravastatin: The usual dose is 10 mg/day; the maximum recommended is 40 mg/day (but it may be no more potent than lovastatin and doses up to 80 mg have been used).

Simvastatin: The usual dose is 10 mg/day; the maximum is 40 mg/day.

Fluvastatin: The usual dose 20 mg/day given at bedtime; the maximum dose is 40 mg/day given either qd or as 20 mg bid.

Liver transaminase levels should be tested initially, every 3 months during the first year, and periodically thereafter. If transaminase levels rise to three times the normal range, the medication should be discontinued.

In patients taking *cyclosporine, gemfibrozil,* or high doses of *nicotinic acid,* the statins should be avoided. If patients have unexplained muscle pain or weakness, creatine kinase should be measured to confirm the diagnosis of myopathy. Therapy should be withheld in the presence of any acute medical or surgical condition that could predispose to rhabdomyolysis or renal failure. A low dose of niacin combined with a statin results in an excellent treatment profile.

Statins may be used in combination with bile acid–binding resins, leading to as much as a 50% reduction in LDL cholesterol levels. The combination of lovastatin with gemfibrozil should be avoided.

Gemfibrozil (Lopid).

Indications: Elevated triglycerides; disorders in which both LDL and triglycerides are elevated; useful as adjunctive therapy for elevated LDL.

Actions: Dose related; 40 to 50% decrease in triglycerides, 20% rise in HDL. Effect on LDL is variable. In patients with isolated hypertriglyceridemia, LDL may increase with therapy. In patients with elevated LDL with or without elevated triglycerides, LDL may decrease by 10%.

Mechanism: Increases the activity of lipoprotein lipase; may inhibit hepatic secretion of VLDL.

Contraindications: Hepatic or severe renal dysfunction; gallbladder disease.

Side effects: Mild GI discomfort (5%), eosinophilia, skin rash, musculoskeletal pain, blurred vision, mild anemia, leukopenia, mild increase in serum glucose, mild elevation in liver enzymes, gallstones.

Drug interactions: Potentiates the effect of warfarin; 5% incidence of myopathy when taken with lovastatin.

Available from pharmacy: 300-mg capsules, 600-mg tablets.

Approach to use: Monitor CBC and liver enzymes periodically. If an elevation in LDL results from treatment of isolated hypertriglyceridemia, consider the addition of bile acid–binding resin or nicotinic acid, or substitution with nicotinic acid, 300 to 600 mg bid before meals.

Combining with other lipid-lowering drugs: May be used in combination with bile acid–binding resins and nitocinic acid. Combination with lovastatin should be avoided.

Probucol (Lorelco).

Indications: Elevated LDL.

Actions: 10 to 15% decrease in LDL, 20 to 30% decrease in HDL.

Mechanism: Probucol increases the catabolism of LDL. Independent of its effect on lipoproteins, probucol inhibits the oxidation of LDL, possibly decreasing the uptake of LDL by endothelial cells. Probucol increases levels of cholesterol ester transfer protein (CETP), increasing the transfer of cholesterol from HDL to other lipoproteins and lowering HDL levels.

Contraindications: Prolonged QT interval (>15% above the upper limit of normal for the resting heart rate); recent MI, serious ventricular arrhythmias, or syncope.

Side effects: Diarrhea, flatulence, abdominal discomfort (10%), QT-interval prolongation; serious arrhythmias have been seen in association with a prolonged QT interval. HDL lowering by probucol has not been determined to be detrimental.

Drug interactions: The addition of a drug that prolongs the QT interval (i.e., tricyclics, quinidine, and phenothiazine) may increase the risk of serious arrhythmia.

Available from pharmacy: 250-mg and 500-mg tablets.

Approach to use: An ECG should be done prior to starting therapy and repeated periodically. If an abnormally long QT interval is observed, therapy should be discontinued or not started. Only use it for patients who have not responded to other therapy.

Dosage: The usual and maximum dose is 500 mg bid.

THE NCEP ADULT TREATMENT PANEL. The Expert Panel on Detection, Evaluation, and Treatment of High Blood Cholesterol in Adults (Adult Treatment Panel II or ATP II) published updated recommendations for cholesterol management from the NCEP [27]. The NCEP is an independent program under the auspices of the NIH that will continue to produce updates.

Rationale. Data (1988–1991) from NHANES III [29] showed that about 31% of the adult U.S. population had total cholesterol levels between 200 and 239 mg/dl, which is considered borderline high. In another 20%, total cholesterol was high, more than 240 mg/dl. High cholesterol was especially evident in men over 35 and in both sexes after age 55. The NCEP emphasized that high-risk postmenopausal women and high-risk elderly patients who are otherwise in good health are candidates for therapy.

The NHANES data also estimate the percentage of Americans with coronary heart disease to be above 7% overall, with the incidence doubling in both sexes after age 55. The NCEP identified these patients as being at the highest risk of further coronary heart disease events and recommended they be treated more aggressively.

Diet and increased exercise are still the mainstays of therapy, and drug therapy is reserved for patients at high risk for coronary heart disease. However, the NHANES estimate of American adults who will need drug therapy for hypercholesterolemia ranges from 5 to 14%, depending on assumptions of efficacy of dietary therapy in lowering LDL cholesterol, ranging from 5 to 15%. This amounts to a total of 12.7 million adults, 4 million of whom have coronary heart disease.

Coronary Heart Disease and Risk Status. The ATP II stressed the presence of coronary heart disease as a guide to type and intensity of cholesterol-lowering therapy, not just as an additional risk factor, as it was in the previous report. Patients with existing coronary heart disease have a substantial risk of new events, and it appears that many patients are not getting the aggressive cholesterol-lowering therapy that is warranted.

Risk Factors and Markers. A distinction is recommended between risk factors and risk markers. The four risk factors specified by the Centers for Disease Control (CDC) and the AHA are hypercholesterolemia, hypertension, cigarette smoking, and physical inactivity [30]. These four factors can be changed by medications or behavior modification and have passed the criteria to be causal rather than just associations. Markers such as age, gender, diabetes, family history, and obesity are associated with atherosclerosis but even when they can be modified, there are no epidemiologic data that they are causal or that modification affects risk. Besides stressing high LDL cholesterol as a risk factor for coronary heart disease, the ATP II updated other risk markers: age over 45 years for men (replaces "male sex" as a risk factor), age over 55 years or after premature menopause without estrogen replacement therapy for women, and family history of premature coronary heart disease (definite MI or sudden death before age 55 in a first-degree male relative, or before age 65 in a first-degree female relative) [31].

Four risk factors and markers continued from the previous report: current cigarette smoking, hypertension (>140/90 mm Hg or on treatment), low HDL cholesterol (<35 mg/dl), and diabetes mellitus. Obesity is no longer an independent risk factor since it operates through other risk factors. This report was presented before physical inactivity was elevated to the status of the fourth risk factor.

Another update is that high HDL cholesterol (>60 mg/dl) is classified as a *negative* risk marker—one that *decreases* the risk of coronary heart disease. It can nullify one risk factor (i.e., subtract one from total for guidelines below).

Future guidelines might better target risk by use of the Framingham risk equation that is utilized by the AHA risk tables (see Table D-1).

Guidelines for Lipoprotein Analysis Based on Total Cholesterol. Total serum cholesterol and HDL cholesterol should be measured in all adults older than 20 years. Lipoprotein analysis is recommended in all patients with evidence of coronary heart disease (Table 5-2).

Treatment Decisions. The NCEP bases treatment decisions in hypercholesterolemia on LDL cholesterol level. If not provided as a specific measurement, LDL cholesterol is calculated by using the following equation:

$$\text{LDL cholesterol (mg/dl)} = \text{total cholesterol} - \left(\frac{\text{triglycerides}}{5} + \text{HDL cholesterol} \right)$$

The LDL cholesterol goal for patients with coronary heart disease or other atherosclerotic diseases is now lower than in previous recommendations (Table 5-3).

Diet and exercise are the first lines of therapy.

Dietary Treatment. The AHA Step I diet resembles NCEP-recommended eating patterns for the general public: saturated fat, 8 to 10% of total calories; total fat, less than 30% of calories; and cholesterol, less than 300 mg/day. The Step II diet, recommended when the Step I diet is inadequate

Table 5-2.   Recommended Lipoprotein Analysis

Classification	Cholesterol Level	Action
Desirable	<200 mg/dl	Retest within 5 yr
Borderline high	200–239 mg/dl	Lipoprotein analysis if patient has coronary heart disease, low HDL,* or >2 other risk factors
High	≥240 mg/dl	Lipoprotein analysis

*An HDL cholesterol level < 35 mg/dl is defined as low.

Table 5-3.   LDL Cholesterol Goals

	Classification	LDL Cholesterol
Patients *without* CHD or other atherosclerotic disease	Desirable	<130 mg/dl
	Borderline high risk	130–159 mg/dl
	High risk	≥ 160 mg/dl
Patients *with* CHD or other atherosclerotic disease	Desirable	<100 mg/dl

CHD = coronary heart disease.

and for patients with coronary heart disease or other atherosclerotic diseases, differs from Step I by reducing saturated fatty acids to less than 7% of calories and cholesterol to less than 200 mg/day.

The treatment decision for initiation of dietary therapy is based on LDL cholesterol levels: above 100 mg/dl for patients with definite coronary heart disease or other atherosclerotic diseases; above 130 mg/dl for patients with no coronary disease but more than two risk factors; and above 160 mg/dl for patients with no coronary disease and less than two risk factors.

NCEP Guidelines for Drug Therapy.   Guidelines for drug therapy feature a new, more aggressive approach to patients with coronary heart disease or other atherosclerotic disease (Table 5-4).

Drug therapy should be initiated only after an adequate trial of diet: 6 to 12 weeks of Step II diet in the coronary heart disease patient, a minimum of 6 months of diet (proceeding to Step II if Step I is inadequate) in others. Dietary therapy should be continued in conjunction with cholesterol-lowering drugs. Drug therapy should be delayed in young adult men (<35 years old) and premenopausal women without other risk factors whose LDL cholesterol levels are in the range of 190 to 220 mg/dl.

Table 5-4. NCEP Guidelines for Drug Therapy

Patients with	LDL Cholesterol Levels for Initiation of Drug	Goal
Definite CHD or other atherosclerotic disease	>130 mg/dl	<100 mg/dl
No CHD but >2 risk factors	>160 mg/dl	<130 mg/dl
No CHD and <2 risk factors	>190 mg/dl	<160 mg/dl

CHD = coronary heart disease.

NCEP Drug Classification. The NCEP used efficacy and safety to classify current agents as "major drugs" and others. Major drugs include bile acid sequestrants, nicotinic acid, and HMG CoA reductase inhibitors (statins). Less effective are fibric acid derivatives and probucol. Estrogen replacement may be considered for postmenopausal women. Niacin (nicotinic acid) is an effective drug (lowering LDL and raising HDL) but patient compliance is a problem because of the skin sensations and headaches. It must be titrated to tolerance doses. Colestipol and cholestyramine are also effective and attractive because they are not absorbed, but they are too difficult for patients to take. The statins are very effective and well tolerated and their price has dropped to about $450/yr. Liver function must be checked quarterly in the first year after starting them and then yearly.

Statin Therapy. Since publication of the Scandinavian Simvastatin Survival Study (4S) and the numerous studies demonstrating regression or cessation of progression of angiographic coronary atherosclerosis, a statin drug is a *must* therapy for the patient with an ischemic syndrome and a cholesterol level above 200 mg/dl. The 4S study randomized 4,444 patients with angina pectoris or previous MI and elevated serum cholesterol on a lipid-lowering diet to double-blind treatment with simvastatin or placebo [32]. Over the 5.4-year median follow-up period, simvastatin produced mean changes in total cholesterol, LDL cholesterol, and HDL cholesterol of −25%, −35%, and +8%, respectively, with few adverse effects. Two hundred fifty-six patients (12%) in the placebo group died, compared with 182 (8%) in the simvastatin group. The relative risk of death in the simvastatin group was 0.70. The 5-year probabilities of survival in the placebo and simvastatin groups were 88% and 91%, respectively. There were 189 coronary deaths in the placebo group and 111 in the simvastatin group (relative risk, 0.58), while noncardio-vascular causes accounted for 49 and 46 deaths, respectively. Six hundred twenty-two patients (28%) in the placebo group and 431 (19%) in the simvastatin group had one or more major coronary events. The relative risk was 0.66, and the respective probabilities of escaping such events were 70% and 80%. This risk was also significantly reduced in subgroups consisting of women and patients of both sexes aged 60 or more. Other benefits of treatment included a 37% reduction in the risk of undergoing myocardial revascularization procedures. This study showed that long-term treatment with simvastatin is safe and improves survival in coronary heart disease patients.

Four drugs that act as specific inhibitors of HMG CoA reductase—lovastatin, pravastatin, simvastatin, and fluvastatin—have been approved by the FDA. The comparative hypocholesterolemic effects of these four drugs based on direct comparative studies that randomized more than 25 patients per treatment group have been analyzed [33]. All studies were conducted in patients with primary hypercholesterolemia and the major end point of efficacy was reduction in the plasma concentrations of LDL cholesterol. Eight comparative trials evaluated the efficacy and safety of lovastatin, simvastatin, or pravastatin, and one trial compared lovastatin and fluvastatin. These trials confirmed the log-linear dose-response curves for all four of these drugs but indicated that on a milligram-for-milligram basis, lovastatin and pravastatin are approximately equipotent, whereas simvastatin is at least twice as effective per milligram of drug administered as lovastatin and pravastatin. Lovastatin at doses of 20 and 40 mg/day was of similar efficacy to fluvastatin at doses of 40 and 80 mg/day, suggesting that on a milligram-for-milligram basis, fluvastatin is half as potent as lovastatin. The side effect profiles of all four drugs appeared similar, and earlier reports that suggested a higher incidence of sleep disorders in patients treated with the more lipophilic drugs, lovastatin and simvastatin, as compared with pravastatin, are not supported.

Cholesterol Lowering Versus Revascularization. Cholesterol lowering decreases the dimensions of atherosclerotic plaques in some patients with coronary artery disease. Because of this observation, there is growing discussion about whether or not cholesterol lowering might be used in place of revascularization (i.e., PTCA and CABG). The available data suggest that cholesterol lowering in place of revascularization may be appropriate for patients with chronic stable angina, for patients who are asymptomatic but have provocable ischemia after MI, and for patients at moderate risk for cardiac events as judged by exercise test or clinical variables [34].

Management of the Patient after Myocardial Infarction

Myocardial Infarction Classification

"Transmural" (Q-wave) MIs are characterized by two contiguous Q waves 40 msec in duration and 25% in amplitude of the following R wave, but are not always transmural at autopsy. "Subendocardial" (non-Q-wave, non-transmural) MIs do not have new Q waves, but changes in ST or T waves only; they still can be transmural at autopsy. The location of a transmural MI is determined by Q waves but the ST or T-wave changes with a non-Q-wave MI do not localize. The acute MI course is complicated by prior infarcts that occurred, but usually anterior (transmural) Q-wave infarcts involve more damage and have a higher complication rate; they are more likely to decrease the ejection fraction and result in shock or CHF. Anterior infarcts usually are associated with tachycardia, and inferior infarcts with bradycardia and heart block. Blocks are usually temporary with inferior MIs and best treated with atropine. Less than half of patients with anterior MIs have multivessel disease, and more than half with inferior MIs have multivessel disease. Non-Q-wave infarcts are usually less complicated unless following prior MIs. Patients should be screened after an uncompleted MI with an exercise test. Calcium antagonist therapy is not preferred over beta-blockers in this or any other subgroup of post-MI patients. Patients with complicated MIs are those with cardiogenic shock, serious arrhythmias (including atrial fibrillation and sinus tachycardia), CHF, cerebrovascular accident, continued ischemia, other illnesses, pericarditis, older age, and prior MI. They should be discharged within 2 weeks. Patients with uncomplicated MIs do not have these other conditions. They should be discharged within 2 weeks, and early ambulation is appropriate.

Treatable causes of hypotension include hypovolemia, right ventricular MI, and acute rupture of the ventricular septum, papillary muscle (mitral regurgitation), and LV free wall. Hypovolemia can be diagnosed by a fluid challenge or Swan-Ganz catheterization. A new murmur and recurrent chest pain suggest a ventricular septal defect or mitral regurgitation. Catheterization demonstrating an oxygen step-up in the right ventricle is diagnostic of ventricular septal defect and a large "V" wave for mitral regurgitation. Myocardial rupture can present with cardiac tamponade. Right ventricular infarctions are a rarity that can complicate an inferior-posterior MI. They show signs of right-sided failure but no rales. When hypotension occurs in this situation, usually fluids can be helpful rather than be avoided. The absence of both an elevated jugular venous pressure and Kussmaul's sign in patients with inferior MI makes the presence of a hemodynamically significant right ventricular MI unlikely. Myocardial rupture accounts for 10% of acute MI deaths and requires early detection and often surgical intervention to alter its course.

Coronary angiography is indicated in patients with persistent ischemia, recurrent damage, or CHF that is difficult to control or explain. However, limited data suggest that prompt (within 6 hours of chest pain onset) catheterization with PTCA may be superior to thrombolysis.

Long-Term Management
All patients who have recovered from an MI should be urged to alter their risk factors. Cigarette smokers should be encouraged to quit (nicotine patches are helpful if accompanied by behavioral modification classes), dietary counseling should be provided, BP should be controlled, and regular walking exercise recommended. *Must-use* medications include an ASA tablet and a beta-blocker in general, and an ACE inhibitor to limit infarction expansion if a large anterior infarction occurred. If available, a formal cardiac rehabilitation program can be helpful. Meta-analysis has demonstrated a 25% mortality reduction in patients in these programs [35].

The management of the post-MI patient depends on the risk stratification of the patient after the infarction. Previous or complicating illnesses including MIs, the type and location of the MI, and prior symptoms must be considered. Patients with angina prior to an MI may do better because they have had time to develop collateral vessels while a prior history of CHF is always ominous. Next, the severity of the MI must be taken into account, particularly in regard to markers of acute MI size including CHF, cardiogenic shock, large amounts of creatine phosphokinase released, chest x-ray signs of CHF, and ECG changes. Whether the patient received thrombolysis and the timing of its administration (within 4 hours of the onset of chest pain is optimal) must also be considered. Lastly, the patient's status after MI must be added into the risk estimation. The risk is higher in the patient who still has ischemic chest pain, is older than 65, or has CHF or serious arrhythmias.

Patients without any of these complicating features can be advised to return to full activities quickly. They should be counseled to start a progressive walking program, stop cigarette smoking, and follow a low-fat diet. Salt restriction is only indicated for patients with high BP or CHF. A standard exercise ECG test can be done at the time of discharge, any time to evaluate symptoms, or when the patient would like to return to full activities. Patients who cannot perform an exercise test have a high mortality. Markers of LV dysfunction such as a systolic BP rise of less than 20 mm Hg and a poor exercise capacity are more predictive of increased risk in patients after a Q-wave MI while exercise-induced ST-segment depression is predictive in those with a non-Q-wave MI. Echocardiography may be helpful in patients with new systolic murmurs or to quantify myocardial damage. Stroke complicates 1 to 2% of MIs and is slightly more frequent in patients receiving thrombolysis.

Little benefit for immediate catheterization of the acute MI patient has been demonstrated, but in selected patients, primary angioplasty can be superior to thrombolysis. Post-MI patients frequently have enough LV damage to put them in the group that has improved survival with CABG compared to medical management (i.e., ejection fraction < 50% and three-vessel or left main coronary disease). Such patients should be considered for CABG if testing results or symptoms suggest it. The timing for surgery depends on the amount of damage and the acuteness of symptoms. In general, it is good to wait several months after the MI to perform surgery.

After their MI, patients begin to be concerned and even frightened by noncardiac chest pains or sensations that they never noticed before their MI. Counseling is necessary to ensure that they do not become cardiac cripples. An exercise test can be very reassuring to both the health care provider and the patient. Regarding chest pain, the chest pain of pericarditis that can accompany or appear 2 weeks after an MI must be distinguished from angina. Pericarditis pain is usually sharp, positional, related to respiration or swallowing, and not worsened by exercise. The pain of pericarditis responds to ibuprofen.

Must-use drug therapy includes ASA, beta-blocker, lipid-lowering drug, and for those with a large anterior MI, an ACE inhibitor and warfarin. Beta-blockers without intrinsic sympathetic activity increase long-term survival and lessen the reinfarction rate. This seems to be mediated by raising the fibrillatory threshold. They should be given for at least 2 years, particularly in patients with complicated MIs. Subgroup analysis has shown beta-blockers to be effective in non-Q-wave MI patients as well as those with severe enough damage to cause CHF. The long-term prognosis also is improved by platelet-active agents, smoking cessation, lipid-lowering drugs, and exercise programs, but not by antiarrhythmics. When mural thrombus is visualized in patients who require echocardiography (those with a large MI or CHF), anticoagulation is indicated. Psychological and vocational counseling may be helpful for some patients and while a formal exercise program can be beneficial, a symptom-limited walking or indoor ergometer program can be more convenient. High-risk patients may require monitoring during exercise. Treatment of ventricular arrhythmias after MI has become controversial because additional drugs can cause arrhythmias. Beta-blockers are the preferred treatment for arrhythmias because they also raise the fibrillatory threshold and are known to improve survival.

Anticoagulation
While anticoagulation is not indicated for all patients with LV damage or MI, it is indicated in subgroups of patients after MI who have mural thrombi or an anterior wall MI, mechanical valve prosthesis, atrial fibrillation, or coronary artery stents (see Table B-1). The management of mural thrombus complicating acute anterior MI remains controversial in part because of the small number of patients in the studies on this topic. A meta-analysis of published studies addressed three questions [36]: (1) What is the embolic risk for mural thrombi after myocardial infarction? (2) What is the impact of systemic anticoagulation in reducing the embolic risk of mural thrombi? (3) What is the impact of systemic anticoagulation, thrombolytic therapy, and antiplatelet therapy in preventing mural thrombus formation? The odds ratio for increased risk of emboli in the presence of echocardiographically demonstrated mural thrombus (11 studies, 856 patients) was 5, and the event rate difference was less than 0.1%. The odds ratio of anticoagulation versus no anticoagula-

tion in preventing embolization (seven studies, 270 patients) was 0.14, with an event rate difference of -0.3. The odds ratio of anticoagulation versus control in preventing mural thrombus formation (four studies, 307 patients) was 0.32, and the event rate difference was -0.2. The odds ratio for thrombolytic therapy in preventing mural thrombus (six studies, 390 patients) was 0.48, with an event rate difference of -0.16, whereas for antiplatelet agents (two studies, 112 patients) the odds ratio was 1.4, with an event rate difference of 0.16. This analysis supported the hypotheses that (1) mural thrombus after MI poses a significantly increased risk of embolization, (2) the risk of embolization is reduced by systemic anticoagulation, and (3) anticoagulation can prevent mural thrombus formation. Thrombolytic therapy may prevent mural thrombus formation, but evidence for a similar benefit of antiplatelet therapy is lacking.

INTERNATIONAL NORMALIZED RATIO. An understanding of the INR, which was developed to standardize reporting of the prothrombin time (PT) and provide consistent regulation of anticoagulation, is important [37]. The recommended therapeutic range for the INR (which is calculated from the patient's PT, a mean control PT, and the international sensitivity index) for oral anticoagulant treatment of most conditions is 2.0 to 3.0. In patients with mechanical cardiac valves, the INR should be at least 2.5 to 3.5. Patients with mechanical cardiac valves who are receiving anticoagulant therapy and are scheduled for noncardiac operations must have a risk-to-benefit assessment of the need for continuous anticoagulation performed preoperatively. Many of these patients can safely discontinue warfarin therapy for several days as outpatients before the surgical procedure. Preoperative heparin therapy and warfarin withdrawal in the hospital are recommended only for patients with cardiac valves at high risk for systemic embolization (with a mitral valve prosthesis, cardiomyopathy, or previous thromboembolism). The optimal frequency of INR monitoring is unknown. Patients in most of the reported trials were followed about every 3 to 4 weeks. A reasonable recommendation is to determine the INR every month on an average, but one should wait up to 2 months to recheck the INR in stable patients.

INTERACTIONS WITH ASPIRIN. Since aspirin is indicated to lessen arterial thrombogenesis (secondary to plaque rupture) and to keep grafts patent, it is often indicated in patients who should also be on warfarin. This combination must be used carefully and usually requires the INR to be slightly lower than usually indicated. Also, the condition with the greatest risk for morbidity and mortality should be targeted for therapy (with warfarin or aspirin).

INTERACTIONS WITH FOODS AND DRUGS.   To evaluate the quality of studies about drugs and food interactions with warfarin and their clinical relevance, a MEDLINE literature review was performed [38]. Of 793 retrieved citations, 120 contained original reports on 186 interactions. Of 86 different drugs and foods appraised, 43 had level 1 evidence. Of these, 26 drugs and foods did interact with warfarin. Warfarin's anticoagulant effect was potentiated by 6 antibiotics (co-trimoxazole, erythromycin, fluconazole, isoniazid, metronidazole, and miconazole); 5 cardiac drugs (amiodarone, clofibrate, propafenone, propranolol, and sulfinpyrazone); phenylbutazone; piroxicam; alcohol (only with concomitant liver disease); cimetidine; and omeprazole. Three patients had a hemorrhage at the time of a potentiating interaction (caused by alcohol, isoniazid, and phenylbutazone). Warfarin's anticoagulant effect was inhibited by 3 antibiotics (griseofulvin, rifampin, and nafcillin); 3 drugs active on the CNS (barbiturates, carbamazepine, and chlordiazepoxide); cholestyramine; sucralfate; foods high in vitamin K (see Appendix A); and large amounts of avocado. Many drugs and foods interact with warfarin, including antibiotics, drugs affecting the CNS, and cardiac medications. Many of these drug interactions increase warfarin's anticoagulant effect.

BLEEDING COMPLICATIONS.   A review of (1) the clinical epidemiology of bleeding during anticoagulant therapy with heparin or warfarin, (2) data useful in estimating the risk for bleeding in individual patients, and (3) the efficacy of methods for its prevention was performed [39]. Relevant literature was identified by a computerized search of the MEDLINE database and by review of the bibliographies of original and review articles. Studies were classified according to their design. Estimates of the risk for bleeding during anticoagulant therapy, compared with the risk without therapy, were obtained from randomized trials. Estimates of the frequency of bleeding during the course of anticoagulant therapy and information about risk factors for bleeding were obtained primarily from longitudinal studies of inception cohorts of patients followed from the start of therapy. The average daily frequencies of fatal, major, and major or minor bleeding during heparin therapy were 0.05, 0.8, and 2.0%, respectively; these frequencies are approximately twice those expected without heparin therapy. The average annual frequencies of fatal, major, and major or minor bleeding during warfarin therapy were 0.6, 3.0, and 9.6%, respectively; these frequencies are approximately five times those expected without warfarin therapy. The risk for anticoagulant-related bleeding is highest at the start of therapy. The risk for major bleeding during the first month of warfarin therapy is approximately 10 times the risk after the first year of therapy. An individual patient's risk for major anticoagulant-related bleeding can be estimated on the basis of specific risk factors such as the intensity of the anticoagulant effect achieved and the presence of serious comorbid diseases, especially cerebrovascular, kidney, heart, and liver disease; older age and concurrent medicines may also be independent risk factors. Major bleeding most often affects the GI tract, soft tissues, and urinary tract. Diagnostic evaluation of GI bleeding and gross hematuria leads to identification of previously unknown lesions in approximately one-third of patients, even when the PT is elevated. Intracranial bleeding is rare, but is frequently fatal. The frequency of bleeding during warfarin therapy is reduced by less-intense therapy achieving a PT with an INR of 2.0 to 3.0, which is efficacious for most indications. Anticoagulant-related bleeding is common and often serious. The risk for bleeding can be estimated in an individual patient, giving the primary physician a quantitative basis for weighing the risks and benefits of therapy and for optimizing patient management. The frequency of anticoagulant-related bleeding is reduced by less-intense warfarin therapy.

Management of the Patient after Intervention for Ischemic Heart Disease

Coronary Artery Bypass Surgery

Patients who have undergone CABG should be counseled to modify the risk factors for coronary atherosclerosis and to return to full functionality including exercise capacity. The latter can usually be accomplished by urging the patient to walk at least ½ hour daily with gradual increasing of the speed. The patient's subsequent treatment should take into consideration the cardiac anatomy established prior to the surgery (i.e., severity of the coronary disease and completeness of revascularization and LV function), whether an MI was sustained perioperatively

(8% of patients will sustain an MI during CABG), the degree of CNS impairment (<1% of patients sustain a cerebrovascular accident but up to 12% may have some degree of temporary memory or cognitive impairment postoperatively), and whether postoperative transient depression occurs. The relatively common symptoms of pericarditis and chest wall tenderness may mimic angina; pleural effusions and pericardial effusions may mimic CHF. Preoperative and postoperative ECGs should be compared, looking for new Q waves or ST-segment changes. Chest x-ray films should be compared if the patient complains of shortness of breath or dullness is percussed at the lung bases. If the patient has not previously had a problem with depression, the postoperative depression is best dealt with by explaining to the patient that it sometimes occurs and is self-limited. A treadmill test is often helpful to reassure a patient regarding exercise and to evaluate the patient for residual ischemia or a failed bypass. Patients should be urged to begin walking 30 minutes every day within 2 weeks of surgery. It is unusual for LV function to improve postoperatively from the preoperative level (except in the case when hibernating myocardium was present) and so diuretics and ACE inhibitors should be continued in patients with LV dysfunction. Low-dose ASA (81 mg) is effective in improving and sustaining venous and left internal mammary artery graft patency, so ASA is a *must-use* drug in these patients.

Percutaneous Transluminal Coronary Angioplasty
After PTCA, patient counseling should focus on modification of the risk factors for coronary atherosclerosis and return to full functionality. The latter can usually be accomplished by urging the patient to walk at least ½ hour daily with gradual increasing of the speed. The patient's subsequent treatment should take into consideration the cardiac anatomy established prior to the PTCA (i.e., severity of the coronary disease and completeness of revascularization and LV function). Reocclusion usually occurs within the first 6 months in 40% of patients, some of whom will be considered for a repeat PTCA. Very often patients remain on their preprocedure antianginal medications because of the fear of reocclusion. They should be taking ASA every day.

Stents
When stents are placed instead of relying on coronary dilation, the same concerns are raised but in addition antico-

agulation is indicated. Also, stent placement usually requires a larger transcutaneous catheter entry site with more arterial damage, and so patients are more likely to have local hematomas and AV fistulas. The latter can be recognized by a bruit and can be associated with high-output CHF and exacerbation of angina. In patients who recently underwent placement of a coronary stent [40, 41], the current recommendation is to use warfarin (INR 3.0–3.5), ASA (325 mg), and dipyridamole (75 mg tid) for the first 2 months, and then ASA alone thereafter.

Treatment/Recognition of Pulmonary Embolus: A Diagnostic Confounder

Because a pulmonary embolism can confound the diagnosis of either myocardial damage or ischemia, it is presented here.

The most common site and source of largest emboli are the calf veins of the legs (90% of emboli, up to 100 cm^3 in volume). Causes include stasis, damage to venous walls, and hypercoagulability. Stasis results from bed rest, pregnancy, and CHF. Damage to veins occurs from trauma and inflammation. Hypercoagulability is due to cancer, genetic defects, and thrombotic thrombocytopenic purpura. Emboli can originate from the right side of the heart or the pelvis but this is less common. When a clot breaks loose, it passes into the lungs, causing pulmonary artery pressure to increase. Pulmonary infarction, acute cor pulmonale, or acute dyspnea with pleuritic pain can occur. Pulmonary embolisms are often recurrent and so a history of prior events increases concern.

The symptoms and signs include elevated temperature, tachycardia, hyperventilation, pleuritic pain, cough, hemoptysis, increased P_2, and right ventricular parasternal lift.

The ECG may show sinus tachycardia, transient right bundle-branch block, atrial arrhythmias, right ventricular hypertrophy with strain, right axis deviation, or P-pulmonale (tall, peaked P waves in leads II and aVF), but the ECG often is normal. The chest x-ray film may at first appear normal or show decreased vascularity; by 18 hours, an infiltrate is seen. Blood gas analysis may show hypoxemia, hypocarbia, alkalosis, or increased A-a gradient. Radionuclide (lung) scans are the diagnostic method of choice; pulmonary angiography is rarely needed.

Treatment involves an IV heparin (5–10,000 units for the loading dose, then 1,000 units/hr) adjusting dose to prolong the partial thromboplastin time (PTT) to two times the control value. Heparin should be changed over to warfarin after 1 week of treatment. Warfarin should then be continued for at least 3 months. Embolectomy is rarely needed. Rarely must the inferior vena cava be clipped or tied, though inferior vena caval filters inserted intravenously are popular again. Fibrinolytic therapy is not effective. Patients followed after a pulmonary embolism should be evaluated for reoccurrences and the consequences of the embolism. Trauma to the legs or stasis should be avoided along with restrictive leg garments. Patients should be counseled to avoid long periods of immobility (for instance, on airplane flights they should get up and walk periodically or if driving on long trips, they should stop and get out of the car at regular intervals). Properly fitted elastic stockings can be helpful. Any signs or symptoms of malignancy should be pursued for a diagnosis.

VALVES: KEY FEATURE 3—
VALVULAR DYSFUNCTION
Treatment of Valvular Heart Disease
The approach to therapy depends on the specific valve or valves involved and whether they are stenotic or regurgitant. Medical therapy is directed at avoiding recurrent episodes of rheumatic carditis or infective endocarditis, management of CHF, and prevention of embolization. The patient should be carefully followed for signs and symptoms of progressive LV dysfunction and dysfunction of the valve. Yearly echocardiography is indicated in many patients with mild to moderate symptoms or borderline LV function; however, many physicians choose only to perform echocardiography when there is a change in symptoms or physical findings. Nifedipine has been recommended for symptomatic patients with severe aortic regurgitation and normal LV function [42]. In aortic regurgitation the follow-up is intensified if the etiology is Marfan's syndrome or cystic medial necrosis, both of which are associated with aortic root distention and rupture. This contrasts with the relatively benign course of the more frequent etiology, bicuspid aortic valve. When medical therapy is no longer effective, surgical intervention is indicated [43]. Dental evaluations, including extractions and other necessary work, should be performed with appropriate antibiotic prophylaxis several weeks before the insertion of prosthetic heart valves. The artificial valves in

general are not as hemodynamically functional as non-diseased valves and require anticoagulation to decrease the risk of emboli. Even tissue valves have this risk, although it is somewhat decreased and anticoagulation is not required. Whenever possible, diseased valves should be surgically repaired rather than replaced. Surgeons are becoming skilled at this and intraoperative echocardiography has made repair more feasible.INRs should be kept at 2.5 to 3.5 to lessen the possibility of embolic cerebrovascular accidents in patients with mechanical valves. Each of the specific valvular disorders is reviewed below along with their treatments.

Aortic Stenosis
Etiologies:
   Senile, calcific, or degenerative aortic stenosis: Accumulation of calcium in pockets of aortic cusps.
   Congenital bicuspid valve: Calcific changes occur earlier in life, presumably secondary to increased turbulence.
   Rheumatic heart disease: Usually not the first or only valve involved; fusion of commissures; thickened leaflets; patient may have a murmur by age 30 but symptoms may not occur until ages 50 to 60.
   Hypertrophic obstructive cardiomyopathy (IHSS or ASH) or subvalvular membrane.
   Supravalvular due to abnormal membrane.
Pathophysiology: The stenotic valve limits cardiac output, causing syncope, angina, and fatigue. The LV gradually fails because of the pressure required to pump blood through the stenotic valve, resulting in CHF.
Clinical manifestations: CHF with dyspnea on exertion, orthopnea, paroxysmal nocturnal dyspnea, fatigue, weakness; angina; exertional syncope or near syncope; complications of bacterial endocarditis.
Physical examination: Delayed upstroke with anacrotic notch, sometimes a shuddering quality; rales may be present if in CHF; LV systolic impulse is forceful and prolonged; palpable S_4. As the LV fails, impulse is displaced downward and to the left; a palpable systolic thrill may be present. As the stenosis becomes more severe, the peak of the ejection murmur occurs later during systole and A_2 becomes softer. The systolic murmur radiates to the carotids. In a patient with a congenital bicuspid valve and mild aortic stenosis, an ejection click may be heard.

Diagnostic tests:
 Chest x-ray: The LV may appear normal or enlarged
  with LV failure. There can be poststenotic aortic
  dilatation and calcification of the aortic valve.
 ECG: LV hypertrophy and strain; left atrial enlargement, intraventricular conduction defect.
 Echocardiography: Decreased excursion of aortic leaflets;
  thickened and calcified aortic leaflets; LV hypertrophy
  and left atrial enlargement; prolonged A-C interval.
 Cardiac catheterization: Systolic aortic-LV gradient
  greater than 50 mm Hg with normal cardiac output is
  considered severe. Aortic valve area is calculated from
  the Gorlin formula; the normal aortic valve area is 2.6
  to 3.5 cm^2; in the adult with critical aortic stenosis,
  the area is less than 0.5 to 0.7 cm^2.
Treatment: Digoxin and diuretics but if still symptomatic,
 surgery should be considered; age of patient is not a
 contraindication; endocarditis prophylaxis for dental
 surgical procedures; treat atrial fibrillation promptly.

Aortic Insufficiency or Regurgitation (AI)
Etiologies (in approximate order of frequency): Congenital
 bicuspid valve, rheumatic heart disease, bacterial endocarditis, cystic medial necrosis (myxomatous degeneration),
 syphilis, ankylosing spondylitis. Infrequent causes include
 trauma, osteogenesis imperfecta, rheumatoid arthritis,
 Reiter's syndrome, Ehlers-Danlos syndrome, aortic dissection, Hurler's aortitis, and other diseases affecting
 the sacroiliac joints.
Pathophysiology:
 Acute: In infective endocarditis, leaflet tissue is rapidly
  destroyed. The LV is suddenly presented with an
  intolerable pressure.
 Chronic: The LV dilates to accept volume load.
Clinical manifestations:
 Acute: Seen in drug addicts and patients with underlying valvular disease with fever and embolic episodes;
  severe dyspnea, tachypnea, orthopnea, hypotension.
 Chronic: Angina from low coronary perfusion pressure
  and elevated LV wall tension; orthopnea more than
  dyspnea on exertion from prolonged diastolic overfill-
  ing; nocturnal angina often with diaphoresis as pulse
  slows and diastolic pressure falls.
Physical examination:
 Acute: Lacks dramatic findings seen in chronic aortic
  insufficiency; may see pulsus alternans.

Chronic: Murmurs—decrescendo diastolic blowing along the sternum to the apex.

Austin Flint—apical middiastolic rumble.

Corrigan's pulse—abruptly rising and falling pulsation.

de Musset's sign—rhythmic nodding of the head with each beat.

Quincke's pulse—transmission of pulses into precapillary arterioles.

Duroziez's sign—to-and-fro murmur over femoral artery with compression.

Hill's sign—systolic pressure more than 60 mm Hg higher in legs than arms.

Pulsus bisferiens—carotid pulse with percussion wave, then exaggerated tidal wave.

Diagnostic tests:

Acute:

ECG LVH shows LV hypertrophy. Chest x-ray may show no enlargement.

Echocardiography shows reduced amplitude of mitral valve opening, premature closure and delayed opening of mitral valve, flail aortic leaflet.

Chronic:

ECG shows left axis deviation, pattern of LV volume overload, LV hypertrophy.

Chest x-ray shows cardiomegaly.

Echocardiography shows increased LV end-diastolic diameter. Systolic shortening is augmented.

Treatment:

Acute: Prompt surgical intervention as soon as patient is stable.

Chronic: Digoxin, diuretics, salt restriction; surgery indicated for severe chronic aortic insufficiency when symptoms worsen.

Mitral Regurgitation
Etiologies:

Rheumatic: More common in females; may have accompanying mitral stenosis and is usually chronic.

Ruptured chordae, acute; papillary muscle dysfunction or rupture, more common in males, often secondary to coronary disease, acute and chronic.

Mitral valve prolapse.

Endocarditis, acute or subacute.

Trauma, acute.

Calcification of the mitral valve annulus, chronic.

Pathophysiology: Part of the cardiac output is propelled backward into the lungs. In order to maintain cardiac output to the periphery, the LV dilates and eventually fails. Venous pressure and pulmonary pressure also rise to maintain forward flow against the elevated LV pressure.

Clinical manifestations: In the chronic form, there may be a long asymptomatic period (20–30 years) followed by dyspnea on exertion, orthopnea, weakness, fatigue, or palpitations. If the regurgitation is severe or chronic, there may be symptoms of right ventricular failure.

Physical examination: Sinus rhythm or atrial fibrillation; rales may be present, hyperdynamic LV impulse except in late phases; if left atrium large and in sinus rhythm there is a late systolic parasternal lift (rocking sensation of cardiac impulse). On auscultation, the systolic murmur has variable timing in the presence of papillary muscle dysfunction but it should be holosystolic and radiating to the apex.

Diagnostic tests:

Chest x-ray:

Chronic: Enlarged left atrium, LV; pulmonary vascular redistribution; signs of CHF; enlarged right ventricle; calcified mitral valve annulus may be present.

Acute: Left atrium not enlarged; signs of CHF and pulmonary edema.

ECG: Left atrium enlargement; LV hypertrophy; atrial fibrillation; right ventricular hypertrophy.

Echocardiography: Left atrial enlargement; dilated and actively contracting LV; if chronic and right side involved, may have right atrial and right ventricular enlargement; may see flail mitral leaflet.

Cardiac catheterization: Left atrial (pulmonary capillary wedge) pressure: tall regurgitant systolic V waves in acute form; increased pulmonary capillary wedge pressure; in chronic form, pulmonary capillary wedge pressure and V waves may not be as high; increased LV end-diastolic pressure.

LV angiography: Visualization of regurgitant stream; severity of regurgitation can be estimated; LV regurgitant fraction greater than 60% indicates severe mitral regurgitation.

Treatment: Low-salt diet: No added salt initially to 2 g of sodium/day, diuretics, afterload reduction, antibiotic prophylaxis.

Mitral Valve Prolapse

Etiologies: Congenital, myxomatous degeneration, Marfan's syndrome.

Pathophysiology: This syndrome has a very wide spectrum. In its most usual form, it is totally benign and best diagnosed by auscultation (i.e., midsystolic clicks and a late systolic murmur). Though linked to neurocirculatory and skeletal abnormalities, its association with chest pain or PVCs is less definite. Though a "gold standard" should be available using either echocardiography or LV angiography, neither have rigorous criteria established for the diagnosis. This most usual form may be present in 10% of the female and 5% of the male normal population. In its rarest form, it is due to myxomatous degeneration of the mitral valve and is associated with marked mitral regurgitation, ventricular tachycardia, and sudden death.

Clinical manifestations: The presentation depends on form. The more severe form can accompany Marfan's syndrome. There is an association with vague neurocirculatory abnormalities (soldier's heart, orthostatic changes) and chest pain. However, it is only rarely associated with or the cause of these symptoms. Generally, mitral valve prolapse should not be used as a diagnosis for the complaint of chest pain.

Physical examination:

Auscultation: Midsystolic click or clicks, late systolic murmur.

Diagnostic tests:

ECG: Very often normal or showing nonspecific ST and T-wave changes.

Chest x-ray: Weak association with skeletal abnormalities such as straight back syndrome, scoliosis, and pectus; findings of mitral regurgitation and dilated aortic root in rare form.

Exercise test: Perhaps 25% false-positive rate (i.e., ST-segment depression not due to coronary heart disease).

Treatment: Beta-blockers can be helpful for neurocirculatory symptoms; antibiotic prophylaxis when murmur and click are present.

Mitral Stenosis

Etiologies: Predominantly rheumatic, rarely congenital. There is a history of rheumatic fever in two-thirds of patients; two-thirds are female. Valve thickened by fibrous tissue and calcium. Commissures fuse, chordae fuse and shorten, cusps become rigid. The initial insult is rheumatic; later changes are due to continued trauma of altered flow. Thrombus and emboli may arise from the valve.

Pathophysiology: The normal valve area is 4 to 6 cm^2. As valve area decreases, left atrial pressure increases, raising pulmonary venous and capillary pressures, causing dyspnea on exertion. As rate of flow increases across the valve (as in tachycardia), the transvalvular gradient increases and left atrial pressure increases. LV end-diastolic pressure is normal in pure mitral stenosis. Coexisting mitral regurgitation, aortic valve disease, rheumatic myocarditis, hypertension, or coronary artery disease may cause LV dysfunction. In pure mitral stenosis, left atrial and pulmonary artery wedge pressures are increased and the left atrial pressure pulse has a prominent a wave (atrial contraction) and a gradual Y descent. In mild mitral stenosis, pulmonary artery wedge pressure may be normal at rest and only increases with exercise. In severe stenosis, pulmonary artery pressure is increased even at rest and may exceed systemic pressure. If pulmonary artery pressure is greater than 60 mm Hg, right ventricular dysfunction may occur. Clinical and hemodynamic features are dictated by the degree of pulmonary hypertension, which is due to passive congestion, arteriolar constriction, or obliterative changes.

Clinical manifestations: Generally there is a long latent period (approximately 2 decades); onset occurs in the fourth decade. Once the patient is symptomatic, death occurs in 2 to 5 years unless surgery is performed. In early stages, the patient is asymptomatic unless under extreme stress (pregnancy, hyperthyroid, anemia, fever). In later stages, dyspnea on exertion, orthopnea, paroxysmal nocturnal dyspnea, pulmonary edema, and atrial arrhythmias can occur. Hemoptysis is due to rupture of bronchial venous connections (pulmonary apoplexy), which is due to a sudden increase in left atrial pressure. As pulmonary hypertension worsens, symptoms due to pulmonary congestion decrease, and right ventricular failure increases. Recurrent pulmonary emboli, late in the course, occur most frequently in patients with right ventricular failure and pulmonary hypertension. Pulmonary infections are complications. Infective endocarditis is rare with pure mitral stenosis, but not uncommon if in the presence of mitral stenosis and regurgitation combined. Chest pain in 10% of patients is due to pulmonary high BP and coronary embolization. Fibrosis in pulmonary alveolar walls due to pulmonary hypertension causes decreased diffusing capacity, and total lung capacity. Thrombi in the left atrium cause arterial emboli, more commonly in the setting of atrial fibrillation.

Physical examination:

Inspection/palpation: Peripheral and central cyanosis when severe. Large jugular venous a wave if sinus rhythm and pulmonary hypertension. With atrial fibrillation, jugular venous C-V wave. Systemic BP normal or slightly decreased. Right ventricle lift/tap and palpable pulmonary valve closure if severe pulmonary hypertension. LV not palpable in pure mitral stenosis. Palpable diastolic thrill in left lateral decubitus position. Often palpable S_1 is present initially, and palpable opening snap later.

Auscultation:

S_1 is accentuated and snapping since mitral valve only closes when LV pressure overcomes left atrial pressure.

P_2 is accentuated if pulmonary hypertension is present. S_1 may be absent if leaflets cannot open or shut.

Opening snap is heard best at the apex during expiration. Follows aortic valve closure by 0.06 to 0.12 second. Occurs at the instant LV pressure falls below left atrial pressure. Interval between A_2 and opening snap shortens in severe mitral stenosis. Intensity correlates with mobility of anterior leaflet.

A low-pitched rumbling diastolic murmur is best heard at the apex in the left lateral decubitus position. Accentuated by exercise. Duration correlates with severity.

If associated right ventricular failure is present, there will be hepatomegaly, edema, ascites, and pleural effusion.

An enlarged left atrium can lead to Ortner's syndrome, which is hoarseness due to recurrent laryngeal nerve compression.

Differential diagnosis: The apical middiastolic murmur of aortic regurgitation (Austin Flint) may be mistaken for mitral stenosis. Significant mitral regurgitation may have a prominent early diastolic murmur at the apex, but there is usually evidence of LV hypertrophy and the systolic murmur of mitral regurgitation will help make the diagnosis. An atrial septal defect will have right ventricular enlargement, accentuated pulmonary vasculature, and a diastolic flow murmur across the tricuspid valve (confused with a mitral diastolic murmur). However, the second heart sound will be widely split and there will be no evidence of left atrial enlargement. Differentiating split S_2 from A_2–opening snap can be aided by sudden standing, which decreases venous return; the split S_2 narrows and A_2–opening snap widens.

Diagnostic tests:

ECG: If pulmonary hypertension is present, right axis deviation and right ventricular hypertrophy appear. LV hypertrophy if associated problem with cardiomyopathy, regurgitation, aortic valve disease.

Echocardiogram: In M-mode, anterior and posterior leaflets do not separate widely in early diastole, posterior leaflet moves in same direction as anterior leaflet, reduction in ejection fraction slope, calcifications present, enlarged left atrium. Two-dimensional echocardiography can estimate valve area.

Chest x-ray: Straightening of left-sided heart border, prominence of main pulmonary arteries, backward displacement of esophagus, pushing upward and straightening of the left main stem bronchus, and double density sign due to left atrial enlargement. Kerley's B lines if left atrial pressure greater than 20 mm Hg. Filling in of space behind sternum on the lateral view due to right ventricular enlargement.

Cardiac catheterization:

Mitral valve area = Cardiac output ÷ 37.8 × Diastolic filling time × Square root of the diastolic gradient between the LV and the left atrium.

2.1 to 2.5 cm²—symptomatic with near-maximal exercise.

1.6 to 2.0 cm²—symptomatic with moderate exercise.

Less than 1.0 cm²—symptoms with minimal activity or at rest.

Treatment:

Asymptomatic adolescent—penicillin or amoxicillin prophylaxis.

Symptomatic—low-sodium diet, maintenance diuretics; digoxin of no use if in sinus rhythm.

Treat hemoptysis with bed rest, salt and water restriction, diuretics.

Anticoagulate if history of emboli or intermittent atrial fibrillation, or low cardiac output and large left atrium.

If atrial fibrillation is of new onset, cardioversion, electrically or medically, following 2 to 3 weeks of anticoagulation and maintain on quinidine/digoxin.

Surgical treatment or catheter dilation is indicated eventually unless specific contraindication; operate in symptomatic pure mitral stenosis if valve area is less than 1.5 cm^2.

Anticoagulation for Mechanical Valves

The rate of thromboembolic events with mechanical valves averages about 4%/yr or 4/100 patient-yr. The optimal intensity of oral anticoagulant therapy for patients with mechanical heart valves (i.e., the level at which thromboembolic complications are effectively prevented without excessive bleeding) was investigated by a Dutch study [44]. Data were collected on all patients with mechanical heart valves who had been seen at four regional Dutch anticoagulation clinics since 1985. The primary outcome events were episodes of thromboembolism or major bleeding. The intensity-specific incidence of each type of event was calculated as the number of events that occurred at a certain intensity of anticoagulation (expressed in terms of the INR divided by the number of patient-years during which the INR was at this level in the total patient population. A total of 1,608 patients were followed during 6,475 patient-years. Cerebral embolism occurred in 43 patients (0.68/100 patient-yr) and peripheral embolism in 2 (0.03/100 patient-yr). Intracranial and spinal bleeding occurred in 36 patients (0.57/100 patient-yr) and major extracranial bleeding in 128 (2.1/100 patient-yr). The optimal intensity of anticoagulation, at which the incidence of both complications was lowest, was achieved when the INR was between 2.5 and 4.9. To achieve this level of anticoagulation, the study recommended a target INR of 3.0 to 4.0 (generally a more conservative target of 2.5 to 3.5 is recommended). *Factors associated with a higher incidence of thromboembolic events included age over 50 years, valve in the mitral rather than aortic position, and caged-ball rather than bileaflet or tilting-disk valve.* The lower the risk by these characteristics, the broader the optimal range of the INR. Patients over 70 years old had a higher risk of bleeding.

Aspirin should be added to the regimen for carefully selected patients who have mechanical valves [45]. Because dual therapy is controversial in such patients, we consider the following factors before adding ASA (81 mg) to the regimen for patients with mechanical valves taking warfarin:

Risk of hemorrhage, especially compliance, alcohol use, and history of bleeding

Valve location—mitral valve replacements more thrombogenic

Valve type—St. Jude's valves less thrombogenic

Comorbid conditions—history of thrombogenic event or atrial fibrillation, MI

Patient preference

Anticoagulation for Tissue Prosthetic Valves or Repaired Valves

Patients with bioprosthetic (e.g., porcine) valves generally do *not* require long-term anticoagulation, particularly those in the aortic position. Such patients usually only receive anticoagulation therapy for several months after surgery. Since these valves have not passed the test of time as have the mechanical valves, they are usually only utilized in older patients and in those in whom anticoagulation might be problematic. Anticoagulation is not required after valve repair.

Antibiotic Prophylaxis To Prevent Bacterial Endocarditis

Transitory bacteremia can be caused by a variety of manipulations or surgical procedures, and in an individual with structural heart disease, such bacteremia may initiate bacterial endocarditis [46]. Certain procedures are associated with a high risk of bacteremia: dental extraction (70%), periodontal surgery (55%), tonsillectomy (35%), and transurethral prostatic resection (40%). The indications for antibiotic prophylaxis for endocarditis are based on two criteria: an increased risk of endocarditis developing on specific cardiac lesions and the likelihood that selected manipulative procedures give rise to bacteremia with organisms that commonly cause endocarditis. Viridans-type streptococci are responsible for most cases of endocarditis originating in the oral cavity; enterococci are responsible for those episodes arising in the genitourinary tract. A statement presenting the rationale and indications for prophylaxis and the specific recommendations for antibiotic use has been prepared by a committee of the AHA. Although amoxicillin, ampicillin, and penicillin show comparable in vitro efficacy against viridans-type streptococci, amoxicillin (3 g PO 1 hour before and 1.5 g PO 6 hours later) has replaced penicillin V as the recommended agent for oral prophylaxis because it is better absorbed from the GI tract and provides higher and more sustained serum antibiotic concentrations. Erythromycin stearate, erythromycin ethylsuccinate, and clindamycin are specifically recommended for use in patients who are allergic to penicillin because these agents are reliably absorbed and their use results in sustained serum concentrations. Tetracyclines and sulfonamides are not recommended for endocarditis prophylaxis.

Prophylaxis is not recommended for the following procedures because they are not considered to be risks for subsequent endocarditis: dental procedures that are not likely to cause gingival bleeding, simple adjustment of orthodontic appliances, injections of intraoral anesthetics (except intraligamentary injections), shedding of primary teeth, endotracheal intubation, bronchoscopy with a flexible bronchoscope, and tympanostomy tube insertion. Similarly, the occurrence of endocarditis after certain procedures involving the GI tract or the genitourinary tract is rare enough that antibiotic prophylaxis is not required in most patients with underlying heart disease. Such low-risk procedures include uncomplicated vaginal delivery or cesarean section, upper GI tract endoscopy without biopsy, percutaneous liver biopsy, proctosigmoidoscopy without biopsy, brief bladder catheterization in patients whose urine is sterile, barium enema, pelvic examination, dilation and curettage of the uterus, and uncomplicated insertion or removal of intrauterine devices. However, when patients are at high risk for endocarditis, physicians may administer prophylactic antibiotics in conjunction with these low-risk procedures. Structural abnormalities requiring prophylaxis include most congenital heart diseases, rheumatic or other acquired valvular heart disease, hypertrophic cardiomyopathy, mitral valve prolapse with mitral insufficiency, prosthetic heart valves, and a previous episode of endocarditis (even in the absence of overt heart disease).

Maintaining optimal dental health is essential if the risk of endocarditis is to be minimized among patients with vulnerable cardiac lesions. Dental evaluations, including extractions and other necessary work, should be performed with appropriate antibiotic prophylaxis several weeks before the insertion of prosthetic heart valves.

Diagnosis and Treatment of Infective Endocarditis

Etiology and Epidemiology

Infective endocarditis is a bacterial, fungal, rickettsial, or chlamydial infection of a cardiac valve or the endocardium. Endocarditis is classified as either subacute (duration > 6 weeks) or acute. Prosthetic valve endocarditis and endocarditis associated with narcotic abuse must be considered separately. Almost all species of bacteria have been implicated in bacterial endocarditis. Viridans and all other streptococci account for 40% of bacterial endocarditis and *Streptococcus pneumoniae* has caused 1 to 2% of cases. *Staphylococcus aureus* is a frequent cause of native valve bacterial endocarditis and is a particularly prominent cause of hospital-acquired bacterial endocarditis as well as that in IV drug abusers. Enterococci, coagulase-negative staphylococci, and gram-negative bacilli each account for 5 to 10% of cases of endocarditis. Endocarditis caused by gram-negative bacilli including *Pseudomonas aeruginosa, Pseudomonas cepacia,* and *Serratia marcescens* occurs among IV drug abusers and occasionally in patients with bacteremia caused by Enterobacteriaceae. Fungal endocarditis occurs in IV drug abusers and in patients with prosthetic valves.

The incidence of infective endocarditis is about 3.8/100,000 person-yr; 50% of patients are older than 50 years and the substrate is usually degenerative valvular disease, such as calcified aortic stenosis or mitral valve annulus, and mitral valve prolapse.

The overall survival rate for patients with infective endocarditis is about 75%. The rate depends on therapy, the infecting organism, comorbid conditions, and age. It approaches 90% when the infecting organism is a viridans-type streptococcus or *Streptococcus bovis* but is about 50% for nonaddicts with endocarditis from *S. aureus*. With the incorporation of earlier surgical intervention into the therapy for endocarditis, CHF is no longer associated with increased mortality. However, major CNS complications (embolic strokes and intracerebral hemorrhage) and uncontrolled infection remain associated with increased mortality. The short-term outlook is relatively good for IV drug addicts with right-sided endocarditis. Endocarditis from fungi or gram-negative organisms is extremely difficult to cure. The overall survival rate for patients with prosthetic valve endocarditis approaches 70%.

Subacute Bacterial Endocarditis
Subacute bacterial endocarditis (SBE), which has a duration of more than 6 weeks, is caused by relatively avirulent bacteria (i.e., indigenous streptococci). These agents lack sufficient invasiveness to initiate infection in normal hearts but can establish a focus on deformed heart valves or at sites of congenital cardiac lesions. The enterococci are important causes of SBE. The portal of entry for *S. bovis* causing endocarditis or bacteremia is often a malignant or premalignant colonic lesion. Most cases of *S. aureus* endocarditis are acute, but *S. aureus* can cause SBE. SBE most commonly involves the left side of the heart and particularly affects regurgitant, leaking valves. The mitral valve is more frequently involved than the aortic valve. A regurgitant jet stream through an incompetent aortic valve typically produces lesions on the ventricular aspect of the aortic valve and on the aortic leaflet of the mitral valve. Right-sided endocarditis, which involves the tricuspid valve more commonly than the pulmonary valve, is usually caused by pyogenic organisms and occurs in IV drug abusers. Valves distorted by calcium and congenital malformations predispose to endocarditis including mitral valve prolapse.

CLINICAL PRESENTATION. The symptoms of SBE are nonspecific and subtle and may persist for months. Anorexia, fevers, sweats, weakness, myalgias, arthralgias, malaise, and fatigability are prominent. Diagnosis can only be made clinically if SBE is considered, because symptoms either are nonspecific or arise primarily from an organ other than the heart. For example, there may be signs of meningitis, cerebral emboli, or glomerulonephritis. The following clinical features should cause consideration of SBE.

CUTANEOUS MANIFESTATIONS. Petechiae occur in the conjunctivas, in the oropharynx, and on the skin; they are particularly common on the extremities and may be present in large numbers on the lower extremities in particular. Petechiae may continue to appear for some weeks during successful antibiotic treatment. Linear subungual splinter hemorrhages in the middle of the nail bed are a feature of SBE; trauma can cause similar hemorrhages in the distal part of the nail bed. Osler's nodes are tender, purplish, subcutaneous nodules that develop in the pulp of the fingers and disappear within several days; they are thought to be caused by septic microemboli. Small, slightly nodular, nonpainful, erythematous or hemorrhagic areas on the palms or soles, called *Janeway lesions*, may occur in SBE but more commonly in acute bacterial endocarditis (ABE).

MUSCULOSKELETAL FEATURES.   Myalgias, arthralgias, arthritis, or low back pain occur in half the patients with endocarditis, and in about half of these patients such symptoms represent either initial or prominent manifestations of the disease. Arthritis may be either monoarticular or polyarticular. Frank joint effusions occur but are less common than the finding of painful, red, warm, tender joints. Septic arthritis may occur in ABE, but it is not a feature of SBE.

EYE FINDINGS.   Petechial and flame-shaped hemorrhages as well as cotton-wool exudates occur in the retina of patients with endocarditis. Roth's spots are oval white areas in the retina that are surrounded by a zone of hemorrhage.

SPLENOMEGALY.   The spleen is palpably enlarged in about one-third of patients with endocarditis; this finding is more common in SBE than in ABE. Rarely, a splenic abscess may be the cause of fever noted after the endocarditis has been treated.

RENAL MANIFESTATIONS.   Microscopic hematuria is observed in half the patients with bacterial endocarditis. Four types of renal lesions occur, including renal infarcts secondary to embolization, diffuse membranoproliferative glomerulonephritis, focal embolic glomerulonephritis, and renal abscesses.

THROMBOEMBOLIC PHENOMENA.   Significant embolic episodes occur in about one-third of patients with endocarditis. Cerebral emboli produce neurologic signs consistent with a stroke syndrome. Sudden monocular blindness may be produced by emboli in the central retinal artery. Mesenteric emboli may produce acute abdominal pain, ileus, and melena. Emboli in the spleen produce left-upper-quadrant abdominal pain with radiation to the left shoulder; pleuritic chest pain and a splenic friction rub may be present, and a small pleural effusion may develop. Peripheral emboli may produce pain in the digits or gangrene of the extremities.

Pulmonary emboli occur with right-sided endocarditis and frequently cause pulmonary infarcts and pneumonia. Septic pulmonary emboli may cause lung abscess, empyema, and pyopneumothorax. Coronary emboli can occur and cause chest pain.

MYCOTIC ANEURYSMS.   Peripheral mycotic aneurysms in SBE may result from embolic occlusion of the vasa vasorum or from deposition of immune complexes in the arterial wall. In ABE, an aneurysm may result from direct bacterial invasion of the arterial wall. In SBE, an aneurysm can develop during the active stage of infection in any artery but may not become evident for months after the valvular infection has been eradicated; at this point, the aneurysm is sterile. Physical examination should include palpation of the peripheral arteries and auscultation for bruits. The clinical features include pain, a pulsatile mass, evidence of pressure on adjacent structures, or the sudden development of an expanding hematoma or signs of major blood loss. Surgical excision to prevent rupture is usually indicated for accessible aneurysms of significant size.

NEUROLOGIC MANIFESTATIONS.   Neurologic complications develop in a third of patients with endocarditis and cerebral embolism is the most frequent complication. Emboli most commonly obstruct the middle cerebral artery or one of its branches, producing a contralateral hemiparesis and hemisensory deficit. Cerebral embolism can be the initial manifestation of endocarditis or even occur during successful treatment. Microscopic embolic infarcts can cause seizures or an altered level of consciousness and focal signs.

Cerebral mycotic aneurysms occur in less than 10% of patients with bacterial endocarditis. They may become clinically apparent as a sudden cerebral or subarachnoid hemorrhage or as an embolic stroke followed by an intracerebral hemorrhage. A persistent focal headache may precede rupture of an aneurysm. Seizures, which are usually triggered by emboli, and toxic encephalopathy are other cerebral complications of endocarditis.

CARDIAC FINDINGS.   The cardiac features in SBE are those of the underlying valvular or congenital lesion. Murmurs are present in more than 90% of patients with SBE, but at least one-third of patients with ABE have no murmur. Changing murmurs represent a major diagnostic finding in ABE while mild changes can occur due to anemia, high fever, or tachycardia. The appearance of a new aortic diastolic murmur suggests dilatation of the aortic annulus or damage to an aortic leaflet. The sudden onset of a loud mitral pansystolic murmur suggests rupture of a chorda tendinea or tearing of a mitral valve leaflet.

Acute Bacterial Endocarditis
ABE is commonly caused by organisms that are more invasive than the agents of SBE. The agents of ABE can attack
normal heart valves and mural endocardium, cause accelerated cardiac valve destruction, and establish suppura-
tive foci at sites of embolic deposition. Such agents include
S. aureus, the most frequent cause of ABE; *S. pneumoniae*;
group A streptococci; *Neisseria gonorrhoeae*; *Salmonella*
species; other members of Enterobacteriaceae; and *P.
aeruginosa*. ABE may develop in an entirely normal heart,
or it may occur on underlying acquired or congenital cardiac lesions. History or examination often reveals an
antecedent pyogenic infection such as pneumococcal pneumonia or meningitis, staphylococcal abscesses, or furuncu-
losis or IV drug abuse.

   CLINICAL MANIFESTATIONS.   The onset of ABE is usually
abrupt, and rigors are common with temperatures reach-
ing 104°F. Cutaneous manifestations, particularly petechiae, may be prominent, especially when *S. aureus* is the
agent. Embolic manifestations, especially in the CNS and
kidneys, are common in ABE. Metastatic infections in the
bones, kidneys, brain, and lungs may arise from either
septic embolization or the bacteremia. Osler's nodes occur,
but less often than in SBE. Janeway lesions occur on the
palms and soles in up to 10% of patients who have *S.
aureus* endocarditis.

Endocarditis Associated with Drug Abuse
The annual incidence of endocarditis among IV drug
abusers is estimated at about 1%. At the time of their initial attack of endocarditis, most drug addicts have no history or findings of preexisting valvular heart disease. The
tricuspid valve is the site of infection more frequently than
the aortic valve or mitral valve. *S. aureus* is responsible for
approximately 50% of cases. Fever (often accompanied by
chills), malaise, cough, and pleuritic chest pain are the
most common presenting complaints in right-sided endocarditis of addicts. Septic pulmonary emboli frequently
arise and cause sputum production, hemoptysis, and initial radiologic infiltrates. Cavitation of embolic pulmonary
lesions is common. One should look for the large V waves
of tricuspid regurgitation. Peripheral emboli are observed
frequently, and neurologic manifestations are common.

Prosthetic Valve Endocarditis
Infection involving mechanical prosthetic valves and
porcine bioprosthetic valves has a cumulative occurrence,

estimated at 3% at 1 year after valve implantation and at 5% at 4 years after surgery. The overall risk of infection is similar for mechanical and bioprosthetic valves and for aortic and mitral placement. Prosthetic valve endocarditis is considered as early prosthetic valve endocarditis (EPVE), occurring within 60 days after valve replacement (one-third of infections), and late prosthetic valve endocarditis (LPVE), which is manifested clinically later and is more common (two-thirds of infections). EPVE is usually a consequence of intraoperative contamination, or the result of a septic complication (wound infection or pneumonia) of surgery, such as sternotomy. The predisposing factors in LPVE are usually dental procedures, genitourinary tract manipulations, and other incidental transient bacteremic events. EPVE has a mortality of 40% and LPVE a mortality of 20%. Persistent fever in spite of antibiotics, changing heart murmurs, worsening CHF, and new conduction abnormalities are associated with mortality. Mortality is highest in those with neurologic complications. These features, particularly CHF, necessitate consideration for emergent surgery.

S. epidermidis and *S. aureus* are responsible for most early and late infections. *Streptococcus viridans* is responsible in 25% of the cases of LPVE. Coagulase-negative staphylococci, which rarely cause native valve endocarditis, are responsible for many cases of prosthetic valve endocarditis so they should not be considered contaminants.

Infection of prosthetic valves is often associated with valvular dysfunction and pathologic changes that cannot be corrected by antibiotic therapy alone. In native valve endocarditis, the infection is commonly restricted to the valve leaflet, but infection on prosthetic valves often invades perivalvular tissues. Necrosis of the annulus because of invasive infection causes partial dehiscence of the prosthesis and hemodynamically significant valvular regurgitation. Deeper invasion leads to myocardial abscess. Infection of porcine and mechanical prosthetic valves is associated with invasion and destructive changes, particularly when valves at the aortic position are infected and when onset occurs during the first postoperative year. Occasionally, vegetations may partially obstruct the valve orifice or restrict valve movement. When infection is restricted to the leaflets of a porcine valve, abnormalities such as leaflet tears and the development of obstructing vegetations cause clinically significant valvular dysfunction.

The clinical features of EPVE differ from those of LPVE. Although EPVE may be initially hidden by coexisting postoperative infectious complications, the disease is generally rapidly progressive. Fever, a prosthetic regurgitant murmur, and prosthetic valve dysfunction with resulting CHF strongly suggest the diagnosis. Unexplained fever during the postoperative period may be the only initial manifestation of EPVE.

Petechiae occur in about half of patients with EPVE, but Roth's spots, Osler's nodes, Janeway lesions, and other peripheral signs of endocarditis are unusual. Conjunctival petechiae are common findings for several days immediately after surgery in patients who have been on cardiopulmonary bypass, and their presence at that time does not indicate EPVE. Emboli are common in EPVE. Emboli that occlude large peripheral arteries suggest fungal endocarditis. This diagnosis must be based on histologic examination or culture of the clot recovered at embolectomy because blood cultures seldom reveal the organism.

The clinical features of LPVE are similar to those of native valve endocarditis. The onset is often gradual and marked by fever, malaise, fatigue, and anorexia. The course is typically slow except when *S. aureus* or group A streptococcus is the cause.

SPECIAL DIAGNOSTIC AND THERAPEUTIC CONSIDERATIONS. The diagnosis of prosthetic valve endocarditis is based on clinical and echocardiographic findings and the demonstration of a continuous bacteremia. Cultures are negative in less than 5% of patients, suggesting fungus or other fastidious organisms. Persistence of bacteremia, bacteremia after therapy, evidence of vegetations on the prosthesis, valvular dysfunction, or paravalvular infection would suggest the diagnosis of prosthetic valve endocarditis. Prosthetic valve dysfunction, identified by auscultatory findings or noninvasive tests, strongly supports a suspected diagnosis of prosthetic valve endocarditis. New conduction disturbances on the ECG suggest extension of a ring abscess into the septum, with involvement of the conduction system. Echocardiography has limited usefulness in the diagnosis because the prosthesis produces echoes that obscure vegetations and abscesses. Doppler echocardiography is useful in the serial evaluation of the function of infected prosthetic valves. Transesophageal and Doppler echocardiography studies are more effective for assessing the prosthetic valve and perivalvular tissue.

Prosthetic valve endocarditis is treated for longer periods than is native valve bacterial endocarditis caused by similar organisms. Follow-up therapy with orally administered antibiotics for several months is not recommended routinely. Surgery is necessary for patients who have invasive perivalvular infection, prosthesis dysfunction causing CHF, or prosthetic valve endocarditis caused by an antibiotic-resistant organism. Surgical intervention is indicated in half the patients and mortality is no higher in those who undergo replacement during acute infection than those who receive medical therapy alone. There is about a 10% risk of recurrent prosthetic valve endocarditis after valve replacement. When valve replacement is indicated, a delay only increases the risk of serious complications such as emboli and CHF.

Diagnosis of Endocarditis

HISTORY/PHYSICAL EXAMINATION.   The diagnosis of infective endocarditis has been traditionally based on four features: *(1) predisposing valvular disease, (2) bacteremia, (3) embolic phenomena, and (4) evidence of an active endocardial process.* "Osler's tetralogy" has served clinicians well for diagnosing bacterial endocarditis but has certain limitations. The premorbid status of the patient is often unknown, blood cultures may be negative in up to 20% of patients, and systemic emboli may be occult or occur only when they have reached a critical size. This led the Duke University endocarditis service to define *two major criteria (typical blood culture and positive findings on echocardiogram) and six minor criteria (predisposition, fever, vascular phenomena, immunologic phenomena, suggestive echocardiogram, and suggestive microbiologic findings)* [47]. To make the diagnosis of endocarditis, a patient must fulfill two major or one major and two minor criteria. Application of the proposed new criteria increases the number of definite diagnoses and makes for more accurate diagnosis and classification of patients with suspected endocarditis.

The diagnosis of infective endocarditis is easy in the patient with fever, heart murmurs, petechiae, anemia, microscopic hematuria, and splenomegaly; however, one should be alert to atypical presentations in which the most prominent clinical findings are in organs other than the heart. Such presentations include cerebrovascular accident (embolic stroke) in an elderly patient whose low-grade fever is attributed to the stroke; meningitis (cerebrospinal fluid pleocytosis and stiff neck), as a result of either true meningeal infection or bland embolic infarction in silent areas of the brain; unexplained renal insufficiency; musculoskeletal disease; apparent pneumonia that is actually septic pulmonary infarcts; and fever of undetermined origin in which the peripheral stigmata of endocarditis may be minimal and a "functional" heart murmur is heard.

The diagnosis of infective endocarditis must be considered in any patient with a heart murmur and fever. In contrast to younger patients, elderly who have endocarditis are less likely to be febrile and are more likely to present with confusion.

A variety of noninfectious illnesses can mimic infective endocarditis including acute rheumatic fever; marantic endocarditis, because it also can give rise to multiple embolic episodes; polyarteritis nodosa; and cardiac myxoma. Neoplasms may mimic infective endocarditis by induction of marantic endocarditis or by their hemodynamic effects.

LABORATORY FINDINGS.   The leukocyte count in SBE is usually normal, whereas a leukocytosis is commonly present in ABE. Normocytic normochromic anemia is often present and the erythrocyte sedimentation rate is usually elevated. Immunoglobulin abnormalities are frequent in infective endocarditis. Rheumatoid factor is found in 50% of patients with endocarditis of more than 6 weeks' duration; it disappears after successful treatment. Circulating immune complexes have been demonstrated in more than 90% of patients with infective endocarditis.

Renal abnormalities are common, and most patients have proteinuria and microscopic hematuria. Elevated levels of creatinine accompany the development of extensive immune deposit glomerulonephritis.

In most patients with SBE, all blood cultures before initiation of antibiotic therapy are positive due to intense bacteremia associated with an infected endothelial surface. Three to four sets of cultures before the start of therapy are adequate for demonstrating the bacteremia. Cultures should be grown in both aerobic and anaerobic media and should be incubated in 5 to 10% carbon dioxide. Isolation of the etiologic agent on blood culture may be delayed or prevented by prior antimicrobial therapy.

In patients with clinically diagnosed endocarditis, echocardiography (with Dopper studies) using the transthoracic and transesophageal approaches can define the location of endocarditis, recognize intracardiac endocarditis-related complications, and possibly identify patients who are at increased risk for arterial embolization. In patients with native valve endocarditis, valvular vegetations can be detected in 60% with transthoracic echocardiography and 90% with transesophageal echocardiography (TEE). Among patients with suspected endocarditis with negative findings on TEE, up to 10% will subsequently have endocarditis. Echocardiography cannot distinguish noninfectious from infectious thrombotic vegetations on native or prosthetic valves or distinguish active from healed vegetations on native valves.

Cardiac Complications of Endocarditis
CHF is the most frequent cardiac complication of infective endocarditis. Aortic valve infection causes more serious hemodynamic consequences than does mitral valve infection. A mycotic aneurysm of a sinus of Valsalva or an aortic ring abscess may rupture through the membranous septum into the right atrium or ventricle. Such rupture causes a sudden rise in the jugular venous pressure and a to-and-fro murmur and thrill along the left sternal border; the lungs remain relatively clear. The murmur produced by rupture into the right atrium is heard closer to the right sternal border.

Conduction abnormalities may signal the extension of valvular infection to the septum and its major conduction tissues. The proximity of the right cusp and the noncoronary cusp of the aortic valve to the conduction system accounts for the development of complicating conduction abnormalities. Extension of infection from the mitral valve can also produce conduction defects, but it is less frequent than from the aortic valve. The development of PR-interval prolongation or the appearance of a new left bundle-branch block or of a new right bundle-branch block with left anterior hemiblock suggests that the infection has spread from the aortic valve into the ventricular septum. The development of new and persistent conduction abnormalities, particularly in patients with infected aortic valves, usually indicates the presence of a deep-seated abscess and the need for debridement and valve replacement. Conduction abnormalities are an indication for pacing. TEE is the most sensitive and preferred noninvasive test for detecting myocardial abscesses in both native and prosthetic valve endocarditis. Pericarditis in the course of active infective endocarditis is usually caused by extension of a valve ring abscess into the epicardium.

Treatment of Endocarditis

Endocarditis requires hospitalization for antibiotic therapy and, when necessary, surgical debridement of infected perivalvular tissue and replacement of the infected valve. Effective treatment of bacterial endocarditis requires definition of the etiologic agent and its antimicrobial susceptibility. When bacterial endocarditis is suspected, antibiotic therapy may be delayed briefly pending the results of blood cultures. If the infection is fulminant or if there is valvular dysfunction that may require urgent surgical intervention, empirical antibiotic therapy must be initiated promptly after blood has been obtained for culture.

SELECTION OF ANTIMICROBIAL AGENTS. Enterococci. The enterococci are relatively resistant to penicillin, ampicillin, and vancomycin and are overtly resistant to cephalosporins [48, 49]. They can be killed by the synergistic interaction of penicillin, ampicillin, or vancomycin with certain aminoglycoside antibiotics. To achieve the bactericidal synergism that is essential for optimal antimicrobial treatment of enterococcal endocarditis, the enterococcus must simultaneously be exposed to a cell wall–active antibiotic (penicillin, ampicillin, or vancomycin) at a concentration at or above the organism's minimum inhibitory concentration (MIC) and an aminoglycoside that will exert a lethal effect. *These agents require referral to an infectious disease consultant since new antibiotics are becoming available and relapses are common.*

Penicillin-Sensitive Streptococci. Two highly effective regimens have been widely used to treat endocarditis caused by *S. viridans* and other types of penicillin-sensitive organisms. One regimen employs parenteral penicillin alone in high doses for 4 weeks, and the second regimen adds streptomycin during the initial 2 weeks of the 4-week course. *The new AHA guidelines call for ceftriaxone, 2 g IV or IM once daily for 4 weeks, which can be done on an outpatient basis.* Since HACEK organisms are acquiring resistance to penicillin, this regimen is recommended for them as well.

Occasionally, strains of *S. viridans* and *S. bovis* that cause endocarditis are highly resistant to streptomycin. Combination therapy with streptomycin and penicillin is not synergistic against these strains. However, the combination of gentamicin and penicillin does act synergistically to kill them.

A penicillinase-resistant penicillin should be the initial agent used to treat *S. aureus* endocarditis, unless the presence of methicillin-resistant *S. aureus* strains is suspected. In the latter case, vancomycin should be used until the susceptibility of the actual strain has been clarified.

Although antibiotic therapy for endocarditis in addicts generally follows the pathogen-specific regimens used for the treatment of nonaddicts, methicillin-susceptible *S. aureus* endocarditis restricted to the tricuspid valve has been successfully treated with a penicillinase-resistant penicillin plus an aminoglycoside given for 2 weeks [50].

Endocarditis caused by gram-negative bacilli should be treated with one of the potent beta-lactam antibiotics, such as a third-generation cephalosporin, with or without an aminoglycoside.

Since the response of fungal endocarditis to therapy is most discouraging, with an 80% mortality, emergent valve debridement and valve replacement should be considered in these patients.

When blood cultures are negative or culture results are not available, the selection of empirical therapy requires careful consideration of the clinical clues and factors predisposing to endocarditis that might suggest the identity of the causative organism. *In the absence of information suggesting a probable cause for native valve SBE, treatment with ampicillin and gentamicin as for enterococcal endocarditis is advised.* If the course is fulminant or *S. aureus* is an etiologic consideration, combined therapy with nafcillin and gentamicin is recommended.

MONITORING CLINICAL RESPONSE. A decrease in fever is usually evident within 1 week of instituting appropriate antibiotic therapy; some patients become afebrile 24 to 48 hours after the start of therapy. Persistent fever during several weeks of appropriate antimicrobial therapy suggests the possibility of intracardiac abscess, metastatic foci of infection, and nosocomial complications of therapy. Petechiae and embolic phenomena may occur for several weeks after initiation of recommended treatment; such findings do not necessarily indicate that therapy is ineffective, particularly if other signs indicate the patient is getting better. Blood for cultures should be obtained on several occasions after antibiotic therapy is initiated if the patient does not become afebrile within a few days.

Antithrombotic Therapy

A decision regarding the use of antithrombotic therapy in patients with native or prosthetic valve endocarditis should be individualized. It should be based on whether the patient has cardiac or extracardiac disease that would warrant use of such therapy in the absence of endocarditis. In patients with prosthetic valves who have cardiac disease that requires long-term warfarin therapy, such therapy should be continued during endocarditis unless there are specific contraindications. The indications for anticoagulant therapy are uncertain when systemic embolism occurs during the course of infective endocarditis involving a native or bioprosthetic heart valve. The therapeutic decision should consider comorbid factors, including atrial fibrillation, evidence of left atrial thrombus, evidence and size of valvular vegetations, and the distribution and severity of embolism. There is an increased risk of hemorrhage in patients with emboli, and there is no evidence that antithrombotic therapy will prevent embolization of vegetations.

Surgical Intervention

Operative intervention to debride infected perivalvular tissue or to replace or reconstruct a dysfunctioning valve has a major role in the management of complicated infective endocarditis that involves either a native or a prosthetic valve. Several observations have prompted the increased use of surgery in the treatment of active endocarditis: (1) The mortality of patients undergoing valve surgery during active endocarditis is not greater than that of patients treated medically, (2) the risk that residual endocarditis from the initial infecting organism will develop on the newly implanted prosthesis is low, and (3) some intracardiac complications of endocarditis that cannot be remedied by antibiotic therapy can be corrected surgically. Long-term survival rates for patients who undergo valve replacement during active endocarditis are satisfactory.

The indications for surgical treatment of active native and prosthetic valve endocarditis have been developed through a retrospective analysis of therapy. Moderate to severe CHF from valve dysfunction or vegetations is the most widely accepted indication for valve replacement. Surgical intervention should also be considered when there is clinical evidence of perivalvular invasion and abscess formation and when infection remains uncontrolled despite maximal antimicrobial therapy. Fungal endocarditis and prosthetic valve endocarditis that occurs within a year after valve implantation caused by coagulase-negative organisms are treated surgically because they respond poorly to medical therapy. Because left-sided native valve endocarditis and prosthetic valve endocarditis caused by *S. aureus* are frequently invasive, early surgery should be considered for patients with these infections who do not show prompt and sustained improvement during antibiotic therapy.

EXERCISE: KEY FEATURE 4—EXERCISE CAPACITY OR EXERCISE INTOLERANCE

Treatment for Poor Exercise Capacity and Fatigue

In general, mild to moderate exercise is a reasonable prescription except when a disease state is acute or unstable. Exercise training has been the most definite way of improving exercise capacity in normal subjects and in patients with either ischemia or LV dysfunction. The concerned health care professional should counsel all patients to increase their dynamic, isotonic, aerobic exercise activity. The exercises that benefit the cardiovascular system are walking, biking, running, and swimming as opposed to isometric exercises like weight lifting. The AHA, American College of Sports Medicine (ACSM), and the CDC just raised physical inactivity to the status of the fourth risk factor (along with cigarette smoking, high BP, and hypercholesterolemia). The emphasis as a public health measure is on physical activity rather than exercise training. *For this reason, counseling patients to walk a continuous ½ hour every day and to progressively increase the speed is safe and appropriate.* Walking is even the best therapy for patients with claudication who should exercise to pain and then start again.

Individuals who want to improve their aerobic activity for higher levels of performance should be given an exercise prescription that is tailored to their state of health. Often an exercise test is the best way of determining the safety and appropriate level of such a prescription. The aerobic exercise should be performed at least three times a week and the training session should last at least ½ hour. The intensity should be set at approximately 70% of maximal effort as determined by the Borg scale or by a percentage of maximal heart rate. If ischemic signs or symptoms occur at this level, then the intensity should be lowered. Interval training where bouts of near-maximal exercise are included has been the way that aerobic capacity is really increased but this should only be included in the prescription for healthy individuals. Remember that training to higher levels does not have a particular health benefit and often leads to orthopedic injuries.

In studying changes in exercise capacity with serial testing, one of the problems is that habituation or learning occurs. Individuals will walk longer and to higher workloads without actually improving their maximal oxygen uptake. However, some of the vasodilators given for the treatment of chronic CHF and some of the antianginal agents have improved treadmill performance. This is not always persistent nor is it consistent. For instance, with long-acting nitrates, the various different preparations have varying rates of release and absorption, resulting in uncertain efficacy. Also, there appears to be a varying induction of tolerance, possibly due to individual variation.

ARRHYTHMIAS: KEY FEATURE 5— ARRHYTHMIAS AND CONDUCTION ABNORMALITIES

Treatment of Arrhythmias

Atrial Fibrillation

Atrial fibrillation is a chaotic atrial rhythm. The ECG's usual discrete atrial activity is replaced by an irregular undulating atrial activity and a variable R-R interval [51]. It increases in prevalence with age and its appearance is associated with a doubling of the expected mortality; the prognosis of "lone" atrial fibrillation is controversial.

SYMPTOMS.   Symptoms can include palpitations, fatigue, dyspnea, dizziness, and decreased exercise capacity.

THERAPEUTIC GOALS.   The three therapeutic goals are as follows:

1. *Rate control:* Quinidine should not be given prior to slowing the rate with digoxin since quinidine and similar agents can speed AV conduction. Diltiazem is preferable to a beta-blocker because exercise capacity is improved rather than impaired.
2. *Cardioversion and maintenance of sinus rhythm:* About 50% of patients presenting with new-onset atrial fibrillation will spontaneously convert within 2 days. Chemical cardioversion is usually 50% successful using quinidine, propafenone, flecainide, sotalol, or amiodarone. Usually two-thirds of treated patients stay in

sinus rhythm for 1 year. Patients with a history or findings of CHF should be hospitalized for chemical cardioversion because of the dangers of proarrhythmias. Unless the atrial fibrillation can be documented as being less than 24 hours' duration, *the patient should receive anticoagulation therapy for 3 weeks prior and 4 weeks after cardioversion.*

3. *Prevention of thromboembolism:* Without anticoagulation, the risk for thromboembolic stroke is about 1%/yr for low-risk patients and more than 5%/yr for high-risk patients. Aspirin is sufficient for low-risk patients while warfarin is needed for all others who do not have a contraindication. Usually one-fourth or more of the patients with atrial fibrillation are at high risk. Markers for high-risk patients are history of hypertension, prior stroke or TIA, diabetes, history of CHF, and age older than 65.

Treatment is determined by the underlying cause and chronicity of this arrhythmia. Figure 5-3 illustrates an approach to treatment dependent on the presentation timing of atrial fibrillation [52]. Infection, fever, hyperthyroidism, metabolic or electrolyte abnormalities, cardiomyopathy, MI, and valvular heart disease are all possibilities, although lone atrial fibrillation is possible. Usually a medical history and physical examination along with appropriate laboratory studies including thyroid function are indicated. Echocardiography including a Doppler study and measurement of chamber size (including the left atrium) is especially indicated. If the patient is at high risk for thrombi (i.e., previous emboli), TEE may be advisable and thrombi should be searched for during the echocardiographic study. Anticoagulation to reach an INR of 2.0 to 3.0 is indicated for 3 weeks prior to attempting cardioversion unless there are convincing data to support the acuteness of the atrial fibrillation or if there is hemodynamic compromise. Rate control can be accomplished by digoxin, diltiazem, or a beta-blocker, or a combination of these. Diltiazem is preferred over a beta-blocker because it preserves exercise capacity. Chemical cardioversion is usually attempted first using quinidine, procainamide (Pronestyl), or sotalol. Procainamide (IV) is the drug of choice if the conduction is over an accessory pathway (with Wolff-Parkinson-White syndrome). Patients with a history of CHF or documented structural heart disease should be admitted to the hospital for drug therapy

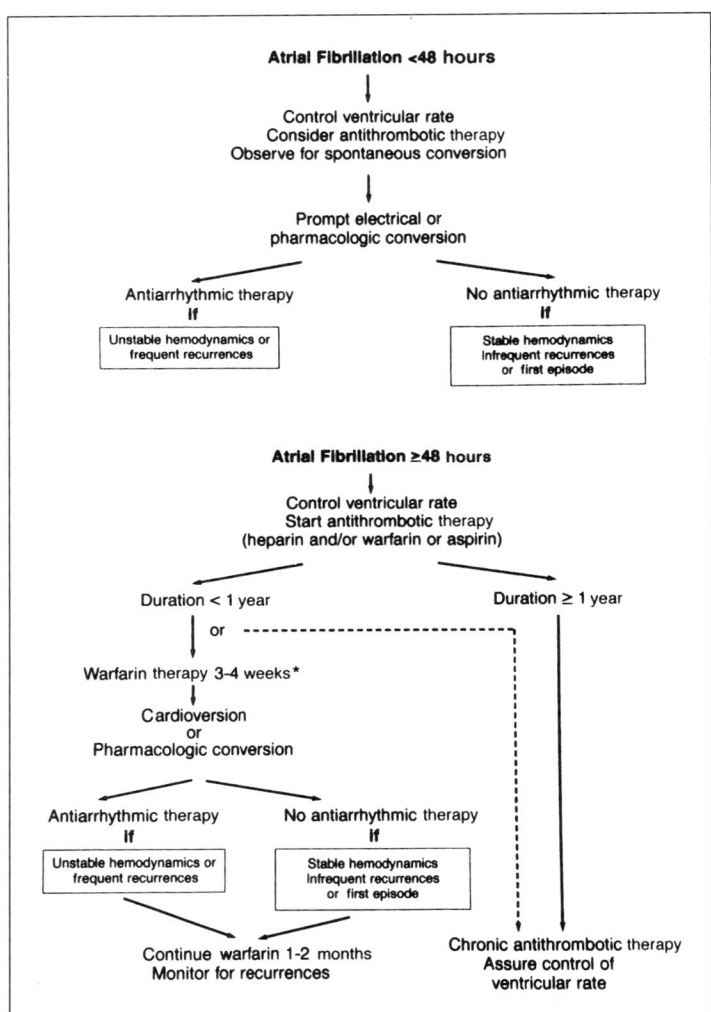

Fig. 5-3.   **Algorithms for the management of atrial fibrillation applicable to patients other than those with recent stroke.** *Consider transesophageal echocardiography; if no intracardiac thrombi are found, proceed directly to cardioversion while continuing anticoagulation therapy. The success rate of cardioversion exceeds that of pharmacologic conversion when the duration of atrial fibrillation is more than 2 or 3 days. (From H Golzari, RD Cebul, and RC Bahler. Atrial fibrillation: restoration and maintenance of sinus rhythm and indications for anticoagulation therapy. *Ann Intern Med* 1996;125:311–323.)

because of the danger of proarrhythmias. If this fails, the patient is admitted for direct electrical cardioversion. Electrical cardioversion is best carried out by an experienced cardiologist working with an anesthesiologist. The defibrillator should be synchronized on the QRS complex so that it does not induce ventricular fibrillation. Back-to-front paddles should be used, starting at 100 joules and progressing to 300 joules.

ETIOLOGY OR ASSOCIATED DISEASES.   The following are causative factors or diseases associated with atrial fibrillation [53]: rheumatic valvular disease (mitral stenosis), valvular heart disease, hypertension, coronary artery disease, hyperthyroidism and hypothyroidism, pericarditis, myocarditis, cardiomyopathy (dilated/hypertrophic), alcohol use (holiday heart syndrome), hemachromatosis, coronary bypass surgery, sick sinus syndrome (post-VVI permanent pacer placement), and pulmonary embolism.

Echocardiography with Doppler is the best test for assessing predictors for converting to or maintaining sinus rhythm. It can give information regarding:

- Left atrial size (diameter or area): an enlarged left atrium has a predisposition to atrial fibrillation but does not rule out the possibility of a successful cardioversion
- LV chamber dimensions and LV function
- LV wall thickness: usually due to high BP, a risk marker for atrial fibrillation
- Valve status (calcification, restricted motion, regurgitation by Doppler): mitral stenosis is particularly associated with atrial fibrillation
- Intracardiac filling abnormalities (i.e., thrombus, myxoma)
- Myocardial appearance: possible amyloid heart disease
- Pericardial effusion and membrane thickening: pericarditis is associated with atrial fibrillation

TEE has the advantages of providing a better imaging window: no lung, no chest wall, and potentially better visualization, particularly of the posterior structures. It provides a better view of the atria, particularly the left atrium which is posterior. Its disadvantages are that it is semiinvasive and expensive, and causes patient discomfort; the patient must be sedated and a physician must be present.

THERAPY.

Cardioversion.

Electrical cardioversion

Chemical cardioversion

Type I: antiarrhythmic drugs (quinidine, procainamide [drug of choice for Wolff-Parkinson-White syndrome], disopyramide)

Type Ic: antiarrhythmic drugs (encainide, flecainide, propafenone)

Type III: antiarrhythmic drugs (amiodarone, sotalol)

Rate Control (AV Nodal Suppressants).

Digoxin for control at rest

Beta-blockers (esmolol, propranolol, and atenolol)

Calcium channel blockers (verapamil, diltiazem)

Amiodarone

Nonmedical Rate Control.

Ablation of the AV node

Surgery (Maze procedure)

Rate-responsive pacing following catheter ablation of the AV node

Anticoagulation.

Warfarin (Coumadin) to INR of 2.0 to 3.0

Aspirin, 325 mg

Oral Dosing of Medications for AV Nodal Suppression.

Digoxin	0.125–0.5 mg qd
Diltiazem	90–360 mg total daily dose (60 mg tid)
Verapamil	120–360 mg total daily dose (40 mg tid)
Atenolol	25–100 mg qd
Metoprolol	25–100 mg qd
Propranolol	10–60 mg q4–6h
Sotalol	80–160 mg q12h
Amiodarone	200 mg qd
Propafenone	150–300 mg q8h
Flecainide	100–200 mg q12h

INTRAVENOUS AV NODAL SUPPRESSANT DRUGS.

Adenosine	6 mg IV push followed by 12 mg IV push
Digoxin	0.25 mg–1.00 mg
Verapamil	5–10-mg bolus; IV infusion by some studies 5–30 mg/hr
Diltiazem	25 mg/kg IV over 2 minutes (20 mg); 0.35 mg/kg IV (25 mg) 15 minutes later, IV maintenance infusion 5–15 mg/hr

Esmolol	0.25 mg/kg (10–20 mg); IV push 2–5 minutes; IV drip 0.050–0.200 mg/kg/min (3.0–12.0 mg/hr)
Metoprolol	5 mg q5min up to 15 mg (oral dosing q12h)
Propranolol	0.1 mg/kg divided into 3 doses q5–10min (follow 1 hour later by 200 mg q4–6h oral dosing)
Atenolol	5–10 mg IV (follow by 100 mg orally a day)

MAINTENANCE OF NORMAL SINUS RHYTHM. A meta-analysis was performed to evaluate the efficacy and safety of quinidine for the suppression of atrial fibrillation after cardioversion, through an analysis of randomized control trials in which the patients were followed for 3 to 12 months [54]. On blinded review, two independent readers agreed to the choice of six studies (of 52 on the topic) that met the following criteria: Patients had chronic atrial fibrillation (lasting > 72 hours), underwent cardioversion, and were randomized to quinidine-treatment or control groups; follow-up of patients allowed evaluation of efficacy at a minimum of 3 months; digoxin was the only other anti-arrhythmic agent allowed. The six trials included 808 patients, aged 15 to 79 years. Duration of atrial fibrillation was up to 10 years. Fifty-two percent of the patients had underlying valvular disease. Dosage and preparation of quinidine and use of placebos varied among the trials. Seven hundred twenty-seven patients (90%) were followed for at least 3 months. Three months after cardioversion, 70% of the patients taking quinidine and 45% of the control subjects were in sinus rhythm. giving a pooled rate difference of 25% in favor of quinidine. The rate differences at 6 months (23%) and 12 months (24%) also favored quinidine. The proportion of patients remaining in sinus rhythm steadily decreased to 50% of patients taking quinidine and 25% of control patients at 12 months. Of 373 patients receiving quinidine, 66 (18%) had side effects including diarrhea, syncope, and pyrexia. Twelve patients on quinidine died, 3 from sudden cardiac death. Three patients assigned to control groups died. The odds of dying for patients taking quinidine were about three times that for the control patients. Be very cautious about using quinidine: it reduces the recurrence of atrial fibrillation but may increase the risk of death. Thus, the value of therapy for maintenance of normal sinus rhythm after electrical cardioversion is controversial.

Amiodarone [55], sotalol [56], and propafenone may be effective for chemical cardioversion and maintenance of normal sinus rhythm but the studies with them are inconclusive. Quinidine and procainamide are both drugs with such irritating side effects that most patients do not tolerate them for long. Quinidine causes diarrhea and procainamide causes joint pains. The risk of torsades appears to be greatest during the early period after cardioversion. When patients should be hospitalized for the initiation of antiarrhythmic drug therapy remains controversial.

RISK OF EMBOLIC STROKE.   Atrial fibrillation is associated with an increased risk of ischemic stroke of about 5%/yr or 5/100 patient-yr. Data on individual patients with atrial fibrillation were pooled from five recently completed randomized trials comparing patients taking warfarin or aspirin with control subjects [57]. For the warfarin-control comparison there were 1,889 patient-yr for the warfarin group and 1,802 for the control group. For the aspirin-placebo comparison there were 1,132 patient-yr for the aspirin group and 1,133 for the placebo group. The daily dose of aspirin was 75 mg in the three trials and 325 mg in another. To monitor warfarin dosage, three studies used prothrombin time ratios and two used INRs. The lowest target intensity was a prothrombin time ratio of 1.2 to 1.5 and the highest target intensity was an INR of 2.8 to 4.2. The primary end points were ischemic stroke and major hemorrhage, as assessed by each study. Patients younger than 65 years who had none of the other predictive factors (15% of all patients) had an annual rate of stroke of 1.0%. The annual rate of stroke was 4.5% for the control group and 1.4% for the warfarin group (risk reduction, 68%). The efficacy of warfarin was consistent across all studies and subgroups of patients. In women, warfarin decreased the risk of stroke by 84%, compared with 60% in men.

The efficacy of aspirin was not as consistent. The risk reduction with 75 mg of aspirin in the Atrial Fibrillation, Aspirin, Anticoagulation Study was 18%, and 44% with 325 mg of aspirin in the Stroke Prevention in Atrial Fibrillation Study. When both studies were combined, the risk reduction was 36%. The annual rates of major stroke were 1.0% for the control group, 1.0% for the aspirin group, and 1.3% for the warfarin group. Thus, warfarin decreases the risk of stroke in patients with atrial fibrillation (a 68% reduction in risk) with no increase in the frequency of major bleeding. The efficacy of aspirin is less consistent than that of warfarin, particularly in the elderly. *Patients with atrial fibrillation younger than 65 years without a history of hypertension, LV dysfunction, previous stroke or TIA, or diabetes are at very low risk of stroke even when not treated.*

TRANSESOPHAGEAL ECHOCARDIOGRAPHY TO RULE OUT EMBOLIZATION. Recent studies proposed that the exclusion of an atrial thrombus by TEE would allow for the safe cardioversion from atrial fibrillation or flutter without the need of prophylactic anticoagulation [58]. Because all of the TEE trials were small, descriptive and lacked randomized, conventionally treated control groups, the pooled risk of embolic events from TEE trials was compared with that of a control group pooled from the literature on cardioversion both with and without conventional anticoagulation. Embolic events were significantly more frequent in the TEE group than in the anticoagulation control group (1.34 vs 0.33%, respectively), whereas there was no significant difference between the TEE group and the nonanticoagulation control group (2%). Thus, TEE screening to exclude patients with atrial thrombi before cardioversion *does not* identify patients who can safely undergo cardioversion without anticoagulation.

ANTICOAGULATION. Warfarin therapy decreases the rate of stroke by about 68% in patients with nonvalvular atrial fibrillation. The efficacy of aspirin is not as defined, but it is known to be less than that of warfarin. A collaborative analysis [59] using a Cox proportional hazards model to analyze data from five of the nonvalvular atrial fibrillation trials identified subgroups of patients with nonvalvular atrial fibrillation at low, medium, and high risk of stroke. The subgroup with the lowest rate (1–3%/yr) of stroke were those patients with lone atrial fibrillation–nonvalvular atrial fibrillation without a history of stroke, TIA, hypertension, diabetes, or heart disease. Patients with nonvalvular atrial fibrillation who had heart disease (defined as angina, CHF, or a prior MI) had a medium rate (3–4%/yr) of stroke. Patients who had the highest rate (≥5%/yr) of stroke had at least one of the following: a history of stroke, TIA, diabetes, or hypertension. In fact, the rate of stroke in these patients is comparable to patients with atrial fibrillation and mitral stenosis. Patients at moderate or high risk of stroke should be offered warfarin therapy if they are good anticoagulation candidates. In contrast, the rate of stroke in patients with lone atrial fibrillation is so low without warfarin therapy that many experts would treat these patients with aspirin therapy (especially patients < 75 years old) or, in some cases, omit prophylaxis entirely.

Treatment of AF is dependent on the age of the patient and other risk factors. Risk factors for CVA with AF include previous TIA or stroke, hypertension, heart failure, diabetes, clinical coronary artery disease, mitral stenosis, prosthetic heart valves, and thyrotoxicosis. Treatment is directed by the guidelines indicated below.

Age	Risk Markers	Recommended Treatment
Age < 65	Risk markers	Warfarin INR 2 to 3
Age < 65	No risk markers	ASA or nothing
Age 65 to 75	Risk markers	Warfarin INR 2 to 3
Age 65 to 75	No risk markers	Warfarin or ASA
Age > 75		Warfarin INR 2 to 3

Premature Ventricular Contractions

BENIGN ARRHYTHMIAS.   Frequent PVCs (>5/hr or 100/24 hr), ventricular couplets, or tachycardia are not common in the normal population. Individuals who have frequent PVCs (>5/hr) or repetitive PVCs (e.g., nonsustained ventricular tachycardia) without underlying structural heart disease may be considered to have primary electrical cardiac disease. These patients have a very low risk for the development of sudden cardiac death. Therapy is directed toward the elimination of symptoms such as palpitations or dizziness, if present. Often, reassurance or use of a minor tranquilizer is sufficient and is to be desired, as the treatment is often more dangerous than the PVCs. We have seen surprising arrhythmias in pilots and athletes that disappear as mysteriously as they appear. There is controversy over the relationship of the more common forms of mitral valve prolapse to PVCs, but a recent finding has been an association with hypertrophied myocardial trabeculations and right ventricular dysplasia. The axiom that the clinical significance of arrhythmias relates to the company they keep (i.e., CHF, ischemia) holds true.

Treatable causes of increased PVCs should be carefully sought [60]. These include electrolyte abnormalities, medications, cardiac dilation due to early CHF, ischemia, a recent infection, increase in caffeine ingestion (carbonated drinks often contain caffeine in addition to coffee and tea), and stress. There are individuals who develop surprising arrhythmias when subjected to psychological stress. Whether or not mitral valve prolapse or trabeculations of hypertrophied LV muscle are associated with an increased prevalence of PVCs is debated. Beta-blockers and verapamil have often been found to be effective for suppressing exercise-induced ventricular tachycardia or PVCs. Beta-blockers are effective in the post-MI period most likely because they raise the electrical threshold for ventricular tachycardia. This action is not present in beta-blockers with intrinsic sympathetic activity. Many of the antiarrhythmic drugs can actually increase the PVC frequency in up to 10% of patients.

LETHAL ARRHYTHMIAS. Patients with paroxysmal sustained ventricular tachycardia can, in general, be considered to have a high risk of sudden death. The vast majority of these patients have a LV ejection fraction of 30% or less. In such patients, even the presence of nonsustained ventricular tachycardia (usually defined as <15 seconds of self-terminating rhythm disturbance) may cause important hemodynamic symptoms. The most important feature of this type of PVC presentation is that the rhythm disturbance can cause severe hemodynamic consequences, usually manifesting itself as syncope, presyncope, unstable angina, or exacerbation of CHF. Patients with good ventricular function may tolerate these rhythms surprisingly well. The indications for treatment of such patients are immediate relief of hemodynamic symptoms and prevention of sudden cardiac death. These patients almost always must be treated in a monitored facility in the hospital. Sudden cardiac death can be prevented by the use of electrophysiologic tests or ambulatory ECG monitoring to properly select the medication that eliminates inducible sustained ventricular tachycardia. Automatic implantable cardioverter-defibrillators (AICDs) or implantable defibrillators can now be placed transvenously and appear to be cost-effective.

COMPLEX OR FREQUENT VENTRICULAR ARRHYTHMIAS. The much more common clinical presentation of PVCs is seen in patients with heart disease but in whom the presence of PVCs causes no important hemodynamic consequence. These patients may occasionally feel palpitations or dizziness, but most are unaware of them. Some of these patients may have frequent episodes of nonsustained ventricular tachycardia or PVC frequency up to 3,000/hr in a 24-hour period. In patients who have such chronic PVCs without hemodynamically important effects or symptoms, there is controversy as to whether therapy will have an impact on preventing sudden cardiac death prevalence.

Ambulatory (Holter) monitoring is the logical approach for diagnostic and therapeutic decisions. Exercise testing is complementary and especially indicated when PVCs are associated with exertion. Exercise-induced ventricular tachycardia has been successfully treated with beta-blockers or verapamil.

IMPLANTABLE DEFIBRILLATORS. Today, nonspecialists more frequently may interact with patients who have implantable defibrillators. The capacity of implantable defibrillators to recognize and treat tachyarrhythmias can be temporarily disabled by placing a magnet on top of the device [61]. General surgery, radiotherapy, lithotripsy, and electroconvulsive therapy can usually be safely done under continuous ECG monitoring in patients with implantable defibrillators. The device should be deactivated before the procedure and reactivated and reassessed immediately afterward. MRI is usually contraindicated in patients with implantable defibrillators. The presence of an implantable defibrillator should not deter standard resuscitation techniques. Multiple defibrillator discharges in a short period of time represent a serious problem. Causes of multiple discharges include ventricular electrical instability, inefficient defibrillation, nonsustained ventricular tachycardia, and inappropriate shocks caused by supraventricular tachyarrhythmias or oversensing of signals. Patients with frequent discharges should be initially evaluated in a setting that allows ECG monitoring and cardiac resuscitation. The defibrillator should be deactivated by a specialist and replaced if inappropriate firing is documented. Infections of implantable defibrillator systems are potentially life-threatening, and empirical oral antibiotic therapy should never be given when this possibility exists. Adjustment disorders specific to the defibrillator, including anxiety with secondary panic reaction; defibrillator dependence, abuse, or withdrawal; and imaginary shocks, are not uncommon.

THE CLINICAL APPROACH TO THE HIGH-RISK PATIENT. Once PVCs are identified, one must be certain that it is not secondary to an easily correctable cause such as a metabolic abnormality (e.g., hypokalemia), a toxic reaction to a drug (e.g., toxic reactions to digoxin), ischemia, hypoxia, or myocardial dilation due to CHF. An associated conduction abnormality or the presence of a long QT-interval syndrome will influence selection of proper therapy. The initiation of oral antiarrhythmic therapy is rational only if its effect on the frequency of the PVCs is monitored. In fact, it is now clear that at least 10% of patients so treated may have an adverse reaction to such therapy in the form of exacerbation of PVCs ("proarrhythmic event"). A therapeutic effect is often difficult to define in view of the extreme daily variability. There is no need to follow antiarrhythmic drug blood levels.

DRUG THERAPY FOR VENTRICULAR ARRHYTHMIAS. Often drug therapy for arrhythmias is more dangerous than effective. The Cardiac Arrhythmia Suppression Trial (CAST) dramatically changed the way cardiologists have treated ventricular arrhythmias [62]. Previously, PVC counts were assessed using ambulatory monitoring to document drug response, and antiarrhythmic drug blood levels were frequently measured to maintain adequate blood levels. In CAST, which was a randomized trial, post-MI patients with PVCs that could be suppressed with encainide or flecainide (both more effective and better tolerated than quinidine or procainamide) were randomized to receive drug or placebo. Mortality was two to three times higher in the treated group. CAST 2 demonstrated a higher mortality with another drug, moricizine, than placebo. Mexiletine and disopyramide have done no better while amiodarone may be beneficial. Beta-blockers clearly reduce mortality after MI but do not necessarily lessen the number of PVCs. Studies have not supported that antiarrhythmic therapy lessens symptoms in patients with PVCs or nonsustained ventricular tachycardia. The more reliable end point is survival and not lessening of the ventricular ectopy.

Antiarrhythmic drugs can exacerbate arrhythmias, as exemplified by atrial flutter with 1 : 1 AV conduction due to quinidine and propafenone and increased PVCs or ventricular tachycardia with many drugs. Even lidocaine given after an MI is associated with increased mortality, probably due to depression of LV function and CHF. Torsades de pointes is a polymorphic ventricular tachycardia associated with prolonged QT interval, and is due to drugs including quinidine and sotalol and can be exacerbated by hypokalemia and bradycardia. Some of the newer antihistamines have been associated with this and should be avoided in patients with heart disease. Other cardiac side effects of antiarrhythmic drugs are heart block and CHF.

The EP versus ECG Monitoring (ESVEM) study demonstrated either electrophysiologic studies or ambulatory monitoring to be effective in choosing drug therapy for patients with sustained ventricular tachycardia/cardiac arrest and that sotalol was more effective than other agents [63]. Studies comparing AICD, amiodarone, and sotalol are in progress.

Heart Block

Heart block and cardiogenic syncope require referral to a cardiologist. *Cardiogenic syncope is usually not associated with the aura and postictal phases of neurogenic syncopy and has both a sudden onset and offset.* Often a pacemaker is required; however, a thorough work-up should be performed. It is very disappointing when a patient with syncope continues to lose consciousness after pacemaker insertion.

Pacemakers

Dual-chamber pacemakers have been in use for more than 15 years. Although they may confer a physiologic advantage over single-chamber ventricular pacemakers, they are more expensive and have a generally shorter service life than do single-chamber devices. While dual-chamber pacing is commonly used, possible contraindications to dual-chamber pacing are chronic atrial fibrillation, atrial tachycardias, poor prognosis or disability, or dominant sinus rhythm.

Data on pacemaker implantation were obtained from the Medical Device Implant Supplement to the 1988 National Health Interview Survey, a nationally representative, population-based survey of 47,485 households (122,310 persons) [64]. The survey yielded an estimate of a half million adults with pacemakers (prevalence, 2.6/1,000). Prevalence rose significantly with age, from 0.4/1,000 among persons ages 18 to 64, to 26/1,000 among those ages 75 or older. Age-adjusted prevalence in males was 1.5 times that in females, and in whites 1.6 times that in nonwhites, although these differences were of borderline statistical significance. Prevalence did not vary significantly by region of residence, educational level, or income, but was significantly increased (more than threefold) in those reporting any activity limitation compared with those with no limitation. Fifteen percent of pacemakers in use were replacements; about one-fifth of these had been replaced more than twice. Sixty percent of previous pacemakers had been in place for at least 5 years. Pacemaker insertion prevalence is almost twice as high in the US as in other developed countries.

INDICATIONS FOR PERMANENT PACEMAKER THERAPY.
Symptomatic bradycardia:
Syncope or near syncope
TIAs, light-headedness
Exercise intolerance or CHF
Heart block with ventricular response less than 40 bpm
and/or asystole for longer than 4 seconds
Hypersensitive carotid sinus with syncope

Heart block is usually temporary with inferior MIs while it can be permanent with anterior MIs. Rare indica-tions are for IHSS, for CHF, and after ablation for atrial fibrillation. Ambulatory ECG monitoring is absolutely necessary to document the relationship of bradycardia to symptoms. Pacemakers are currently rarely used for tachyarrhythmias because catheter radiofrequency abla-tion is usually successful.

PULSE WIDTH AND THRESHOLD.   Pulse width and thresh-old voltage are inversely related. Threshold voltage is low initially, then increases only to stabilize at a lower level several months after lead wire placement. Current models are characterized by a pulse width of 0.1 to 2.0 msec with a constant current voltage limit. There is no increase in impedance due to fibrous tissue growth at the pacemaker wire contact point. A temporary pacemaker should not be used to determine the threshold for permanent pacemak-ers. Little improvement in threshold occurs with a pulse width greater than 0.6 msec and no improvement occurs with a width greater than 1.2 msec.

EXTERNAL PROGRAMMING.   External programming with pulsed magnetic or radiofrequency signals can accomplish the following:

1. Decreasing either the pulse width or voltage can lengthen battery life and avoid complications like pec-toral muscle twitching and diaphragmatic pacing.
2. The sensitivity can be programmed for voltage and slew rate.
3. The refractory period of sensing can be set so that the T wave is not sensed (nor the QRS or afterpotential sensed either).
4. The refractory period can be shortened to allow sensing of PVCs.
5. The atrial refractory period of a dual-chamber pace-maker can be lengthened to avoid endless loop pacemaker-mediated tachyarrhythmias.

6. Hysteresis programmability can maintain sinus rhythm longer in a patient who becomes bradycardiac periodically but requires an initial faster rate.
7. The mode is programmable as ventricular demand, ventricular triggered, or asynchronous.

PACEMAKER FUNCTION CODE. The pacemaker function code is provided by the manufacturers by the following letters in five positions:

First: chamber paced—V for ventricular, A for atrial, D for dual for both atrial and ventricular, and 0 for none
Second: chamber sensed
Third: response to a sensed beat—T for triggered, I for inhibited, D for double (AT/VI or AI/VI), 0 for none or asynchronous
Fourth: programmability—P for simple, M for multiple, C for communicating (telemetry), R for rate modulation, and 0 for none
Fifth: antitachycardia function—P for pacing, S for shock and dual

Types of Pacemakers. The types of pacemakers commercially available are listed below:

VVI: ventricular demand
VVIR: ventricular demand with rate responsiveness
VVT: ventricular triggered
AAI: atrial demand
AAIR: atrial demand with rate responsiveness
VAT: P-wave synchronous
VDD: modern P-wave synchronous
DVI: AV sequential—dual-chamber paced, sensing only in the ventricle
DDD: fully automatic (optimal, physiologic, and universal), currently the most commonly used
DDDR: fully automatic rate responsive
DDIR and DVIR: unusual mode for patients with sinus node dysfunction and with questionable AV conduction

PACEMAKER-MEDIATED TACHYCARDIA. Retrograde AV conduction of ventricular pacing can cause an inverted P wave and an endless loop or circus tachycardia. This can be stopped by blocking ventricular-atrial conduction (do not use drugs!) or by blocking sensing in the atria (apply a magnet) or programming prolongation of the atrial refractory period.

PACEMAKER FOLLOW-UP. Follow-up must be conducted by someone who understands the technical function of the pacemaker and who is capable of diagnosing and dealing with complex arrhythmias. Patients should understand their pacemaker and carry a card providing information regarding brand, model, serial number, rate, and pulse width settings. Household appliances no longer interfere with pacemaker function but electrical generators and MRI machines can be a problem. Formal follow-up in a clinic or via telephone is advantageous because

1. Notification of recalls will be sooner and less stressful. It is much better for the patient to hear about this from his or her care provider rather than in the news.
2. Rare asymptomatic malfunctions will be noted.
3. The patient can be reassured and questions can be answered.
4. Pacemaker site infection or hemorrhage can be recognized.

PACEMAKER INTERROGATION.   Measurement and manipulation of pulse width threshold as a basis for establishing the pulse width are unnecessary, making telephone monitoring preferable. This is easily performed with the available simple devices. The transtelephonically recorded ECG strip is used to evaluate function by distinguishing between complexes initiated by the pacemaker and by the patient. By placing a magnet (usually specific for a particular model) over the generator in the office, the sensing circuit is disabled and the pacemaker becomes asynchronous, regularly firing and ignoring the patient's intrinsic electrical activity. Theoretically, a pacemaker spike on a T wave could cause ventricular fibrillation but this has not happened in clinical use. Some models have very complex magnet responses. Telemetry can be used to program and interrogate most modern pacemakers. If a very low impedance is found by interrogation, a break in insulation is likely and a high impedance suggests a lead wire break or connection problem.

PHYSICAL EXAMINATION.   Physical examination including carotid massage, pressure over the pacemaker, and arm movements may be helpful in diagnosing pacemaker problems. Rarely are pacemaker wire sounds heard that imitate clicks or systolic ejection sounds.

ECG FINDINGS.   There is a wide QRS complex with ventricular pacers that makes ECG interpretation impossible. Often, computerized ECG machines do not recognize the pacemaker spikes and print out undetermined rhythm with intraventricular conduction defect. ECG abnormalities consistent with pacemaker malfunction that require diagnosis and action include lack of or intermittent capture, no pacemaker spikes, rate change, lack of appropriate sensing, and intermittent or erratic prolongation of the pacing spike interval. A pacemaker-mediated tachycardia may also be demonstrated on the ECG. Complex arrhythmias require consultation with an expert but placement of the magnet over the device may resolve an emergency.

PACING COMPLICATIONS NOT RELATED TO ECG ABNORMALITIES.

1. *Pacemaker syndrome.* This is when the following symptoms occur or worsen after initiation of pacing (usually ventricular): light-headedness, shortness of breath, CHF, syncope associated with hypotension, neck fullness, vagal symptoms, and pounding in the head. The most striking symptoms occur when retrograde AV nodal conduction occurs. AV sequential pacing avoids this syndrome.

2. *Diaphragmatic stimulation.* This can be due to right ventricular perforation, which surprisingly may not necessitate removal. Regardless, reprogramming of the pacemaker can stop this from occurring.

3. *Pectoral muscle stimulation.* This can be due to unipolar pacing or a lead break but usually can be stopped by reprogramming of the pacemaker.

4. *Infection.* A pacemaker does not necessitate antibiotic prophylaxis before dental or surgical procedures. Infection can occur usually shortly after implantation and necessitates removal. Gentle, constant traction has been recommended to pull out the leads but surgical removal has been reported. Antibiotics naturally should be tried first, but the infection is difficult to eradicate. An infectious disease expert should be consulted.

5. *Erosion.* The pacemaker can erode the overlying skin but fortunately this is a rare problem that requires consultation with a plastic surgeon.

6. *Thrombosis.* The vein containing the electrode lead wire usually thromboses but this should not cause a problem nor be treated.

7. *Manipulation by the patient.* Twiddler's syndrome is when a patient rotates the pacemaker, causing hemorrhage or lead breaks.

8. *Runaway pacemaker.* Pacemaker-induced tachycardia rarely occurs but could necessitate skin incision and cutting the leads.

9. *Allergic reactions*. These are rare and simulate an infection.

INTERFERENCE WITH PACEMAKERS CAN COME FROM THE FOLLOWING ELECTRICAL ENERGY SOURCES:

1. Galvanic—Direct Contact Required.

Electrocautery. Surgery in pacemaker patients should not present problems but electrocautery may cause sensing problems. A cardiologist and the pacemaker's manufacturer should be consulted.

Cardioversion/defibrillation. The lowest effective energy and anterior-posterior paddles should be used with the anterior paddle as far from the pacemaker as possible.

2. Electromagnetic—Direct Contact Not Required.

Electroconvulsive therapy. This is less likely to cause a problem but again consultation is necessary.

MRI. The intense magnetic fields generated by these devices can damage pacemakers so MRI studies are contraindicated unless the pacemaker manufacturer says otherwise.

Radiation therapy. Standard x-ray imaging is not a problem but therapeutic radiation devices can damage a pacemaker.

MI diagnosis. It is better to rely on other techniques than the ECG, including technetium pyrophosphate imaging.

Lithotripsy. Consultation with a cardiologist and the manufacturer is indicated.

The following can cause interference rarely but not damage. They should be considered when associated with pacemaker failure:

Catheter ablation.
Diathermy.
Arc welding.
Transcutaneous nerve stimulation.
Weapon detectors.
Very large stereo speakers.

RECOMMENDATIONS FOR PACEMAKERS AND IMPLANTED CARDIOVERTER-DEFIBRILLATORS IN THE OPERATING ROOM.

1. It is important that the pacemaker manufacturer and model number be identified prior to any elective operative procedure.

2. Older pacemakers (in general, >5 years old) should be scheduled for evaluation preoperatively.

3. If electrocautery is to be used, every effort should be made to use bipolar cautery. If this is unacceptable,

unipolar cautery should be used cautiously, with the grounding placed far away from the pacemaker site (i.e., the leg). No electrocautery should be used within 6 cm of the implanted pacemaker [65].

Syncope

Syncope is a brief sudden loss of consciousness and muscle tone secondary to cerebral ischemia or inadequate oxygen or glucose delivery to the brain. Syncopal episodes are relatively common [66]. The causes of syncope may be benign and require very little in the way of evaluation or treatment. Micturition syncope and vasovagal syncope after the sight of blood are common in healthy young individuals. However, syncope may be the harbinger of sudden death, and extensive evaluation and monitoring may be appropriate. The history is the most important clue when attempting to identify which patient with syncope is at risk for sudden death, including use of medications such as vasodilators or antidepressants. Cardiogenic syncope is usually not associated with the aura and postictal phases of neurogenic syncopy and has both a sudden onset and offset. A careful cardiac and neurologic examination should be performed in any patient presenting with syncope, including the measurement of orthostatic BP. Selective use of laboratory testing and cardiac monitoring may assist the practitioner in making the diagnosis. Most often patients with syncope will have a benign cause such as vasovagal events, hyperventilation, or orthostatic hypotension. The cause is frequently problematic if the diagnosis is not quickly made after the initial clinical and laboratory evaluation. The periodic and unpredictable frequency of events with days to years separating spells and a high remission rate are obstacles to diagnosis.

Patients with a cardiac condition causing their syncope are at increased risk for sudden death [67]. The ominous, cardiac-related causes of syncope in the younger population include hypertrophic cardiomyopathy, aberrant coronary arteries, and aortic dissection secondary to Marfan's syndrome or cystic medial necrosis. In the older population, coronary or cerebral atherosclerosis may present as syncope. Dysrhythmias may be the cause of syncope in both populations.

Etiologies of Syncope

A variety of etiologies can underlie syncope, and the cause is often multifactorial. Prodromal symptoms often accompany fainting of vasovagal origin, while the occurrence of syncope without warning in a patient with cardiac problems suggests arrhythmia. Many medications, including antihypertensive drugs, antidepressant drugs, and digitalis, may be responsible for episodes of fainting. The physical examination of a patient with a history of syncope includes measurement of orthostatic BP, as well as careful cardiovascular and neurologic evaluations. The decision to use ancillary laboratory and ECG testing is guided by the patient's history and the findings on physical examination. Although new technologies can aid in the diagnosis of syncope, they should not be used routinely.

DIFFERENTIATION OF ETIOLOGIES.   A study was undertaken to identify and quantitate the symptoms associated with neurocardiogenic syncope, syncope due to ventricular tachycardia, and syncope resulting from AV block [38]. Eighty patients referred for evaluation of syncope in whom a diagnosis of neurocardiogenic syncope, AV block, or ventricular tachycardia was established were studied. Each patient was interviewed using a standard questionnaire. The clinical histories were then compared to identify which variables best differentiated the cause of syncope. The clinical histories of patients with syncope due to ventricular tachycardia or AV block were similar. Only age, the duration of prodromal symptoms, diaphoresis prior to syncope, and fatigue following syncope differed. In contrast, the clinical history in patients with neurocardiogenic syncope differed greatly from that in patients with syncope due to AV block or ventricular tachycardia. Features of the clinical history that were predictive of syncope due to AV block or ventricular tachycardia were *male gender, age older than 54 years, two or fewer episodes of syncope, and a duration of warning of less than 5 seconds*. Features of the clinical history predictive of syncope not due to ventricular tachycardia or AV block were palpitations, blurred vision, nausea, warmth, diaphoresis, or light-headedness prior to syncope, and nausea, warmth, diaphoresis, or fatigue following syncope.

NEURALLY MEDIATED SYNCOPE (COMMON FAINT OR VASOVAGAL RESPONSE).   Neurally mediated syncope is the most frequent cause of syncope in patients who do not have structural heart disease [69]. Precipitating factors include heat, hunger, emotional upset, and venipuncture. It is associated with prodromal symptoms such as palor, sweating, nausea, and blurry vision. Neurally mediated syncope is believed to be a reflex triggered by excessive afferent discharge from mechanoreceptors located in the arterial tree or viscera, particularly the LV. In response to these signals, a CNS-mediated sudden rise in parasympathetic efferent activity occurs, causing relative or absolute bradycardia and sympathetic inhibition with arterial vasodilation and hypotension. Although the understanding of the pathophysiology of this syndrome is still incomplete, it is well established that sympathetic nerve activity and norepinephrine release decrease inappropriately during neurally mediated syncope, whereas appropriate increases in plasma concentrations of epinephrine, angiotensin II, vasopressin, and endothelin-1 occur. The diagnosis of neurally mediated syncope can be made with acceptable levels of specificity and sensitivity by the upright tilt test.

HEAD-UP TILT TEST. Head-up tilt testing has gained broad acceptance as a reliable diagnostic method for the assessment of patients with recurrent unexplained syncope. *A positive test result is defined as syncope, near syncope or extreme light-headedness associated with hypotension or bradycardia, or both.* The development of head-up tilt testing has provided a method for studying the mechanisms, clarifying the diagnosis, and evaluating treatment of neurocardiogenic syncope, or what was formerly described as vasovagal or vasodepressor syncope. The triggering event for an episode of neurocardiogenic syncope is thought to be an increase in adrenergic tone resulting in activation of cardiopulmonary mechanoreceptors that may overwhelm or reverse normal compensatory mechanisms and result in paradoxical hypotension, bradycardia, or both. Therefore, the rationale for the use of beta-adrenergic blocking agents is to block the initial increase in adrenergic tone and thus interrupt the cascade of inappropriate and exaggerated neurocardiac and peripheral vascular adjustments that lead to syncope.

Once the diagnosis of neurocardiogenic syncope is established, there is no consensus on treatment. The efficacy of drug therapy in preventing a recurrence of symptoms in such patients is not entirely clear, and controversies exist regarding the need to confirm the effects of pharmacologic interventions. Clinical follow-up was obtained in 303 patients with a history of syncope and positive results on head-up tilt testing [70]. After the diagnostic head-up tilt, patients were assigned to different therapeutic approaches according to their preference or logistic impediments. Of 303 patients, 44 received empiric therapy,

210 were treated with medications proved effective during repeated head-up tilt testing, and 49 refused or discontinued medical therapy. The three groups were similar with regard to age, sex, and clinical presentation. The mean follow-up time was 3 years. Among the patients treated according to head-up tilt–guided therapy, 130 were on beta-blockers; 35, on theophylline; 10, on ephedrine; 31, on disopyramide; and 4, on miscellaneous regimens. Empiric treatment consisted of beta-blockers in 37 of 44 patients and other drugs in the remaining patients. During the follow-up, recurrence of symptoms was experienced in 12 (6%) of the 210 patients receiving the head-up tilt–guided therapy, 16 (36%) of 44 in the empirical therapy group, and 33 (67%) of 49 in the no-therapy group. Recurrence of symptoms in patients on empirical or no therapy was significantly more frequent as compared to the head-up tilt–guided therapy group. In patients with unexplained syncope and positive results on upright tilt testing, therapeutic strategies based on the response during the head-up tilt were effective in reducing symptoms during follow-up.

In another study, IV propranolol was effective in preventing neurocardiogenic syncope diagnosed during head-up tilt testing and predicted the response to oral beta-blocker therapy. Oral beta-blocker therapy prevented recurrent syncope in the majority of patients. Recurrence of syncope was lowest when efficacy of oral beta-blocker therapy was confirmed by repeat head-up tilt testing [71].

To demonstrate the prognosis of patients manifesting prolonged asystole during head-up tilt testing, 209 consecutive patients with a history of syncope and positive results on the head-up tilt test were studied [72]. Nineteen patients had asystole lasting longer than 5 seconds (mean duration, 15 seconds). When compared with patients without asystole, these patients were younger (32 vs 47 years), but clinical manifestations were not any more dramatic (both reported seven or eight episodes) and injuries during syncope (2 vs 13 patients) were similar. During follow-up (mean, 2 years), with the patients taking pharmacologic therapy such as beta-blockers, ephedrine, theophylline, or disopyramide, the recurrence rate was about 10% in both groups. No patient in the asystole group underwent pacemaker implantation. Additionally, of 75 normal volunteers with no history of syncope undergoing tilt tests to define its specificity, 3 had asystole with a mean duration of 10 seconds. During follow-up, despite no treatment, all

3 remained symptom free. Thus, asystole during head-up tilt testing does not predict either a more malignant outcome or a poor response to pharmacologic therapy. Moreover, an asystolic response does not enhance the specificity of the head-up tilt test because it may be present in asymptomatic "normal" volunteers.

ELECTROPHYSIOLOGIC STUDY FOR EVALUATION OF SYNCOPE. To validate a model for predicting the outcome of electrophysiologic testing in patients with unexplained syncope, 141 consecutive patients (96 men; mean age, 59 years) who had electrophysiologic testing for syncope were studied [73]. Six clinical predictors (three for ventricular tachyarrhythmias and three for bradyarrhythmias) were compared with the test results. Audit of medical charts gave historical, physical, and investigative findings for organic heart disease. ECG abnormalities noted were PVCs (>3 PVCs/min, multiform or salvos of PVCs), first-degree heart block (PR interval >0.2 second), bundle-branch block, and sinus bradycardia (<50 bpm). Nonsustained ventricular tachycardia was assessed from 24-hour Holter monitoring. The gold standard was electrophysiologic testing. Ventricular tachyarrhythmias were defined as sustained ventricular tachycardia longer than 30 seconds or requiring cardioversion because of hemodynamic compromise; nonsustained, reproducible ventricular tachycardia of more than 6 beats with severe symptoms or compromise; or ventricular fibrillation induced by ventricular extrastimuli. Bradyarrhythmic outcomes were defined as AV nodal effective refractory period longer than 425 msec, prolonged His-ventricular interval longer than 90 msec, prolonged corrected sinus node recovery time longer than 1,000 msec, or spontaneous infra-Hisian block or Mobitz type II AV block during incremental atrial pacing. Electrophysiologic studies identified 18 patients (12%) with ventricular tachyarrhythmic outcomes and 28 (20%) with bradyarrhythmic outcomes. *Ventricular tachyarrhythmia was predicted by organic heart disease (odds ratio [OR] 9), frequent PVCs on ECG (OR, 2), and nonsustained ventricular tachycardia on Holter monitoring (OR, 3). Bradyarrhythmia was predicted by sinus bradycardia (OR, 6), first-degree heart block (OR, 2), and bundle-branch block (OR, 3).* The sensitivity of the presence of more than one tachyarrhythmic predictor was 100% and of more than one bradyarrhythmic predictor was 79%. Thus, electrophysiologic testing provides useful information in patients with one or more clinical predictors. For patients without these predictors, electrophysiologic testing has little diagnostic benefit. The most important practice recommendation that can be derived from this is that electrophysiologic tests for inducible ventricular tachyarrhythmias generally should not be necessary in patients with syncope who have no evidence of organic heart disease and no substantial ventricular ectopy (frequent PVCs or nonsustained ventricular tachycardia) on Holter monitoring. An important point is that patients with unexplained syncope should probably be assessed by Holter monitoring for at least 48 hours before it is concluded that no substantial ventricular ectopy exists. Electrophysiologic testing has a moderately high yield of inducible ventricular tachyarrhythmias in patients with syncope and organic heart disease, substantial ventricular ectopy, or both on ECG monitoring, and a high yield of bradyarrhythmic outcomes in patients with first-degree heart block, bundle-branch block, or sinus bradycardia of less than 50 bpm on initial ECG.

Electrophysiologic testing has its highest yield and is most cost-effective in patients with heart disease. Patients with inducible ventricular tachycardia have a poorer prognosis than those without it. The prognosis has not been universally improved by therapy guided by electrophysiologic testing, possibly because the action of the antiarrhythmic drugs is different when acutely and chronically administered.

MISCELLANEOUS CARDIAC EVALUATIONS: PREOPERATIVE AND FOR ATHLETICS

Evaluation of Cardiac Risk for Patients Undergoing Noncardiac Surgery

Coronary artery disease represents an important risk in patients undergoing elective noncardiac surgical procedures because the stress of surgery and postoperative recovery can cause ischemia and CHF [74, 75]. The new algorithmic, stepwise approach presented by the American College of Cardiology/American Heart Association Task Force should be referred to by all health care practitioners evaluating such patients (Fig. 5-4). Preoperative cardiac assessment should be based on the prevalence of coronary artery disease (if known) in the population undergoing the procedure and the institutional event rate for the procedure.

Procedural Risk

HIGH. Procedures considered high risk (cardiac risk greater than 5%) are vascular, intraabdominal or thoracic;

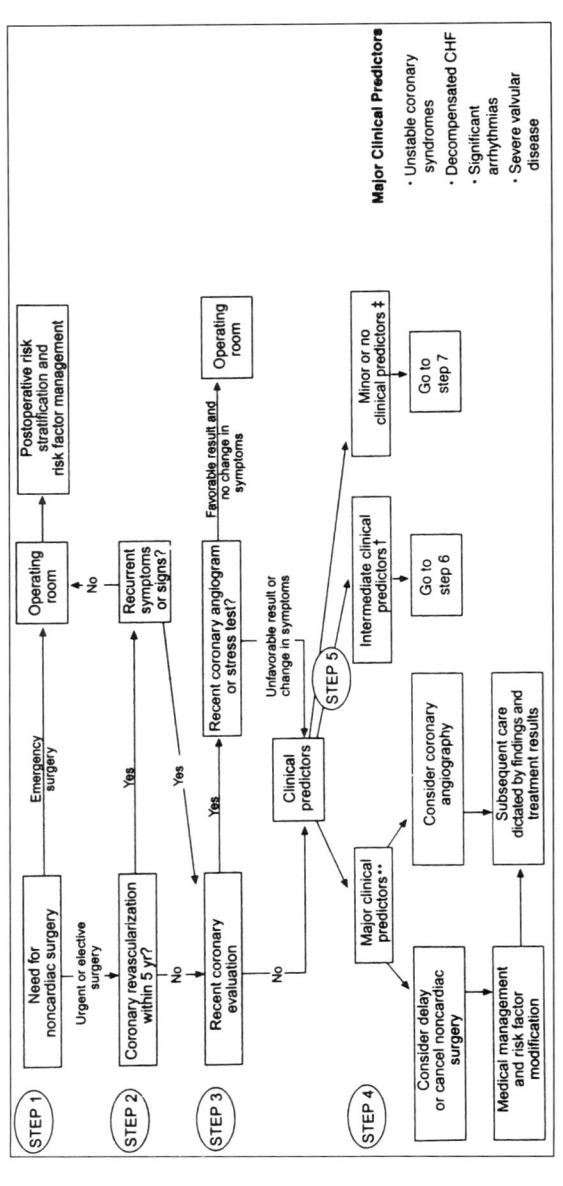

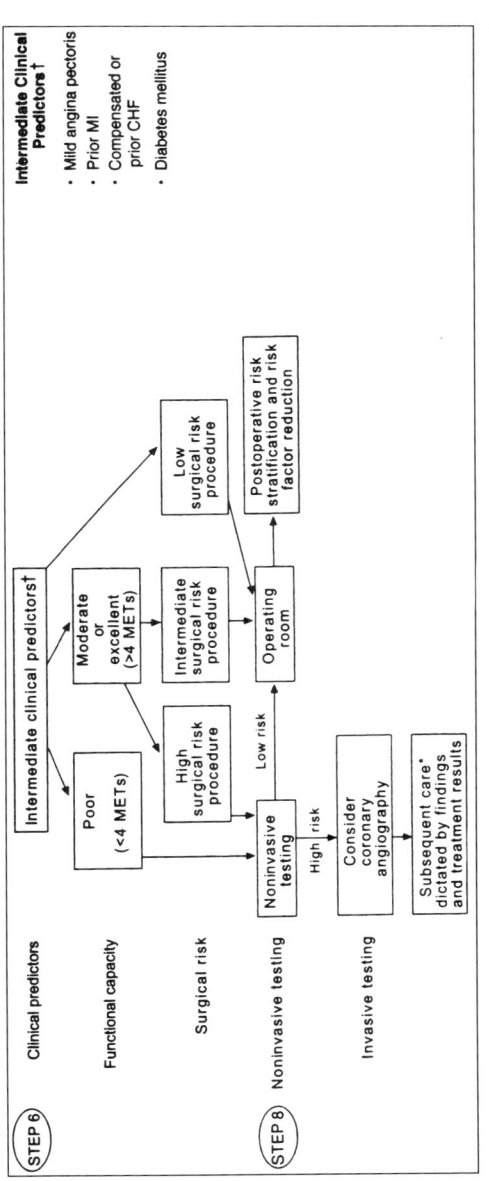

continued

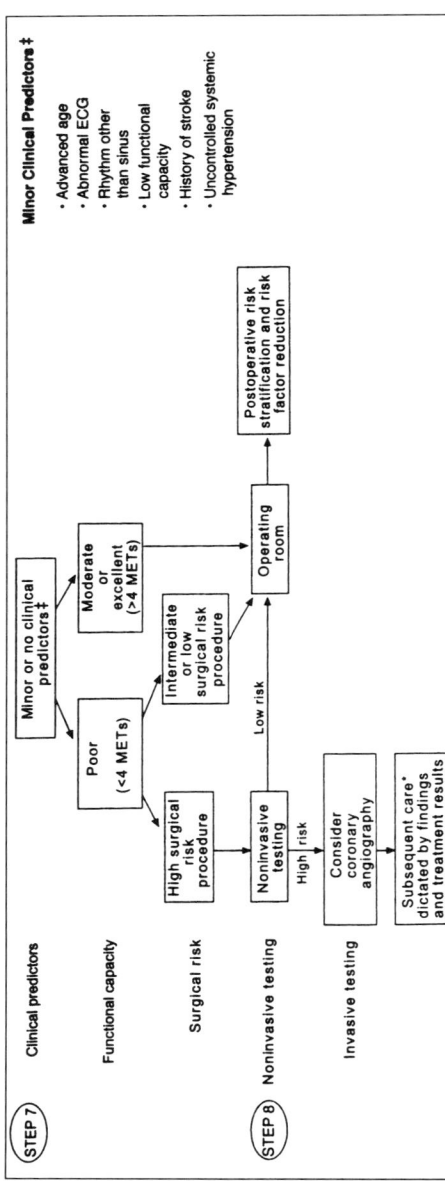

Fig. 5-4.   The American College of Cardiology/American Heart Association Task Force flow diagram for preoperative work-up for noncardiac surgery. (Reproduced with permission from KA Eagle et al. Guidelines for Perioperative Cardiovascular Evaluation for Noncardiac Surgery. ACC/AHA Task Force Report. *Circulation* **1996;93:1278–1317.)**

major orthopedic; prolonged procedures associated with large fluid shifts or blood loss; and any emergency proce-dures, particularly in the elderly.

INTERMEDIATE. Procedures with an estimated cardiac risk of less than 5% include carotid endarterectomy, head and neck surgery, and intraperitoneal and intrathoracic, orthopedic, and prostate procedures.

LOW. Procedures with an estimated cardiac risk of less than 1% include endoscopy, superficial surgery, and cat-aract and breast procedures.

Clinical Predictors

The following are clinical predictors of increased perioper-ative cardiovascular risk (MI, CHF, death).

MAJOR.

Unstable coronary syndromes including complicated MI and severe angina

Decompensated CHF

Severe valvular disease

Significant arrhythmias (high-grade block, supraventric-ular tachycardia with uncontrolled rate, ventricular arrhythmias causing syncope)

INTERMEDIATE.

Mild angina pectoris

Prior MI

CHF, compensated or by history

Diabetes mellitus

MINOR.

Advanced age

ECG with LV hypertrophy, left bundle-branch block, ST-T abnormalities

Rhythm other than sinus

Low exercise capacity

Cerebrovascular accident

Uncontrolled high BP

Exercise capacity is an important factor for assessment of perioperative surgical risk per the new guidelines. Good exercise or functional capacity is the ability of a 50- to 70-year-old patient to achieve 100% of age-predicted METs without significant symptoms of dyspnea or angina. Exer-cise capacity can be assessed by treadmill testing or by a questionnaire such as the Duke physical activity score. Preoperative testing may include treadmill testing, ambu-latory ECG monitoring, echocardiographic stress testing with dobutamine or exercise, or nuclear perfusion imaging but *the guidelines specify the standard exercise test as the first choice.* Assessing the severity of an abnormality results in a small percentage of positive test results yielding a high positive predictive value for events. Therefore, more aggressive interventions should be reserved for the most abnormal noninvasive test results, and the severity of the risk assessment should impact the timing of any coronary revascularization procedure, not the decision to proceed to more invasive testing and therapies. In summary, it is important to realize that most of the patients being screened, even vascular surgery patients (with high prevalence of coronary artery disease and procedural risk), will be found suitable to go to surgery without additional invasive intervention and cardiac revascularization. Thus, good exercise capacity and absence of cardiac risk factors should allow 30 to 40% of this population to proceed to elective surgery without further evaluation. The high-risk perfusion scan abnormalities are usually found in less than one-fourth of those patients being recommended for further noninvasive testing.

Indications for Coronary Angiography
in Perioperative Evaluation
This procedure is definitely indicated for patients with suspected or proven coronary artery disease with high-risk results during noninvasive work-up, angina unresponsive to therapy, or unstable angina, or when the findings of a noninvasive work-up are uncertain in a clinically high-risk patient undergoing a high-risk procedure.

Detsky Nomogram
A multifactorial cardiac risk index has been demonstrated to assess patients undergoing noncardiac surgery [76]. A bayesian approach to assessing cardiac risks by converting average risks for patients undergoing particular surgical procedures (pretest probabilities) to average risks for patients with each index score (posttest probabilities) is presented in a simple nomogram (Fig. 5-5).

   This nomogram was prospectively studied in 455 consecutive patients referred to the general medical consultation service for cardiac risk assessment prior to noncardiac surgery [77]. For patients undergoing major surgery, the original index performed less well in the validation dataset than in the original derivation set, but still added predictive information. The modified index also added predictive information for patients undergoing both major and minor surgery, predicting correctly 75% of the time. It is recommended that clinicians estimate local overall

Cadiac Evaluation of the Patient Undergoing Noncardiac Surgery

Discussion

The purpose of evaluating a patient for cardiac risk is to identify the patient who will need more effective perioperative management in order to decrease perioperative morbidity and mortality. We prefer to use the multifactorial risk index approach of Detsky et al. [76]. After calculating a risk factor score, one can arrive at an individual patient's risk for that surgery (posttest probability) by conversion on a likelihood ratio nomogram (right). Specifically, you determine the pretest probability (from table B), then calculate your risk factor score (from A) and draw a line through those points on the nomogram to arrive at your posttest probability.

A. Modified Multifactorial Index

MI within 6 mo	10
MI more than 6 mo	5
Class III angina (Canadian)	10
Class IV angina (Canadian)	20
Unstable angina < 6 mo	10
Alveolar pulm. edema	
Within 1 wk	10
Ever	5
Suspected critical AS	5
Rhythm other than sinus +	
APBs on last ECG	5
> 5 PVCs prior to surgery	5
Poor general medical status	5
Age > 70	5
Emergency operation	10

B. Pretest Probabilities for Surgery Types

Surgery	Severe*	All**
Vascular	13.2%	21%
Aortic	15.6%	25%
Peripheral	5.8%	17.6%
Orthopedic	13.6%	18.2%
Intrathoracic/peritoneal	8%	12.55%
Head and neck	2.6%	7.8%
Minor surgery (TURP)	1.6%	2.1%

*Cardiac death, MI, pulmonary edema.
** Above plus coronary insufficiency and new or worsened CHF without alveolar pulmonary edema.

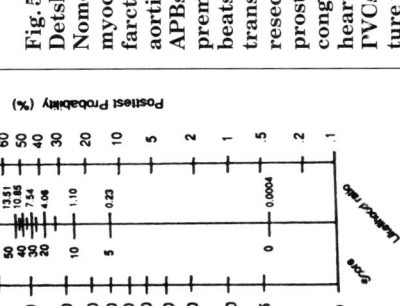

Fig. 5-5. The Detsky Index Nomogram. MI = myocardial infarction; AS = aortic stenosis; APBs = atrial premature beats; TURP = transurethral resection of the prostate; CHF = congestive heart failure; PVCs = premature ventricular contractions.

complication rates (pretest probabilities) for the clinically relevant populations in their settings before they apply the predictive properties (likelihood ratios) demonstrated in this study, in order to calculate cardiac risks for individual patients (posttest probabilities).

Evaluation of Patients for Surgery
with Peripheral Vascular Disease

A meta-analysis was performed to evaluate the accuracy of clinical risk indexes, exercise testing, dipyridamole-thallium scanning, gated blood pool ejection fraction measurement, and ECG ST-segment monitoring in the preoperative cardiac risk stratification of patients having peripheral vascular surgery [78]. Data extracted included the criteria for inclusion and exclusion of study patients, the techniques used for testing, the definitions of positive results, and the clinical outcomes. A bayesian conceptual framework was used to determine the accuracy of the various stratification techniques. The three clinical indexes (Goldman, Detsky, and Eagle) were limited by their inability to predict postoperative complications in patients with low or moderately low scores (low sensitivity). Exercise testing failed as a general screening test, primarily because many patients (approximately 70%) failed to reach their target heart rate. A negative test result did not significantly lower posttest probability of cardiac complications (low sensitivity), particularly in patients with limited exercise capacity. Patients identified clinically to be at high risk for cardiac complications after peripheral vascular surgery are unlikely to benefit from further risk stratification. Dipyridamole-thallium scanning and ST-segment monitoring may be helpful in risk stratification for those patients with intermediate clinical risk, but are unreliable for those patients at low clinical risk. Exercise testing has a limited role in preoperative cardiac risk assessment because patients requiring peripheral vascular surgery frequently cannot achieve the necessary workload because of claudication.

CONCLUSION OF META-ANALYSIS FOR PREOPERATIVE EVALUATION OF VASCULAR PATIENTS.   High-risk patients can be recognized by the following clinical risk factors:

1. Angina
2. Diabetes mellitus
3. Diagnostic Q waves
4. Symptomatic ventricular tachyarrhythmias
5. Age older than 70 years
6. Poor exercise capacity

If two or more of these factors are present, then a nonexercise stress test is indicated. If the stress test shows only one area of stress-induced ischemia, then the surgery can usually be performed, perhaps with beta-blocker therapy. If multiple areas are found, then perhaps cardiac catheterization is required before surgery. If none or only one is present, then the risk is so low that further evaluation is not indicated. Perioperative care as well as preoperative risk stratification require collaboration among the internist, the cardiologist, the anesthesiologist, and the surgeon.

Evaluation of Athletes:
Cardiology for Sports Medicine

The causes of sudden cardiac death in young competitive athletes are displayed in Figure 5-6.

Distinguishing Hypertrophic Cardiomyopathy
from Athletic Heart Syndrome

CHARACTERIZING HYPERTROPHIC CARDIOMYOPATHY.   Physical examination, family history, 12-lead ECG, and echocardiography (most definitive method) are necessary for the diagnosis of hypertrophic cardiomyopathy. When maximum diastolic LV wall thickness is larger than 15 mm, hypertrophic cardiomyopathy is considered to be present; 13 to 14 mm is a "gray zone." The septum–posterior free wall ratio usually is above 1.3. Possible risk should be resolved with other echocardiographic or clinical features but there is no certainty as to what predicts risk (outflow gradient, arrhythmias, exercise capacity, or symptoms do not appear to be predictive).

SCREENING IN THE FUTURE.   Deconditioning leading to a reduction in the septal thickness of an athlete's heart may distinguish it from hypertrophic cardiomyopathy [79]. Echocardiographic Doppler indices of LV filling may also help distinguish these two similar syndromes.

American College of Cardiology / American College
of Sports Medicine Task Force Guidelines
on Screening for Sports Participation

Prior to the development of these guidelines [80], the physician was often subjected to incredible pressures and forced by athletes, families, schools, or other sports organizations into making decisions or changing decisions. These guidelines provide the physician with a formal scientific expert statement that can support the decision he or she has made for an individual athlete.

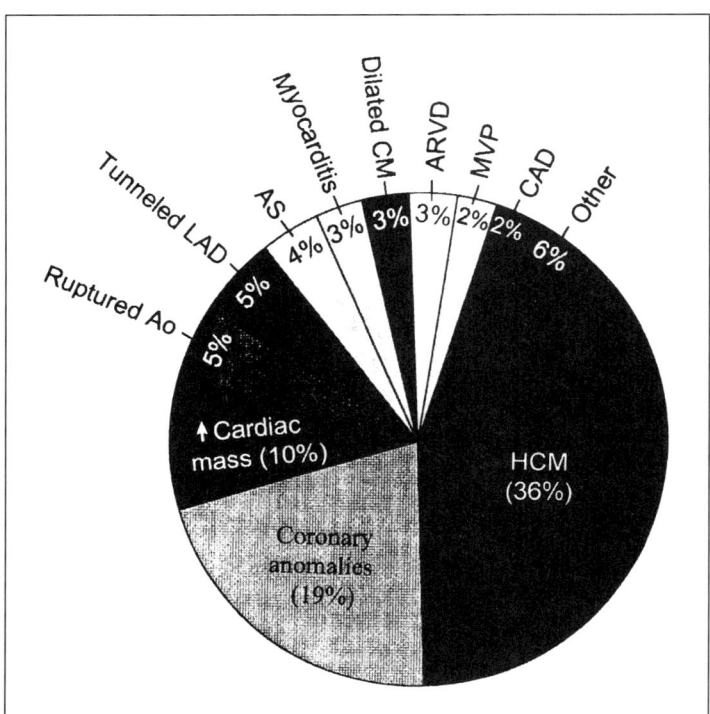

Fig. 5-6.   Causes of sudden cardiac death in young competitive athletes, based on systematic tracking of 158 athletes (with a median age of 17), primary from 1985 to 1995. Ao = aorta; LAD = left anterior descending coronary artery; AS = aortic stenosis; CM = cardiomyopathy; ARVD = arrhythmogenic right ventricular dysplasia; MVP = mitral valve prolapse; CAD = coronary artery disease; HCM = hypertrophic cardiomyopathy. (Reproduced with permission from BJ Maron et al. Cardiovascular preparation screening of competitive athletes: a statement from the American Heart Association. *Circulation* **1996;94:850–856.**

HYPERTROPHIC CARDIOMYOPATHY.   If the diagnosis is un-equivocal, the individual should participate only in low-intensity competitive sports (including those athletes with and without symptoms or LV outflow obstruction). If the individual is *older than 30 years*, the physician can use individual judgment if the following are absent:

Ventricular tachycardia
Family history of sudden cardiac death due to hyper-
    trophic cardiomyopathy
History of syncope

Severe hemodynamic abnormalities
Exercise-induced hypotension
Moderate to severe mitral regurgitation
Evidence of abnormal myocardial perfusion
Mitral valve prolapse

The presence of any of the following criteria suggests participation in only low-intensity sports:

History of syncope (arrhythmogenic in origin)
Family history of sudden cardiac death associated with
    mitral valve prolapse
Repetitive forms of sustained and nonsustained supraventricular tachycardias or complex ventricular arrhythmias
Moderate to marked mitral regurgitation
Associated embolic event

MYOCARDITIS.   Athletes judged to probably have myocarditis should be withdrawn from all competitive sports, with a subsequent convalescent period (6 months). Return to competition should be allowed when ventricular function and cardiac dimensions are normalized, and clinically relevant arrhythmias are absent. There is no basis for strong recommendation of an endomyocardial biopsy as a precondition for return to competition.

PERICARDITIS.   The athlete with pericarditis should not participate in sports during the acute episode! The individual can return to competition when the disease is no longer active. Remember that recurrences are relatively frequent.

REFERENCES

1. Konstam MA, et al. *Heart Failure: Clinical Practice Guideline No. 11*. Publication AHCPR 94-0612. Rockville, MD: Agency for Health Care Policy and Research, 1994.
2. Singh S, et al. Amiodarone in patients with congestive heart failure and asymptomatic ventricular arrhythmia. *N Engl J Med* 1995;333:77–82.
3. Figge H, Figge J. The effects of amiodarone on thyroid hormone function: A review of the physiology and clinical manifestations. *J Clin Pharmacol* 1990;30:588–595.
4. Gheorghiade M. Digoxin: resolved and unresolved issues. *ACC Educational Highlights* 1996;11:1–6.

5. McKelvie R, McConachie D, Yusuf S. Role of angiotensin converting enzyme inhibitors in patients with left ventricular dysfunction and congestive heart failure. *Eur Heart J* 1994;15(Suppl B):9–13.

6. Cody RJ, Kubo SH, Pickworth KK. Diuretic treatment for the sodium retention of congestive heart failure. *Arch Intern Med* 1994;154:1905–1914.

7. Kirklin JW, et al. ACC/AHA guidelines and indications for coronary artery bypass graft surgery. *J Am Coll Cardiol* 1991;17:543–589.

8. Coronary Angioplasty vs. Bypass trial investigation participants. Comparison of results. *Lancet* 1995; 346:1176–1184.

9. Taylor AJ, Bergin JD. Cardiac transplantation for the cardiologist not trained in transplantation. *Am Heart J* 1995;129:578–592.

10. Dalen JE, Hirsch J. Fourth ACCP Consensus Conference on Antithrombotic Therapy. *Chest* 1995;108 (Suppl.):225–522.

11. Wheeler HB, et al. Diagnostic tests for deep vein thrombosis. *Arch Intern Med* 1994;154:1921–1928.

12. Ginsberg JS, et al. Reevaluation of the sensitivity of impedance plethysmography for the detection of proximal deep vein thrombosis. *Arch Intern Med* 1994;154:1930–1933.

13. Pradoni P, et al. The long-term clinical course of acute deep venous thrombosis. *Ann Intern Med* 1996;125:1–6.

14. Calhoun DA. Hypertension: Initial evaluation. *ACC Curr J Rev* 1996;6:61–62.

15. The Fifth Joint National Committee on Detection, Evaluation, and Treatment of High Blood Pressure (JNC V). High blood pressure treatment guidelines. *Arch Intern Med* 1993;153:154–183.

16. Insua JT, et al. Drug treatment of hypertension in the elderly: a meta-analysis. *Ann Intern Med* 1994; 121:355–362.

17. Siscovick DS, et al. Diuretic therapy for hypertension and the risk of primary cardiac arrest. *N Engl J Med* 1994;330:1852–1857.

18. Cook NR, et al. Implications of small reductions in diastolic blood pressure for primary prevention. *Arch Intern Med* 1995;155:701–709.

19. Spirito P, et al. Morphology of the "athlete's heart" assessed by echocardiography in 947 elite athletes

representing 27 sports. *Am J Cardiol* 1994;74:802–806.

20. Maron BJ, Isner JM, McKenna WJ. 26th Bethesda Conference: Recommendations for determining eligibility for competition in athletes with cardiovascular abnormalities. Task Force 3: Hypertrophic cardiomyopathy, myocarditis and other myopericardial diseases and mitral valve prolapse. *Med Sci Sports Exerc* 1994;26(Suppl):S261–S267.

21. Agency for Health Care Policy and Research. *Unstable Angina: Diagnosis and Management. Clinical Practice Guideline #10.* Rockville, MD: AHCPR Publication #94-0604, 1994.

22. Patrono C. Aspirin as an antiplatelet drug. *N Engl J Med* 1994;330:1287–1294.

23. Abrams J. The role of nitrates in coronary heart disease. *Arch Intern Med* 1995;155:357–364.

24. Kendall MJ, et al. Beta-blockers and sudden cardiac death. *Ann Intern Med* 1995;123:358–367.

25. American College of Physicians. Guidelines for using serum cholesterol, HDL, and triglyceride levels as screening tests for preventing coronary heart disease in adults. *Ann Intern Med* 1996;124:515–517.

26. The AHA Task Force on Risk Reduction. Cholesterol screening in asymptomatic adults. No cause to change. *Circulation* 1996;93:1067–1068.

27. The Expert Panel: Summary of the second report of the National Cholesterol Education Program (NCEP) Expert Panel on Detection, Evaluation, and Treatment of High Blood Cholesterol in Adults (Adult Treatment Panel II). *JAMA* 1993;269:3015–3023.

28. Gray DR, et al. Efficacy and safety of controlled-release niacin in dyslipoproteinemic veterans. *Ann Intern Med* 1994;121:252–258.

29. Sempos CT, et al. Prevalence of high blood cholesterol among US adults: An update based on guidelines from the second report of the National Cholesterol Education Program Adult Treatment Panel. *JAMA* 1993;269:3009–3014.

30. ACHPR Smoking Cessation Guideline Panel. Smoking cessation clinical practice guideline. *JAMA* 1996; 275:1270–1280.

31. Pearson TA, Fuster V. 27th Bethesda Conference: matching the intensity of risk factor management with the hazard for coronary disease events. *J Am Coll Cardiol* 1996;27:957–1047.

32. Randomised trial of cholesterol lowering in 4444 patients with coronary heart disease: The Scandinavian Simvastatin Survival Study (4S). *Lancet* 1994; 344:1383–1389.

33. Illingworth DR, Tobert JA. A review of clinical trials comparing HMG-CoA reductase inhibitors. *Clin Ther* 1994;16:366–385.

34. Havranek EP. Is cholesterol lowering an alternative to revascularization in some patients with coronary artery disease? *Arch Intern Med* 1995;155:670–676.

35. Agency for Health Care Policy and Research. *Cardiac Rehabilitation. Clinical Practice Guideline #17.* Rockville, MD: AHCPR Publication #96-0672, 1995.

36. Vaitkus PT, Barnathan ES. Embolic potential, prevention and management of mural thrombus complicating anterior myocardial infarction: A meta-analysis. *J Am Coll Cardiol* 1993;22:1004–1009.

37. Litin SC, Gastineau DA. Current concepts in anticoagulant therapy. *Mayo Clin Proc* 1995;70:266–272.

38. Wells PS, et al. Interactions of warfarin with drugs and food. *Ann Intern Med* 1994;121:676–683.

39. Landefeld CS, Beyth RJ. Anticoagulant-related bleeding: Clinical epidemiology, prediction, and prevention. *Am J Med* 1993;95:315–328.

40. Fischman D, et al. A randomized comparison of coronary-stent placement and balloon angioplasty in the treatment of coronary artery disease. *N Engl J Med* 1994;331:496–501.

41. Serruys PW, et al. A comparison of balloon-expandable-stent implantation with balloon angioplasty in patients with coronary artery disease. *N Engl J Med* 1994;331:489–495.

42. Scognamiglio R, et al. Nifedipine in asymptomatic patients with severe aortic regurgitation and normal left ventricular function. *N Engl J Med* 1994;331: 689–694.

43. Tornos MP, et al. Clinical outcome of severe asymptomatic chronic aortic regurgitation: a long-term prospective follow-up study. *Am Heart J* 1995;130: 333–339.

44. Cannegieter SC, et al. Optimal oral anticoagulant therapy in patients with mechanical heart valves. *N Engl J Med* 1995;333:11–17.

45. Turpie A, et al. A comparison of aspirin with placebo in patients treated with warfarin after heart valve replacement. *N Engl J Med* 1993;329:524–529.

46. Durack DT. Prevention of infective endocarditis. *N Engl J Med* 1995;332:38–44.

47. Durak DT, Lukes AS, Bright DK. New criteria for diagnosis of infective endocarditis: Utilization of specific echocardiographic findings. *Am J Med* 1994;96: 200–209.

48. Kaye D. Treatment of infective endocarditis. *Ann Intern Med* 1996;124:606–607.

49. Wilson WR, et al (AHA Writing Group). Antibiotic treatment of adults with infective endocarditis. *JAMA* 1995;274:1706–1713.

50. Chambers HF, Miller RT, Newman MD. Right sided *Staphylococcus* endocarditis in IV drug abusers. *Ann Intern Med* 1988;109:619–624.

51. Prystowsky EN, et al. Management of patients with atrial fibrillation. AHA medical/scientific statement. *Circulation* 1996;93:1262–1277.

52. Golzari H, Cebul RD, Bahler RC. Atrial fibrillation: restoration and maintenance of sinus rhythm and indications for anticoagulation therapy. *Ann Intern Med* 1996;125:311–323.

53. Sawin CT, et al. Low serum thyrotropin concentrations as a risk factor for atrial fibrillation in older persons. *N Engl J Med* 1994;331:1249–1252.

54. Coplen SE, et al. Efficacy and safety of quinidine therapy for maintenance of sinus rhythm after cardioversion. A meta-analysis of randomized control trials. *Circulation* 1990;82:1106–1116.

55. Podrid P. Amiodarone: Reevaluation of an old drug. *Ann Intern Med* 1995;122:689–700.

56. Hohnloser S, Woosley R. Sotalol. *N Engl J Med* 1994; 331:31–38.

57. Atrial Fibrillation Investigators. Risk factors for stroke and efficacy of antithrombotic therapy in atrial fibrillation. Analysis of pooled data from five randomized controlled trials. *Arch Intern Med* 1994; 154:1449–1457.

58. Moreya E, Finkelhor RS, Cebul RD. Limitations of transesophageal echocardiography in the risk assessment of patients before nonanticoagulated cardioversion from atrial fibrillation and flutter: An analysis of pooled trials. *Am Heart J* 1995;129: 71–75.

59. Laupacis A, et al. Risk factors for stroke and efficacy of antithrombotic therapy in atrial fibrillation. *Arch Intern Med* 1994;154:1449–1457.

60.   Roden D. Risks and benefits of antiarrhythmic therapy. *N Engl J Med* 1994;331:785–791.

61.   Pinski SL, Trohman RG. Implantable cardioverter-defibrillators: Implications for the nonelectrophysiologist. *Ann Intern Med* 1995;122:770–777.

62.   Echt DS, et al. Mortality and morbidity in patients receiving encainide, flecainide, or placebo. The Cardiac Arrhythmia Suppression Trial. *N Engl J Med* 1991;324:781–788.

63.   Mason JW. A comparison of electrophysiologic testing with Holter monitoring to predict antiarrhythmic drug efficacy for ventricular tachyarrhythmias. Electrophysiologic Study Versus Electrocardiographic Monitoring. *N Engl J Med* 1993;329:445–451.

64.   Silverman BG, et al. The epidemiology of pacemaker implantation in the United States. *Public Health Rep* 1995;110:42–46.

65.   Snow J, et al. Implanted devices and electromagnetic interference: Case presentations and review. *J Invas Cardiol* 1995;7:25–32.

66.   Hart GT. Evaluation of syncope. *Am Fam Physician* 1995;51:1941–1948, 1951–1952.

67.   Williams CC, Bernhardt DT. Syncope in athletes. *Sports Med* 1995;19:223–234.

68.   Calkins H, et al. The value of the clinical history in the differentiation of syncope due to ventricular tachycardia, atrioventricular block, and neurocardiogenic syncope. *Am J Med* 1995;98:365–373.

69.   Kaufmann H. Neurally mediated syncope: Pathogenesis, diagnosis, and treatment. *Neurology* 1995; 45(Suppl 5):S12–S18.

70.   Natale A, et al. Efficacy of different treatment strategies for neurocardiogenic syncope. *Pacing Clin Electrophysiol* 1995;18:655–662.

71.   Cox M, et al. Acute and long term beta-adrenergic blockade for patients with neurocardiogenic syncope. *J Am Coll Cardiol* 1995;26:1293–1298.

72.   Dhala A, et al. Relevance of asystole during head-up tilt testing. *Am J Cardiol* 1995;75:251–254.

73.   Bachinsky WB, et al. Usefulness of clinical characteristics in predicting the outcome of electrophysiologic studies in unexplained syncope. *Am J Cardiol* 1992;69:1044–1049.

74.   Eagle KA, et al. Guidelines for perioperative cardiovascular evaluation for noncardiac surgery. ACC/

AHA Task Force Report. *Circulation* 1996;93:1278–1317.

75.   Leppo JA. Preoperative cardiac risk assessment for noncardiac surgery. *Am J Cardiol* 1995;75:42D–51D.

76.   Detsky AS, et al. Cardiac assessment for patients undergoing noncardiac surgery. A multifactorial clinical risk index. *Arch Intern Med* 1986;146:2131–2134.

77.   Detsky AS, et al. Predicting cardiac complications in patients undergoing non-cardiac surgery. *J Gen Intern Med* 1986;1:211–219.

78.   Wong T, Detsky AS. Preoperative cardiac risk assessment for patients having peripheral vascular surgery. *Ann Intern Med* 1992;116:743–753.

79.   Maron B. Screening athletes for competitive sports: Hypertrophic cardiomyopathy. *Br Heart J* 1993;69:125–128.

80.   Maron BJ, et al. Cardiovascular preparation screening of competitive athletes: a statement from the American Heart Association. *Circulation* 1996;94:850–856.

Appendices

Dietary

In chronic congestive heart failure, in order for diuretics to be effective, sodium and fluids must be restricted. Note the following:

1. Table salt is about 40% sodium.
2. Americans consume about 20 times more salt than their bodies need.
3. About three-fourths of the salt consumed is already in foods and drinks.
4. One teaspoon of salt contains 2 g (2,000 mg) of sodium—the recommended daily amount for people with high BP.
5. Intake to this level can be reduced simply by not salting food during cooking or before eating.
6. Some people are so sensitive to salt that even a moderate amount causes their BP to rise.
7. The more salt one eats, the more medication one will need to control BP if one is a salt-sensitive hypertensive.

TIPS FOR REDUCING SALT INTAKE
Reducing salt intake to a teaspoon or less a day is easy if one:

1. Reads labels on over-the-counter medicine and foods.
2. Puts away the salt shaker, or if one must use salt, uses "light salt" that contains half the sodium of ordinary table salt.
3. Buys fresh meats, fruits, and vegetables instead of canned, processed, and convenience foods.
4. Substitutes spices and lemon juice for salt.
5. Watches out for hidden sodium, for example, in carbonated beverages, nondairy creamers, cookies, and cakes.
6. Avoids salty foods, such as bacon, sausage, pretzels, potato chips, mustard, pickles, and some cheeses.
7. Knows sodium sources.
8. Avoids canned, prepared, and "fast" foods, which are high in sodium, as are condiments such as ketsup. Some foods that do not taste salty contain high amounts of sodium. Consider the values below:

Food	Sodium (mg)
1 can tomato soup	872
1 hot dog	639
1 cheeseburger	709
1 tablespoon ketchup	156
1 dill pickle	928
1 cup corn flakes	256
1 teaspoon table salt	2,000

Other high-sodium sources include baking powder, baking soda, barbeque sauce, bouillon cubes, celery salt, chili sauce, cooking wine, garlic salt, onion salt, softened water, and soy sauce.

Many over-the-counter medicines and other nonfood items contain sodium, such as alkalizers for indigestion, laxatives, aspirin, cough medicine, mouthwash, and toothpaste.

POTASSIUM CONTENT OF COMMON FOODS

For the patient on diuretics, 300 to 400 mg of potassium is the daily recommendation. The following foods contain the following amounts of potassium per 3.5-oz serving.

Meats	mg
Beef	370
Chicken	411
Lamb	290
Liver	380
Pork	326
Turkey	411
Veal	500

Fish	mg
Bass	256
Flounder	342
Haddock	348
Halibut	525
Oysters	203
Perch	284
Salmon	421
Sardines, canned	590
Scallops	476
Tuna	301

Fruits	mg
Apricots	281
Bananas	370
Dates	648
Figs	152
Nectarines	294
Oranges	200
Peaches	202
Plums	299
Prunes	262
Raisins	355

Vegetables	mg
Asparagus	238
Brussels sprouts	295
Cabbage	233
Carrots	341
Endive	294
Lima beans	394
Peppers	213
Potatoes	407
Radishes	322
Spinach	324
Sweet Potatoes	300

Juices	mg
Orange, fresh	200
Orange, reconstituted	186
Tomato	227

Other Foods	mg
Gingersnap cookies	462
Graham crackers	334
Oatmeal cookies with raisins	370
Ice milk	195
Milk, dry (nonfat solids)	1,745
Molasses (light)	917
Peanuts	674
Peanut butter	670

VITAMIN K CONTENT OF COMMON FOODS

The estimated range of daily dietary intake of vitamin K is 70 to 140 µg. If a patient eats excessive amounts of foods high in vitamin K content, the effect of warfarin is lessened. Reduction of vitamin K intake increases the effect of warfarin. A diet containing a consistent vitamin K content within the adequate daily dietary range is recommended.

Food	Vitamin K µg/100 g	Rank of Vitamin K Content*
Fruits		
Applesauce	2	L
Banana	2	L
Orange	1	L
Peach	8	L
Raisin	6	L
Strawberry	10	L
Fats		
Corn oil	3	L
Safflower oil	3	L
Soybean oil	193	H
Eggs		
Hen (whole)	11	L
Meat and meat products		
Bacon	46	M
Beef liver	92	H
Chicken liver	7	L
Ground beef	7	L
Ham	15	L
Pork liver	25	L
Pork tenderloin	11	L

*L = low content of vitamin K (increases effectiveness of warfarin) M = moderate content of vitamin K; H = high content of vitamin K.

Food	Vitamin K μg/100 g	Rank of Vitamin K Content*
Milk and milk products		
Butter	30	M
Cheese	35	M
Milk (cow)	1	L
Cereals and grain products		
Bread	4	L
Maize	5	L
Oats	10	L
Rice	3	L
Wheat flour	4	L
Whole wheat	17	L
Beverages		
Coffee	38	M
Cola	2	L
Tea, black	—	L
Tea, green	712	H
Vegetables		
Asparagus	57	M
Beans, green	40	M
Broccoli	175	H
Brussels sprouts	800–3,000	H
Cabbage	125	H
Califlower-flowerbuds	191	H
Kale	729	H
Lettuce	129	H
Peas, green	29	M
Potato	1	L
Pumpkin	2	L
Spinach	415	H
Tomato	10	L
Turnip greens	650	H
Watercress	80	M

*L = low content of vitamin K (increases effectiveness of warfarin); M = moderate content of vitamin K; H = high content of vitamin K.

DIETARY FORMULAS

LDL cholesterol (mg/dl) = total cholesterol (mg/dl)

$$-\left(\frac{\text{triglyceride (mg/dl)}}{5} + \text{HDL cholesterol (mg/dl)}\right)$$

1 gram fat = 9 calories

If a serving has 5 grams of fat then:

$5 \times 9 = 45$ calories from fat

If the total calories of the serving are 100 then:

$\frac{45}{100} = 45\%$ of calories from fat

DIETARY THERAPY FOR HIGH BLOOD CHOLESTEROL

The chart below indicates the recommended intake of various nutrients for the patient with high blood cholesterol [1].

Nutrient	Recommended Intake	
	Step-One Diet	**Step-Two Diet**
Total fat	Less than 30% of total calories	
Saturated fatty acids	<10% of total calories	<7% of total calories
Polyunsaturated fatty acids	Up to 10% of total calories	
Monounsaturated fatty acids	10 to 15% of total calories	
Carbohydrates	50 to 60% of total calories	
Protein	10 to 20% of total calories	
Cholesterol	<300 mg/d	<200 mg/d
Total calories	To achieve and maintain desirable body weight	

SERVING SIZE AND AVERAGE COMPOSITION FOR FOOD GROUPS IN STEP-ONE AND STEP-TWO DIETS

Food Group	Serving Size*	Average Food Group Composition* Step-One Diet	Step-Two Diet
Fats and oils	1 tsp oil, margarine, or shortening 2 tsp diet margarine, peanut butter, or mayonnaise 1 tbsp nuts, seeds, or salad dressing	41 kcal, 5.0 g fat, 1.0 g saturated fat, 0.1 mg cholesterol	39 kcal, 4.0 g fat, 0.7 g saturated fat, 0.1 mg cholesterol
Breads, cereals, pasta, and starchy vegetables	1 slice bread 1 cup flake cereal ½ cup pasta, peas ⅓ cup rice, dried beans	86 kcal, 1.0 g fat, 0.1 g saturated fat, 0.1 mg cholesterol	
Fruits	½ cup 1 medium-sized piece	55 kcal, 0.3 g fat, negligible saturated fat, no cholesterol	
Vegetables	1/2 cup cooked or raw	24 kcal, 0.2 g fat, negligible saturated fat, no cholesterol	
Optional foods Sweets	6 oz carbonated beverage ¾ oz candy ⅓ cup sherbet	75 kcal, 0.3 g fat, 0.1 g saturated fat, 0.1 mg cholesterol	

SERVING SIZE AND AVERAGE COMPOSITION FOR FOOD GROUPS IN STEP-ONE AND STEP-TWO DIETS (Continued)

Food Group	Serving Size*	Average Food Group Composition*	
		Step-One Diet	Step-Two Diet
Modified fat desserts	White cake with frosting, low sodium; oatmeal cookie, low sodium	153 kcal, 5.0 g fat, 0.7 g saturated fat, 0.1 mg cholesterol	112 kcal
Alcoholic beverages	12 oz beer ½ oz 80-proof liqueur 4 oz wine		

*Data from American Heart Association [2].

REFERENCES
1. The Expert Panel. Summary of the second report of the National Cholesterol Education Program (NCEP) Expert Panel on Detection, Evaluation, and Treatment of High Blood Cholesterol in Adults (Adult Treatment Panel II). *JAMA* 1993;269:3015–3023.
2. American Heart Association. *Dietary Treatment of High Blood Pressure and High Blood Cholesterol.* Dallas: American Heart Association, 1990.

Treatment with Medications

Table B-1. Chronic Anticoagulation and Antithrombotic Recommendations

Diagnosis	No Treatment	Aspirin	Warfarin	INR
Myocardial damage/dysfunction				
Dilated cardiomyopathy	X			
Dilated cardiomyopathy with LV thrombus			X	2.5–3.5
Dilated cardiomyopathy with atrial fibrillation			X	2.0–3.0
Dilated cardiomyopathy with thrombus/CAD		X (81 mg)	X	2.5–3.5
Dilated cardiomyopathy with systemic/ pulmonary emboli				2.0–3.0
Confounder: venous thromboembolism			X (6 mo)	2.0–3.0
Myocardial ischemia				
Known CAD		X (81 mg)		
Post MI (uncomplicated)		X (81 mg)		
Anterior MI (with wall motion abnormality)		X (81 mg)	X	2.0–3.0
MI with LV thrombus		X (81 mg)	X	2.5–3.5
Post CABG		X (81 mg)		
Post PTCA		X (325 mg)		
Coronary stents		X (325 mg)	Stent specific	
Confounder: pulmonary embolism			X (6 mo)	2.0–3.0
Valvular status				
Mitral stenosis	X		Only in atrial fibrillation	
Mitral regurgitation	X			
Aortic stenosis	X			
Aortic regurgitation	X			
Mechanical valves		X (81 mg)	X	2.5–3.5 (? higher dose/ dipyridamole)
Prosthetic tissue valve			X (3 mo)	2.0–3.0
Valve repair	X			

Continued

Table B-1. Chronic Anticoagulation and Antithrombotic Recommendations (Continued)

Diagnosis	No Treatment	Aspirin	Warfarin	INR
Exercise capacity				
Consider primary diagnosis				
Arrhythmias				
Atrial fibrillation (lone, low risk)		X (325 mg)		
Atrial fibrillation (high risk, more than 75 years old)			X	2.0–3.0
Atrial fibrillation (history MI, uncomplicated)		X (325 mg)		
Atrial fibrillation (history MI, complicated)		X (81 mg)	X	2.0–3.0
Atrial fibrillation (precardioversion)			X (1 mo)	2.0–3.0
Atrial fibrillation (post conversion to NSR)			X (1 mo)	2.0–3.0
Vascular disease				
TIA		81/325 mg		
Stroke		81/325 mg		
TIA/stroke (if fails aspirin or contraindicated)			X	2.0–3.0
Peripheral vascular disease		X (81 mg)		
Asymptomatic carotid stenosis		X (325 mg)		
Prevention of CAD (only 2 studies available)		?		

Moving or protruding LV thrombus definitely requires warfarin. During pregnancy, since warfarin is fetopathic, heparin must be utilized and the PTT maintained 1½ to 2 times normal.

MUST CARDIAC MEDICATIONS FOR AMBULATORY CARE

Beta-blockers

Indications:
    After MI for at least a year
    High BP
    Typical and unstable angina
    To decrease ventricular response in atrial fibrillation
      (though they can decrease exercise capacity)
    To decrease episodes of paroxysmal atrial tachycardia

Evidence: 25% decrease in mortality in the first year after MI, also lowers mortality when given IV acutely, decreases morbidity and mortality with high BP (but no decrease in MIs), lessens pain with ischemia and protects myocardium

Side effects: can worsen claudication, lipid pattern and bronchospastic lung disease; can cover up the catecholamine surge warning of a hypoglycemic insulin reaction; can cause depression and erectile sexual dysfunction; can decrease 10-km time in healthy runners

Dose: 25 mg propranolol qid, 50 mg atenolol qd (cardioselective and does not cross blood-brain barrier), 12.5 mg IV metoprolol for MI

ASA

Indications:
    Primary and secondary prevention of coronary artery disease
    Acute MI
    Unstable angina
    Lone atrial fibrillation (if low risk for emboli)
    Stents, percutaneous transluminal coronary angioplasty (PTCA)
    Prosthetic valves to lessen probability of emboli if warfarin contraindicated
    After CABG to maintain graft potency
    CVAs, TIAs

Evidence: for acute MI, decreases immediate mortality by 12%; for unstable angina, decreases mortality 20%; decreases embolic events in patients with atrial fibrillation but still not as effective as warfarin (except in patients with low-risk atrial fibrillation); increases coronary vein graft patency

Side effects: gastritis, bleeding

Dose: 81–325-mg enteric coated tablet once a day

**Vasoactive Calcium Antagonists
(Nifedipine, Nicardipine)**
Indications: specific for vasospastic, Prinzmetal's angina;
   not first line for high BP
Evidence: empirical
Side effects: pedal edema, nausea, light-headedness,
   nausea
Dose: 10–30 mg tid or qid; or long-acting qd

ACE Inhibitors (Captopril, Enalapril, Lisinopril)
Indications:
   Dilated cardiomyopathy
   Acute transmural anterior wall MI
Evidence: 15% decreased mortality in dilated cardiomy-
   opathy, lessens expansion of anterior wall MIs, and
   improves survival 10%
Side effects: hypotension, cough, renal dysfunction, rash
Dose: titrated beginning low because of hypotension; cap-
   topril, 12.5 mg tid up to 150 mg tid; enalapril, 2.5–20 mg
   bid; lisinopril, 10–40 mg once a day

**Diuretics (Thiazides, Loop Agents,
Potassium Sparing)**
Indications:
   High BP
   Dependent edema of CHF
   Volume overload due to CHF or renal disease
Evidence: decreases morbidity and mortality with high BP
   (but not MI incidence) except potassium-wasting diuretics; along with salt and fluid restriction, results in a
   diuresis
Side effects: electrolyte abnormalities, ototoxicity, hypotension, hyperglycemia rare; potassium-sparing agents
   can cause gynecomastia and must be used carefully
   with ACE inhibitor
Dose: hydrochlorothiazide, 25–50 mg bid; furosemide,
   20–80 mg bid; metolazone, 5–20 mg a day; spironolactone, 25–200 mg a day in one or two doses; triamterene,
   100–300 mg in one or two doses

Digoxin
Indications:
   Traditional management of CHF from dilated car-
   diomyopathy (no mortality data yet!)
   Resting rate control of atrial fibrillation (plus diltiazem
   for control of heart rate response to exercise)

Evidence: empirical and observational
Side effects: arrhythmias, nausea, yellowing vision
Dose: 0.25 mg; 0.125 mg in patients older than 65 or with
    liver, renal or lung disease

Warfarin
Indications:
    Large transmural anterior MIs
    Atrial fibrillation (high risk)
    Prosthetic valves, mechanical only
    Coronary stents
    Deep venous thrombosis
    LV thrombus
    Pulmonary embolus
Evidence: 60% decline in cerebral emboli in patients with
    atrial fibrillation, less LV thrombus/emboli after large
    transmural anterior MIs per meta-analysis, less stroke
    than placebo (4–5%/yr on placebo vs less than 1% on
    warfarin) in patients with prosthetic valves
Side effects: bleeding
Dose: depends on INR and specific condition

Antilipidemics
Indications: prevention of the morbidity and mortality
    associated with coronary artery disease in patients with
    coronary artery disease and hypercholesterolemia
Evidence: statins decrease mortality and morbidity; oth-
    ers with weaker effect
Side effects: liver dysfunction, rhabdomyolitis
Dose:
    Lovastatin: Usual starting dose 1 tablet (20 mg) with
        dinner; for very elevated cholesterol (i.e., > 300 mg/dl),
        start with 40 mg; maximum dose, 80 mg/day in a sin-
        gle or divided dose
    Pravastatin: usual dose 10 mg/day; maximum recom-
        mended, 40 mg/day
    Simvastatin: usual dose is 10 mg/day; maximum, 40
        mg/day
    Fluvastatin: usual dose, 20 mg/day given at bedtime;
        maximum dose, 40 mg/day

Nitroglycerin (NTG) and Nitrates
Indications:
    Angina of any type
    Long-acting NTG along with hydralazine for CHF

Evidence: empirical and observational for angina because tolerance develops to long-acting NTG when given for angina but probably not in CHF; improved survival in dilated cardiomyopathy but ACE inhibitors superior

Side effects: headaches, hypotension, tolerance

Dose: 10–40 mg long-acting qid or sublingual prn angina; paste or spray also available

Diltiazem

Indications:

Exercise rate control in atrial fibrillation

Antianginal in patients who cannot tolerate beta-blockers (particularly patients with bronchospastic lung disease, claudication, hypoglycemic reactions with diabetic medications)

Angina with a vasospastic component

Not specific for non-Q-wave MIs; beta-blockers only drugs to decrease morbidity and mortality

Not first-line drug for high BP

Evidence: randomized, blinded controlled trials

Side effects: headache, AV block, constipation

Dose: sustained release capsules 180–300 mg qd or other divided doses

Thrombolysis

Indications: for acute MI

Evidence: decreases mortality 25% if given soon after onset of chest pain and ST elevation

Side effects: bleeding, stroke, allergic reaction to streptokinase if previously given streptokinase

Dose: refer elsewhere

PREVENTION OF BACTERIAL ENDOCARDITIS (RECOMMENDATIONS BY THE AMERICAN HEART ASSOCIATION)

Surgical and dental procedures and instrumentations involving mucosal surfaces or contaminated tissue commonly cause transient bacteremia that rarely persists for more than 15 minutes. Blood-borne bacteria may lodge on damaged or abnormal heart valves or on the endocardium or the endothelium near congenital anatomic defects, resulting in bacterial endocarditis or endarteritis. Although bacteremia is common following many invasive procedures, only a limited number of bacterial species commonly cause endocarditis. It is impossible to predict which patient will develop this infection or which particular procedure will be responsible.

Certain cardiac conditions are more often associated with endocarditis than others.

Cardiac conditions for which endocarditis prophylaxis is recommended:

Prosthetic cardiac valves, including bioprosthetic and homograft valves

Previous bacterial endocarditis, even in the absence of heart disease

Most congenital cardiac malformations

Rheumatic and other acquired valvular dysfunction, even after valvular surgery

Hypertrophic cardiomyopathy

Mitral valve prolapse with valvular regurgitation

Endocarditis prophylaxis is not recommended for:

Isolated secundum atrial septal defect

Surgical repair without residua beyond 6 months of atrial or ventricular septal defect or patent ductus arteriosus

Previous CABG surgery

Mitral valve prolapse without valvular regurgitation

Physiologic, functional, or innocent heart murmurs

Previous Kawasaki's disease without valvular dysfunction

Previous rheumatic fever without valvular dysfunction

Cardiac pacemakers and implanted defibrillators

Furthermore, certain dental and surgical procedures are much more likely to initiate the bacteremia that results in endocarditis than are other procedures.

Dental and surgical procedures for which endocarditis prophylaxis is recommended:

Dental procedures known to induce gingival or mucosal bleeding, including cleaning

Tonsillectomy or adenoidectomy

Surgical operations that involve intestinal or respiratory mucosa

Bronchoscopy with a rigid bronchoscope

Sclerotherapy for esophageal varices

Esophageal dilation, gallbladder surgery, cystoscopy, urethral dilation

Urethral catheterization if urinary tract infection is present

Urinary tract surgery if urinary tract infection is present

Prostatic surgery

Incision and drainage of infected tissue

Vaginal hysterectomy and vaginal delivery in the presence of infection

Endocarditis prophylaxis not recommended for:

Dental procedures not likely to induce gingival bleeding, such as simple adjustment of orthodontic appliances or fillings above the gum line

Injection of local intraoral anesthetic (except intraligamentary injections)

Shedding of primary teeth

Tympanostomy tube insertion

Endotracheal intubation

Bronchoscopy with a flexible bronchoscope, with or without biopsy

Cardiac catheterization

Endoscopy with or without GI biopsy

Cesarean section or other gynecologic procedures

Prophylactic antibiotics are recommended for patients at risk for developing endocarditis who are undergoing procedures most likely to produce bacteremia with organisms that commonly cause endocarditis.

Prophylaxis is most effective when given perioperatively in doses that are sufficient to ensure adequate antibiotic concentrations in the serum during and after the procedure. To reduce the likelihood of microbial resistance, it is important that prophylactic antibiotics be used only during the perioperative period. They should be initiated shortly before a procedure (1–2 hours), and should not be continued for an extended period (no more than 6–8 hours). In the case of delayed healing, or of a procedure that involves infected tissue, it may be necessary to provide additional doses of antibiotics.

Standard Prophylactic Regimen for Dental, Oral, and Upper Respiratory Tract Procedures

Poor dental hygiene and periodontal or periapical infections may produce bacteremia even in the absence of dental procedures. Individuals who are at risk for developing bacterial endocarditis should establish and maintain the best possible oral health to reduce potential sources of bacterial seeding.

Antibiotic prophylaxis is recommended with all dental procedures likely to cause gingival bleeding, including routine professional cleaning. If a series of dental procedures is required, it may be prudent to observe an interval of 7 days between procedures to reduce the potential for the emergence of resistant strains of organisms. If possible, a combination of procedures should be planned in the same period of prophylaxis.

Alpha-hemolytic (viridans) streptococci are the most common cause of endocarditis following dental procedures, and prophylaxis should be specifically directed against these organisms. Certain upper respiratory tract procedures, such as tonsillectomy and adenoidectomy, bronchoscopy with a rigid bronchoscope, and surgical procedures that involve the respiratory mucosa, may also cause bacteremia with organisms that commonly cause endocarditis and have similar antibiotic susceptibilities to those producing bacteremia following dental procedures. Therefore, the same regimen is recommended for these procedures as is recommended for dental procedures. Endocarditis has not been reported in association with insertion of tympanostomy tubes.

The recommended standard prophylactic regimen for all dental, oral, and upper respiratory tract procedures is *amoxicillin (3.0 g orally 1 hour before procedure; then 1.5 g 6 hours after initial dose*. Allergic patients: erythromycin, 1.0 g orally 2 hours before procedure, then half the dose 6 hours after initial dose; or clindamycin, 300 mg orally 1 hour before procedure and 150 mg 6 hours after initial dose).

The antibiotics amoxicillin, ampicillin, and penicillin V are equally effective in vitro against hemolytic streptococci; however, amoxicillin is now recommended because it is better absorbed from the GI tract and provides higher and more sustained serum levels. Penicillin V can be used rather than amoxicillin as prophylaxis against hemolytic streptococcal bacteremia following dental, oral, and upper respiratory tract procedures. Individuals who are allergic to penicillins (such as amoxicillin, ampicillin, or penicillin) should be treated with the provided alternative oral regimens. Erythromycin ethylsuccinate and erythromycin stearate are recommended because of more rapid and reliable absorption than other erythromycin formulations, resulting in higher and more sustained serum levels. For individuals who cannot tolerate either penicillins or erythromycin, clindamycin hydrochloride is the recommended alternative. Tetracyclines and sulfonamides are not recommended for endocarditis prophylaxis.

Regimens for Genitourinary and Gastrointestinal Procedures

Surgery, instrumentation, or diagnostic procedures that involve the genitourinary or GI tracts may cause bacteremia. The rate of bacteremia that is found following urinary tract procedures is high if urinary tract infection is present. Although the risk that any particular patient will develop endocarditis is low, the genitourinary tract is second only to the oral cavity as a portal of entry for organisms that cause endocarditis. The instrumented GI tract seems to be less important as a portal of entry for organisms that cause bacterial endocarditis than the oral cavity or genitourinary tract.

Bacterial endocarditis that occurs following genitourinary and GI tract surgery or instrumentation is most often caused by *Enterococcus faecalis* (enterococci). Although gram-negative bacillary bacteremia may follow these procedures, gram-negative bacilli are only rarely responsible for endocarditis. Thus, antibiotic prophylaxis to prevent endocarditis that occurs following genitourinary or GI procedures should be directed primarily against enterococci.

Specific Situations and Circumstances

Rheumatic Fever

Antibiotic regimens used to prevent the recurrence of acute rheumatic fever are inadequate for the prevention of bacterial endocarditis. Individuals who take an oral penicillin for secondary prevention of rheumatic fever or for other purposes may have *Streptococcus viridans* in their oral cavities that are relatively resistant to penicillin, amoxicillin, or ampicillin. In such cases, the physician or dentist should select erythromycin.

Patients Who Undergo Cardiac Surgery

Patients who have cardiac conditions that predispose them to endocarditis are at risk for developing bacterial endocarditis when undergoing open heart surgery. Similarly, patients who undergo surgery for placement of prosthetic heart valves or prosthetic intravascular or intracardiac materials are also at risk for the development of bacterial endocarditis. Because the morbidity and mortality of endocarditis in such patients are high, perioperative prophylactic antibiotics are recommended.

Endocarditis associated with open heart surgery is most often caused by *Staphylococcus aureus,* coagulase-negative staphylococci, or diphtheroids. Streptococci, gram-negative bacteria, and fungi are less common. No single antibiotic regimen is effective against all these organisms. Furthermore, prolonged use of broad-spectrum antibiotics may predispose to superinfection with unusual or resistant microorganisms.

Prophylaxis at the time of cardiac surgery should be directed primarily against staphylococci and should be of short duration. "First-generation" cephalosporins are most often used, but the choice of an antibiotic should be influenced by the antibiotic's susceptibility patterns at each hospital. For example, high prevalence of infection by methicillin-resistant *S. aureus* in a particular institution should prompt consideration of vancomycin for perioperative prophylaxis. Prophylaxis with the chosen antibiotic should be started immediately before the operative procedure, repeated during prolonged procedures to maintain levels intraoperatively, and continued for no more than 24 hours postoperatively to minimize emergence of resistant microorganisms. The effects of cardiopulmonary bypass and compromised postoperative renal function on antibiotic levels in the serum should be considered, and doses timed appropriately before and during the procedure.

A careful preoperative dental evaluation is recommended so that required dental treatment can be completed before cardiac surgery whenever possible. Such measures may decrease the incidence of late postoperative endocarditis.

Status Following Cardiac Surgery
The same precautions should be observed in the years following most heart or valvular surgery that have been outlined for the patient who has not undergone a surgical procedure but is undergoing dental, GI, genitourinary, or other procedures. The risk of developing endocarditis appears to continue indefinitely and is particularly significant for patients who have prosthetic heart valves. Furthermore, the morbidity and mortality that result from prosthetic valve endocarditis are high. Patients who have an isolated secundum atrial septal defect that has been surgically repaired, a ventricular septal defect, or patent ductus arteriosus do not seem to be at risk of developing endocarditis following a 6-month healing period after surgery. Data are insufficient to allow recommendations

for prophylactic therapy after closure of these lesions by nonsurgical devices. There is no evidence that CABG surgery introduces a risk for developing endocarditis. Therefore, antibiotic prophylaxis is not needed for this condition.

Cardiac Transplantation
There are insufficient data to support specific recommendations for patients who have had heart transplantation.

Exercise Capacity Evaluation

WORKSHEET FOR EXERCISE TESTING

I. Preliminary Patient Preparation
- [ ] 1. Consent signed (less than 4 in 10,000 event rate; less for death)
- [ ] 2. SAQ Questionnaire completed
- [ ] 3. No food intake or smoking for 3 hours

II. Patient Interview: Ask specific questions regarding the following and review records.

- [ ] 1. Past Medical History (with dates)

    A. Cardiovascular

[ ] CHF	[ ] Stroke	[ ] Sudden death
[ ] MI	[ ] Congenital	[ ] Valve disease
[ ] PVD	[ ] Syncope	[ ] Cardiac catheter
[ ] HTN	[ ] Arrhythmia	[ ] Atrial fibrillation
[ ] PTCA	[ ] Pacemaker	

    B. Cardiovascular Surgery

[ ] CABG	[ ] Aorto femoral	[ ] Mitral V repair
[ ] Carotid	[ ] Aortic valve replacement	[ ] Mitral V replacement

    C. Other Medical Disease

[ ] Diabetes mellitus	[ ] COPD
[ ] Musculoskeletal disease	[ ] Anemia
[ ] Cancer	[ ] Thyroid disease

- [ ] 2. Family History

[ ] Family history (CAD in blood relative < 65 years)	
[ ] Heart muscle disease	[ ] Sudden death

- [ ] 3. Risk Factors

[ ] HTN	[ ] Sedentary	[ ] Tobacco smoking
[ ] DM	[ ] Obesity	[ ] Cholesterol

- [ ] 4. Current Symptoms

[ ] PND	[ ] Palpitation	[ ] Claudication
[ ] Orthopnea	[ ] Angina	[ ] GI symptoms
[ ] Edema	[ ] Wheezing	[ ] Neurological symptom
[ ] Weight change	[ ] LOC/syncope	[ ] Noncardiac chest pain

- [ ] 5. Chest Pain History

[ ] Typical angina	[ ] Variant angina
[ ] Atypical angina	[ ] Unstable angina
[ ] Noncardiac chest pain	[ ] None

- [ ] 6. Medication Review

[ ] Digoxin	[ ] Anti-HTN	[ ] Beta-blocker
[ ] Calcium antagonist	[ ] Nitrates	[ ] Antiarrhythmic
		[ ] Diuretics
[ ] ASA	[ ] Coumadin	[ ] Lipid agent
[ ] ACE	[ ] Insulin	

- [ ] 7. Activity Status
  - [ ] Review SAQ questionnaire
  - [ ] Previous treadmill experience and complications
  - [ ] Complications with activity

III.   Patient Examination
[   ] 1. Vital Signs—Heart Rate, BP (BP Controlled)
[   ] 2. Cardiovascular Examination
    [   ] JVP   [   ] Systolic murmur
    [   ] Carotid   [   ] Cardiomegaly
    [   ] Heart (R/O Aortic Stenosis)
[   ] 3. Pulmonary
[   ] 4. Periphery
    [   ] Peripheral pulses   [   ] Carotid bruits
    [   ] Edema   [   ] Femoral bruits
[   ] 5. Musculoskeletal
    [   ] Gait assessment

IV.   Reason for Exercise Test
1. [   ] Diagnosis   [   ] Exercise capacity
   [   ] Prognosis   [   ] Treatment
                                           assessment

2. [   ] Pretest probability determined

V.   Data Review
[   ] Review medical chart
[   ] Review PFT
[   ] Review previous tests
    [   ] ETT   [   ] Cath   [   ] Holter
    [   ] Echo   [   ] MUGA   [   ] Perfusion scan
[   ] Compare Serial ECG
    [   ] Prior ECG   [   ] LBBB   [   ] LVH
    [   ] Baseline   [   ] RBBB   [   ] ST depression
         supine ECG
    [   ] Baseline   [   ] WPW
         standing ECG

VI.   Equipment Check
[   ] Estimate METs, enter target
[   ] Check ECG leads/tracing for artifact
[   ] Check emergency equipment

VII.   Patient Instruction
[   ] Chest pain scale
[   ] Borg scale
[   ] Explain procedure during testing (frequent BP, symptom
       assessment)
[   ] Explain getting on and off of the treadmill
[   ] Demo walk

ACE = angiotensin-converting enzyme; ASA = acetylsalicylic acid; CABG = coronary artery bypass graft; CAD = coronary artery disease; CHF = congestive heart failure; COPD = chronic obstructive pulmonary disease; DM = diastolic murmur; ETT = exercise tolerance test; HTN = hypertension; JVP = jugular venous pulse; LBBB = left bundle branch block; LOC = loss of consciousness; LVH = left ventricular hypertrophy; MI = myocardial infarction; MUGA = multi-gated acquisition; PFT = pulmonary function test; PND = paroxysmal nocturnal dyspnea; PTCA = percutaneous transluminal coronary angioplasty; PVD = peripheral vascular disease; RBBB = right bundle branch block; SAQ = specific activity questionnaire; WPW = Wolff-Parkinson-White.

Table C-1. Functional Classification—
New York Heart Association (NYHA)

Class I	Patients with cardiac disease but without resulting limitations of physical activity. Ordinary physical activity does not cause undue fatigue, palpitation, dyspnea, or anginal pain.
Class II	Patients with cardiac disease resulting in slight limitation of physical activity. They are comfortable at rest. Ordinary physical activity results in fatigue, palpitation, dyspnea, or anginal pain.
Class III	Patients with cardiac disease resulting in marked limitation of physical activity. They are comfortable at rest. Less than ordinary physical activity causes fatigue, palpitation, dyspnea, or anginal pain.
Class IV	Patients with cardiac disease resulting in inability to carry on any physical activity without discomfort. Symptoms of cardiac insufficiency or of the anginal syndrome may be present even at rest. If any physical activity is undertaken, discomfort is increased.

Table C-2. Grading of Angina Pectoris by the Canadian
Cardiovascular Society Classification System

Class	Description of Stage
Class I	Ordinary physical activity does not cause angina, such as walking, climbing stairs. Angina occurs with strenuous, rapid, or prolonged exertion at work or recreation.
Class II	Slight limitation of ordinary activity. Angina occurs on walking or climbing stairs rapidly, walking uphill, walking or climbing stairs after meals, or in cold, or in wind, or under emotional stress, or only during the few hours after awakening, or walking more than two blocks on the level and climbing more than one flight of ordinary stairs at a normal pace and in normal condition.
Class III	Marked limitations of ordinary physical activity. Angina occurs on walking one or two blocks on the level and climbing one flight of stairs in normal conditions and at a normal pace.
Class IV	Inability to carry on any physical activity without discomfort— anginal symptoms may be present at rest.

Table C-3. The Goldman Specific Activity Scale—
Activities That Correspond to Classes I to IV of the
Specific Activity Scale (SAS)

Class I (≥7 METs)	A patient can perform any of the following activities:
	    Carrying 24 lb up eight steps
	    Carrying an 80-lb object
	    Shoveling snow
	    Skiing
	    Playing basketball, touch football, squash, or handball
	    Jogging/walking 5 mph

Class II (≥5 METs)	A patient does not meet class I criteria but can perform any of the following activities to completion without stopping:
	    Carrying anything up eight steps
	    Having sexual intercourse
	    Gardening, raking, weeding
	    Walking 4 mph

continued

**Table C-3.   The Goldman Specific Activity Scale—
Activities That Correspond to Classes I to IV of the
Specific Activity Scale (SAS) (Continued)**

Class III (≥2 METs)	A patient does not meet class I or class II criteria but can perform any of the following activities to completion without stopping:
	     Walking down eight steps
	     Taking a shower
	     Changing bed sheets
	     Mopping floors, cleaning windows
	     Walking 2.5 mph
	     Pushing a power mower
	     Bowling
	     Dressing without stopping

Class IV (≤2 METs)	None of the above

Table C-4.   The Duke Activity Scale Index (DASI)

Activity	Weight
Can you	
1. Take care of yourself (i.e., eating, dressing, bathing, using the toilet)?	2.75
2. Walk indoors, such as around your house?	1.75
3. Walk a block or two on level ground?	2.75
4. Climb a flight of stairs or walk up a hill?	5.50
5. Run a short distance?	8.00
6. Do light work around the house like dusting or washing dishes?	2.70
7. Do moderate work around the house like vacuuming, sweeping floors, or carrying in groceries?	3.50
8. Do heavy work around the house like scrubbing floors or lifting or moving heavy furniture?	8.00
9. Do yard work like raking leaves, weeding, or pushing a power mower?	4.50
10. Have sexual relations?	5.25
11. Participate in moderate recreational activities such as golf, bowling, dancing, or doubles tennis or throw a basketball or football?	6.00
12. Participate in strenuous sports such as swimming, singles tennis, football, basketball, or skiing?	7.50

Notes: The index equals the sum of weights for "yes" replies.
V_{O_2} (oxygen uptake) = $0.43 \times DASI + 9.6$.

Veterans Specific Activity Questionnaire (VSAQ)

Before beginning your treadmill test today, we need to estimate what your usual limits are during daily activities. The following is a list of activities that increase in difficulty as you read down the page. Think carefully, then underline the first activity that, if you performed it for a period of time, would typically cause fatigue, shortness of breath, chest discomfort, or otherwise cause you to want to stop. If you do not normally perform a particular activity, try to imagine what it would be like if you did.

1 MET:	—	Eating, getting dressed, working at a desk.
2 METs:	—	Taking a shower, shopping, cooking.
	—	Walking down eight steps.
3 METs:	—	Walking slowly on a flat surface for one or two blocks.
	—	A *moderate* amount of work around the house, like vacuuming, sweeping the floors or carrying groceries.
4 METs:	—	Light yard work, i.e., raking leaves, weeding, sweeping, or pushing a power mower; painting or light carpentry.
5 METs:	—	Walking briskly.
	—	Social dancing, washing the car.
6 METs:	—	Play nine holes of golf carrying your own clubs. Heavy carpentry, mow lawn with push mower.
7 METs:	—	Carry 60 lb, perform heavy outdoor work, i.e., digging, spading soil, etc.
	—	Walking uphill.
8 METs:	—	Carry groceries upstairs, move heavy furniture.
	—	Jog slowly on flat surface, climb stairs quickly.
9 METs:	—	Bicycling at a moderate pace, sawing wood, jumping rope (slowly).
10 METs:	—	Brisk swimming, bicycle up a hill, jog 6 mph.
11 METs:	—	Carry a heavy load (i.e., a child or firewood) up two flights of stairs.
	—	Cross country ski, bicycling briskly, continuously.
12 METs:	—	Running briskly, continuously (level ground, 8 min/mile).
13 METs:	—	Any competitive activity, including those that involve intermittent sprinting.
	—	Running competitively, rowing competitively, bicycle racing.

METs from VSAQ: ———— Maximal Speed: ———— mph

METs Achieved: ———— Maximal Grade: ———— %

METs from Nomogram: ———— Maximal Exercise
Time: ———— (min ± sec)

Patient Name _____

Social Security Number _____

Date _____

Fig. C-1. **The Veterans Specific Activity Questionnaire.**

Appendix D

Risk Factors

Risk Intervention	Recommendations
Smoking: **Goal** **complete cessation**	Strongly encourage patient and family to stop smoking. Provide counseling, nicotine replacement, and formal cessation programs as appropriate.
Lipid management: **Primary goal** **LDL <100 mg/dL** **Secondary goals** **HDL >35 mg/dL;** **TG <200 mg/dL**	Start AHA Step II Diet in all patients: ≤30% fat, <7% saturated fat, <200 mg/d cholesterol. Assess fasting lipid profile. In post-MI patients, lipid profile may take 4 to 6 weeks to stabilize. Add drug therapy according to the following guide:

LDL <100 mg/dL	LDL 100 to 130 mg/dL	LDL >130 mg/dL	HDL <35 mg/dL
No drug therapy	Consider adding drug therapy to diet, as follows:	Add drug therapy to diet, as follows:	Emphasize weight management and physical activity. Advise smoking cessation. If needed to achieve LDL goals, consider niacin, statin, fibrate.

Suggested drug therapy

TG <200 mg/dL	TG 200 to 400 mg/dL	TG >400 mg/dL
Statin Resin Niacin	Statin Niacin	Consider combined drug therapy (niacin, fibrate, statin)

If LDL goal not achieved, consider combination therapy.

Physical activity: Minimum goal 30 minutes 3 to 4 times per week	Assess risk, preferably with exercise test, to guide prescription. Encourage minimum of 30 to 60 minutes of moderate-intensity activity 3 or 4 times weekly (walking, jogging, cycling, or other aerobic activity) supplemented by an increase in daily lifestyle activities (eg, walking breaks at work, using stairs, gardening, household work). Maximum benefit 5 to 6 hours a week. Advise medically supervised programs for moderate- to high-risk patients.
Weight management:	Start intensive diet and appropriate physical activity intervention, as outlined above, in patients >120% of ideal weight for height. Particularly emphasize need for weight loss in patients with hypertension, elevated triglycerides, or elevated glucose levels.
Antiplatelet agents/ anticoagulants:	Start aspirin 80 to 325 mg/d if not contraindicated. Manage warfarin to international normalized ratio=2 to 3.5 for post-MI patients not able to take aspirin.
ACE inhibitors post-MI:	Start early post-MI in stable high-risk patients (anterior MI, previous MI, Killip class II [S₃ gallop, rales, radiographic CHF]). Continue indefinitely for all with LV dysfunction (ejection fraction≤40%) or symptoms of failure. Use as needed to manage blood pressure or symptoms in all other patients.
Beta-blockers:	Start in high-risk post-MI patients (arrhythmia, LV dysfunction, inducible ischemia) at 5 to 28 days. Continue 6 months minimum. Observe usual contraindications. Use as needed to manage angina, rhythm, or blood pressure in all other patients.
Estrogens:	Consider estrogen replacement in all postmenopausal women. Individualize recommendation consistent with other health risks.
Blood pressure control: Goal ≤140/90 mm Hg	Initiate lifestyle modification—weight control, physical activity, alcohol moderation, and moderate sodium restriction—in all patients with blood pressure>140 mm Hg systolic or 90 mm Hg diastolic. Add blood pressure medication, individualized to other patient requirements and characteristics (ie, age, race, need for drugs with specific benefits) if blood pressure is not less than 140 mm Hg systolic or 90 mm Hg diastolic in 3 months or if initial blood pressure is >160 mm Hg systolic or 100 mm Hg diastolic.

Fig. D-1.   Guide to comprehensive risk reduction for patients with coronary and other vascular diseases. ACE = angiotensin-converting enzymes; MI = myocardial infarction; TG = triglycerides. (Reproduced with permission from Smith, et al. Preventing heart attack and death. Circulation 1996;94:850–856. Copyright 1996 by American Heart Association.)

Table D-1. Framingham Heart Study Coronary Heart Disease Risk Prediction Chart

1. Find points for each risk factor

Age (if female) (yr)	Points	Age	Points
30	-12	41	1
31	-11	42-43	2
32	-9	44	3
33	-8	45-46	4
34	-6	47-48	5
35	-5	49-50	6
36	-4	51-52	7
37	-3	53-55	8
38	-2	56-60	9
39	-1	61-67	10
40	0	68-74	11

Age (if male) (yr)	Points	Age	Points
30	-2	48-49	9
31	-1	50-51	10
32-33	0	52-54	11
34	1	55-56	12
35-36	2	57-59	13
37-38	3	60-61	14
39	4	62-64	15
40-41	5	65-67	16
42-43	6	68-70	17
44-45	7	71-73	18
46-47	8	74	19

HDL cholesterol	Points	HDL	Points
25-26	7	67-73	-4
27-29	6	74-80	-5
30-32	5	81-87	-6
33-35	4	88-96	-7
36-38	3		
39-42	2		
43-46	1		
47-50	0		
51-55	-1		
56-60	-2		
61-66	-3		

Table D-1. Framingham Heart Study Coronary Heart Disease Risk Prediction Chart (Continued)

1. Find points for each risk factor (cont.)

Total cholesterol (mg/dl)

Chol	Points	Chol	Points
139–151	−3	220–239	2
152–166	−2	240–262	3
167–182	−1	263–288	4
183–199	0	289–315	5
200–219	1	316–330	6

Systolic blood pressure (mm Hg)

SBP	Points	SBP	Points
98–104	−2	150–160	4
105–112	−1	161–172	5
113–120	0	173–185	6
121–129	1		
130–139	2		
140–149	3		

Other Factors	Points Yes	Points No
Cigarette smoking	4	0
Diabetes		
Male	3	0
Female	6	0
ECG-LVH	9	0

2. Add points for all risk factors

____ + ____ + ____ + ____ + ____ + ____ + ____ = ____
(Age) (Total chol) (HDL) (SBP) (Smoking) (Diabetes) (ECG-LVH) (Total)

Note: Minus points subtract from total.

3. Look up risk corresponding to point total

Points	Probability (%) 5 yr	Probability (%) 10 yr	Points	Probability (%) 5 yr	Probability (%) 10 yr	Points	Probability (%) 5 yr	Probability (%) 10 yr	Points	Probability (%) 5 yr	Probability (%) 10 yr
≤1	<1	<2	9	2	5	17	6	13	25	14	27
2	1	2	10	2	6	18	7	14	26	16	29
3	1	2	11	3	6	19	8	16	27	17	31
4	1	2	12	3	7	20	8	18	28	19	33
5	1	3	13	3	8	21	9	19	29	20	36
6	1	3	14	4	9	22	11	21	30	22	38
7	1	4	15	5	10	23	12	23	31	24	40
8	2	4	16	5	12	24	13	25	32	25	42

4. Compare with average 10-year risk

Age (yr)	Probability (%) Women	Probability (%) Men	Age (yr)	Probability (%) Women	Probability (%) Men
30–34	<1	3	60–64	13	21
35–39	<1	5	65–69	9	30
40–44	2	6	70–74	12	24
45–49	5	10			
50–54	8	14			
55–59	12	16			

SBP = systolic blood pressure; ECG-LVH = left ventricular hypertrophy by electrocardiography.
Source: Anderson, et al. AHA Statement: updated coronary risk profile. *Circulation* 1991;83:356–362. Copyright 1991 by American Heart Association.

Appendix E

Pacemaker Patient Education

**Guidelines for the Patient with a Cardiac
Pacemaker or Automatic Implantable
Cardiac Defibrillator (AICD)**

1. Wear a medialert bracelet to identify yourself as a pacemaker or AICD patient.
2. Keep an identification card containing pacemaker or AICD information in your wallet.
3. Avoid contact with large magnetic fields, such as power plants or around running car engines, motorcycles, chainsaws, etc., because this energy could discontinue or alter pacemaker or AICD function. Smaller magnetic fields, such as microwaves, small electrical tools, and garage-door openers, are acceptable.
4. Patients should not pick up stereo speakers or hold portable compact disc or cassette players next to pacemakers or AICDs because they contain magnets.
5. Avoid MRI testing unless the specific instructions are reviewed with a cardiologist.
6. If beeping is heard from an AICD, contact a physician immediately. This warning sound can be emitted from the AICD before the function turns off.
7. Driving should be discussed with your health care provider. A temporary waiting period may be advisable before driving to allow an adjustment to the pacemaker or AICD. If function remains stable and limited shocks are received, driving can be safe.
8. Patients should avoid magnetic wand detectors, such as those used at airport security checkpoints. Patients should request a manual search instead.
9. Patients and family members should learn CPR. Cough CPR can be effective for direct current (DC) tachyrhythm.
10. Some dental procedures may need prophylactic antibiotics even if there is no other valvular disease present. Normal teeth cleaning does not require special treatment.
11. Activities should be increased slowly; a normal activity level should be achieved 1 to 2 weeks after pacemaker or AICD insertion. If a pacemaker is placed in the left mid-clavicular region, limit left arm move-

ment for approximately 2 weeks following surgery in order to promote healing and prevent swelling. With normally functioning pacemakers, heart rate should increase with level of exertion.

12. New or exacerbated symptoms, such as chest pain, fatigue, dyspnea, or syncope, should be reported immediately. Multiple repetitive (more than 3) shocks from an AICD should be reported to a cardiologist immediately.

13. Both clinic visits and telephone monitoring may be necessary to ensure proper battery function.

Appendix F

Key Features: Differential Diagnosis in the ADVIsE Approach

Table F-1.   Differential Diagnosis in the ADVIsE Approach

Dysfunction	Ischemia	Valves	Exercise	Arrhythmias
Primary				
Dilated cardiomyopathy (systolic dysfunction)	Coronary artery disease (including spasm and silent ischemia)	Aortic stenosis Aortic regurgitation Mitral stenosis Mitral regurgitation	Exercise intolerance	Atrial fibrillation Ventricular tachy-cardia Premature ventricular contractions Heart block
Confounders				
Anxiety Diastolic dysfunction (hypertrophic cardiomyopathy) Athletic heart Pulmonary disease (COPD) Pericardial effusion/cardiac tamponade Venous thrombosus	Esophageal reflux Pulmonary high BP Aortic stenosis Pericarditis Pulmonary embolus Costochondritis	Endocarditis Functional murmur Obstructive hyper-trophic cardio-myopathy	Deconditioning Pulmonary disease (COPD)	Anxiety Vasomotor syncope
Rare confounders				
Radiation heart disease High output cardiac failure Right ventricular infarct	Spasm with normal coronary arteries Dissecting aortic aneurysm	Marfan's syndrome	None	Long QT interval Right ventricular dysplasia

Table F-2. Myocardial Damage/Dysfunction: History and Physical Examination

Myocardial Damage/Dysfunction	History	Physical Examination
Primary		
Dilated cardiomyopathy (systolic dysfunction)	Right sided Edema Ascites Abdominal discomfort Nausea Weight gain Left sided Dyspnea Dyspnea on exertion Orthopnea Paroxysmal nocturnal dyspnea Cough Fatigue Nocturia Night sweats	Vital signs—tachycardia, decreased systolic BP Pulses—pulsus alternans, paradoxical pulse JVP—elevated, positive HJR, V-wave of TR Carotid—decreased amplitude Heart Decreased S_1, presence of S_3/S_4 Murmur of MR/TR Dyskinetic LV impulse Parasternal lift Displaced, enlarged point of maximal impulse Lungs—rales, effusions (dullness at bases) Abdomen—hepatomegaly, ascites Extremities—peripheral edema
Confounders		
Anxiety	Hyperventilation History of psychological problems	Normal
Diastolic dysfunction (hypertrophic cardiomyopathy)	Dyspnea Hypertension Renal disease	JVP—no elevated JVP Heart—S_4, sustained hyperdynamic precordial movement
Athletic heart	Training	Heart—cardiomegaly, S_3, bradycardia

Pulmonary disease (COPD)	Dyspnea Wheezing Industrial exposure Cough Cigarette smoking	Pulses—pulsus paradoxus Lungs—wheezing
Venous thrombosis	Leg pain Leg swelling Malignancy, disability	Unilateral pedal edema; calf tenderness (Homan's sign)
Cardiac tamponade/pericardial effusion	Dyspnea Syncope Sweating Dizziness	Vital signs—tachycardia, decreased BP Pulses—pulsus paradoxus Heart—distant heart sounds
Rare confounders Right ventricular infarct	Dyspnea Chest pain Inferior wall MI	JVP—elevated JVP Heart—parasternal "lift," right-sided S_3 Lungs—no rales
High output CHF	Anemia Hyperthyroidism Arteriovenous fistula	Tachycardia
Radiation heart disease	Radiation therapy Weight gain Chest pain	Neck vein distention Normal heart size

JVP = jugular venous pulse; HJR = hepatojugular reflux; TR = tricuspid regurgitation; MR = mitral regurgitation.

Table F-3. Myocardial Damage/Dysfunction: ECG and Chest X-Ray

Myocardial Damage/Dysfunction	ECG	Chest X-Ray
Primary		
Dilated cardiomyopathy (systolic dysfunction)	LBBB LV hypertrophy with strain Q waves Low voltage Left atrial abnormality	Effusions Increased vascular markings Kerley's B lines
Confounders		
Anxiety	Normal	Normal
Diastolic dysfunction (hypertrophic cardiomyopathy)	LV hypertrophy with strain LBBB	Normal-size heart or mildly enlarged
Athletic heart	Sinus bradycardia LV hypertrophy voltage	Normal
Pulmonary disease (COPD)	$S_1 S_2 S_3$ Right ventricular hypertrophy Low voltage Right axis abnormality Right axis deviation	Hyperinflation Low, flat diaphragms
Venous thrombosis	Normal	Normal
Cardiac tamponade/pericardial effusion	Drop in QRS voltage	Enlarged heart silhouette
Rare confounders		
Right ventricular infarct	ST elevation in right-sided precordial leads Inferior Q waves	Lateral view filled in behind sternum
High output CHF	Normal	Normal
Radiation heart disease	Low voltage	Pulmonary fibrosis

LBBB = left bundle-branch block.

Table F-4. Myocardial Damage/Dysfunction: Diagnostic Tests

Myocardial Damage/Dysfunction	Exercise Test	Echocardiography	Nuclear Tests	Nonexercise Stress Test	Holter Monitoring	Catheterization
Primary						
Dilated cardiomyopathy (systolic dysfunction)	Helpful Standard Gases	Necessary	Helpful MUGA	Unnecessary	Unnecessary	Helpful Ventriculography
Confounders						
Anxiety	Unnecessary	Helpful	Unnecessary	Unnecessary	Unnecessary	Usually unnecessary
Diastolic dysfunction (hypertrophic cardiomyopathy)	Unnecessary	Necessary	Unnecessary	Unnecessary	Unnecessary	Helpful Ventriculography
Athletic heart	Helpful Standard	Helpful	Unnecessary	Unnecessary	Unnecessary	Helpful Ventriculography
Pulmonary disease* (COPD)	Helpful Standard Gases	Helpful	Unnecessary	Unnecessary	Unnecessary	Unnecessary
Venous thrombosis	Unnecessary	Necessary (peripheral)	Unnecessary	Unnecessary	Unnecessary	Unnecessary
Cardiac tamponade/pericardial effusion	Unnecessary	Necessary	Unnecessary	Unnecessary	Unnecessary	Helpful Ventriculography Hemodynamics
Rare confounders						
Right ventricular infarct	Unnecessary	Necessary	Unnecessary	Unnecessary	Unnecessary	Helpful Hemodynamics
High output CHF	Unnecessary	Helpful	Unnecessary	Unnecessary	Unnecessary	Helpful Hemodynamics
Radiation heart disease	Unnecessary	Necessary	Unnecessary	Unnecessary	Unnecessary	Helpful Hemodynamics

*Diagnosis of pulmonary disease requires resting pulmonary function tests.

Table F-5.   Myocardial Ischemia: History and Physical Examination

Myocardial Ischemia	History	Physical Examination
Primary		
Coronary artery disease	Typical angina Claudication Multiple risk factors	Carotid bruits Femoral bruits Xanthelasma, tendon xanthoma
Silent ischemia	Multiple risk factors Claudication Coronary artery disease Elderly	Carotid bruits Femoral bruits Xanthelasma, tendon xanthoma
Variant angina (spasm around fixed lesions)	Substernal chest pain Cyclic; same time each day At rest	Normal
Confounders		
Esophageal reflux	Substernal burning chest pain Nausea	Abdomen—Midepigastric tenderness
Pulmonary high BP	Substernal chest pain Dyspnea	Jugular venous pulse—giant A waves

Aortic stenosis	Substernal chest pain/typical angina Dyspnea Fatigue Syncope	See Valvular
Pericarditis	Precordial chest pain (sharp) Fever Dyspnea	Heart—friction rub
Costochondritis	Chest pain at 2nd costochondral cartilage	Normal
Rare confounders		
Variant angina (spasm in normal coronaries)	Substernal chest pain At rest Raynauld's phenomena Cyclic; same time each day	Normal
Dissecting aortic aneurysm	High BP	Vital signs—systolic BP different between arms

Table F-6. Myocardial Ischemia: ECG and Chest X-Ray

Myocardial Ischemia	ECG	Chest X-Ray
Primary		
Coronary artery disease (including silent ischemia and variant angina around fixed lesions)	Serial ECGs for comparison Q waves (evidence of ischemic damage) T-wave inversion ST depression	Normal
Confounders		
Esophageal reflux	Nonspecific changes or normal	Normal
Pulmonary high BP	$S_1 S_2 S_3$ Right ventricular hypertrophy Right atrial abnormality	Increased size of pulmonary artery Decreased vascular markings
Aortic stenosis	LV hypertrophy with strain	Prominent aortic root Increased cardiac silhouette
Pericarditis	PR depression ST elevation Low amplitude T waves	Normal until effusion gathers
Costochondritis	Normal	Normal
Rare confounders		
Variant angina (spasm in normal coronaries)	ST elevation without diagnostic Q waves Cyclic; same time each day	Normal
Dissecting aortic aneurysm	LV hypertrophy	Widened aortic root

Table F-7. Myocardial Ischemia: Diagnostic Tests

Myocardial Ischemia	Exercise Test	Echocardiography	Nuclear Tests	Nonexercise Stress Test	Holter Monitoring	Catheterization
Primary						
Coronary artery disease	Necessary Perfusion Standard Gases Echo	Helpful Resting study	Helpful Perfusion scan	Helpful Dipyridamole perfusion Dobutamine echocardiography	Unnecessary	Helpful Coronary angiography Ventriculography
Confounders						
Esophageal reflux	Helpful Standard	Unnecessary	Helpful Perfusion scan	Helpful Dipyridamole perfusion Dobutamine echocardiography	Unnecessary	Unnecessary
Pulmonary high BP	Helpful Standard Gases	Unnecessary	Unnecessary	Unnecessary	Unnecessary	Helpful Hemodynamics
Aortic stenosis	Helpful Standard Gases	Necessary	Helpful Perfusion scan	Helpful Dipyridamole perfusion Dobutamine echocardiography	Unnecessary	Helpful Hemodynamics Coronary angiography Ventriculography
Pulmonary embolus	Unnecessary	Helpful	V/Q scan	Unnecessary	Unnecessary	Helpful Pulmonary angiogram
Pericarditis	Unnecessary	Helpful	Helpful Perfusion scan	Helpful Dipyridamole perfusion Dobutamine echocardiography	Unnecessary	Unnecessary

continued

Table F-7. Myocardial Ischemia: Diagnostic Tests (Continued)

Myocardial Ischemia	Exercise Test	Echocardiography	Nuclear Tests	Nonexercise Stress Test	Holter Monitoring	Catheterization
Confounders (continued)						
Costochondritis	Helpful Standard	Unnecessary	Helpful Dipyridamole scan	Unnecessary	Unnecessary	Unnecessary
Rare confounders						
Variant angina (spasm in normal coronaries)	Necessary Standard Gases Echo	Unnecessary	Helpful Perfusion	Unnecessary	Helpful	Necessary Coronary angiography Ergotamine stress
Dissecting aortic aneurysm	Unnecessary	Helpful	Unnecessary	Unnecessary	Unnecessary	Necessary Coronary angiography

Table F-8. Valvular Status: History and Physical Examination

Valvular Status	History	Physical Examination
Primary		
Aortic stenosis	Chest pain Syncope Dyspnea Fatigue	Pulses—narrow pulse pressure Carotids—slow carotid upstroke, decreased amplitude, anacrotic notch, carotid bruit Heart—soft S_2, S_4, systolic ejection murmur
Aortic regurgitation	Palpitations Fatigue Dyspnea Orthopnea Paroxysmal nocturnal dyspnea	Pulses—wide pulse pressure Carotids—increased carotid amplitude Heart—diastolic blow, soft S_1

Mitral stenosis	Dyspnea Fatigue Palpitations Hemoptysis	Heart—loud S_1, presystolic accentuation of diastolic murmur, opening snap
Mitral regurgitation	Dyspnea Fatigue Orthopnea Paroxysmal nocturnal dyspnea Palpitations	Heart—holosystolic murmur, S_3 common, soft S_1
Confounders Endocarditis	Valvular heart disease IV drug use	Murmurs CHF Embolic phenomenon
Functional murmur	Asymptomatic	No other findings than moderate to soft systolic murmur
Obstructive hypertrophic cardiomyopathy	Sudden death CHF in family	Heart—systolic murmur that increases with Valsalva's maneuver Cardiomegaly
Rare confounder Marfan's syndrome	Family history	Arm range to height ratio Appearance Ocular findings

Table F-9. Valvular Status: ECG and Chest X-Ray

Valvular Status	ECG	Chest X-Ray
Primary		
Aortic stenosis	LV hypertrophy with strain Left atrial abnormality	Aortic valve calcification Poststenotic dilation of aorta
Aortic regurgitation	LV hypertrophy	Cardiomegaly Aortic root dilation
Mitral stenosis	Right axis Right ventricular hypertrophy Atrial fibrillation	Prominent pulmonary arteries Kerley's B lines Small heart Enlarged left atrium pushing into esophagus
Mitral regurgitation	LV hypertrophy IVCD Left atrial abnormality Infarction Q waves	Cardiomegaly Vascular redistribution Large left atrium
Confounders		
Endocarditis	Changes consistent with diseased valve	Pulmonary infiltrates Changes consistent with diseased valve
Functional murmur	Normal	Normal
Obstructive hypertrophic cardiomyopathy	LV hypertrophy LBBB WPW	Normal
Rare confounder		
Marfan's syndrome	Nonspecific	Normal or widened aortic root or enlarged left atrium

IVCD = intraventricular conduction defect; LBBB = left bundle-branch block; WPW = Wolff-Parkinson-White syndrome.

Table F-10. Valvular Status: Diagnostic Tests

Valvular Status	Exercise Test	Echocardiography	Nuclear Tests	Nonexercise Stress Test	Holter Monitoring	Catheterization
Primary						
Aortic stenosis	Helpful Standard Gases	Necessary	Unnecessary	Unnecessary	Unnecessary	Necessary Coronary angiography Ventriculography Hemodynamics
Aortic regurgitation	Helpful Standard Gases	Necessary	Unnecessary	Unnecessary	Unnecessary	Necessary Coronary angiography Ventriculography Hemodynamics
Mitral stenosis	Helpful Standard Gases	Necessary	Unnecessary	Unnecessary	Unnecessary	Necessary Coronary angiography Ventriculography Hemodynamics
Mitral regurgitation	Helpful Standard Gases	Necessary	Unnecessary	Unnecessary	Unnecessary	Necessary Coronary angiography Ventriculography Hemodynamics
Confounders						
Endocarditis	Unnecessary	Necessary TEE	Unnecessary	Unnecessary	Unnecessary	Unnecessary
Functional murmur	Unnecessary	Helpful	Unnecessary	Unnecessary	Unnecessary	Unnecessary
Obstructive hypertrophic cardiomyopathy	Unnecessary	Necessary	Unnecessary	Unnecessary	Unnecessary	Necessary Ventriculography Hemodynamics

continued

Table F-10.   Valvular Status: Diagnostic Tests (Continued)

Valvular Status	Exercise Test	Echocardiography	Nuclear Tests	Nonexercise Stress Test	Holter Monitoring	Catheterization
Rare confounder Marfan's syndrome	Unnecessary	Necessary	Unnecessary	Unnecessary	Unnecessary	Necessary Coronary angiography Ventriculography Hemodynamics

TEE = transesophageal echocardiography.

Table F-11.   Exercise Capacity: History and Physical Examination

Exercise Capacity	History	Physical Examination
Primary Exercise intolerance	See Tables F-2, F-5, F-8, F-14	See Tables F-2, F-5, F-8, F-14
Confounders Deconditioning	Fatigue Sedentary lifestyle	Specific for illness-limiting exercise
Pulmonary disease (COPD)	Dyspnea Wheezes Cough Cigarette smoking Industrial exposure	Pulses—pulsus paradoxus Lungs—wheezes, prolonged expiration
Rare confounders None		

Table F-12.   Exercise Capacity: ECG and Chest X-Ray

Exercise Capacity	ECG	Chest X-Ray
Primary Exercise intolerance	Depends on diagnosis Can be normal	Depends on diagnosis Can be normal
Confounders Deconditioning Pulmonary disease (COPD)	Normal S_1, S_2, S_3 Right ventricular hypertrophy Low voltage Right axis deviation Right atrial abnormality	Normal Hyperinflation Low, flat diaphragms
Rare confounders None		

Table F-13. Exercise Capacity: Diagnostic Tests

Exercise Capacity	Exercise Test	Echocardiography	Nuclear Tests	Nonexercise Stress Test	Holter Monitoring	Catheterization
Primary						
Exercise intolerance	Necessary Standard Gas exchange	Helpful	Helpful MUGA	Unnecessary	Unnecessary	Unnecessary
Confounders						
Deconditioning	Necessary Standard Gas exchange	Helpful	Helpful MUGA	Unnecessary	Unnecessary	Unnecessary
Pulmonary disease* (COPD)	Helpful Standard Gas exchange	Helpful	Helpful MUGA of right ventricle	Unnecessary	Unnecessary	Unnecessary
Rare confounders						
None						

MUGA = multigated acquisition.
*Diagnosis of pulmonary disease requires pulmonary function tests.

Table F-14. Arrhythmias: History and Physical Examination

Arrhythmias	History	Physical Examination
Primary		
Atrial fibrillation	Palpitations Fatigue Dyspnea	Vital signs—irregular pulse Heart—no S_4
Ventricular tachycardia	Palpitations Syncope Dyspnea	Pulses—pulsus alternans JVP—cannon A waves
Premature ventricular contractions	Palpitations	Pulses—pulsus alternans JVP—cannon A waves
Heart block	Syncope	JVP—cannon A waves Heart—soft S_1
Confounders		
Anxiety	Hyperventilation History of psychological problems	Normal
Vasomotor syncope	Syncope Pallor Nausea Sweating	Vital signs—bradycardia, hypotension
Rare confounders		
Long QT syndrome	Syncope	Normal
Right ventricular dysplasia	Family with sudden death, syncope	Normal

JVP = jugular venous pressure.

Table F-15.   Arrhythmias: ECG and Chest X-Ray

Arrhythmias	ECG	Chest X-Ray
Primary		
Atrial fibrillation	Arrhythmias (no P waves, irregularly irregular rhythm, chaotic baseline) plus underlying disease process	Normal or changes of underlying disease process
Ventricular tachycardia	Arrhythmias (wide complex tachycardia) plus underlying disease process	Normal or changes of underlying disease process
Premature ventricular contractions	Arrhythmias (wide irregular complexes) plus underlying disease process	Normal or changes of underlying disease process
Heart block	Arrhythmias (arteriovenous dissociation) plus underlying disease process	Normal or changes of underlying disease process
Confounders		
Anxiety	Tachycardia	Normal
Vasomotor syncope	Normal	Normal
Rare confounders		
Long QT syndrome	QT > 50% R-R interval	Normal
Right ventricular dysplasia	Premature ventricular contractions	Normal

Table F-16.   Arrhythmias: Diagnostic Tests

Arrhythmias	Exercise Test	Echocardiography	Nuclear Tests	Nonexercise Stress Test	Holter Monitoring	Catheterization
Primary						
Artial fibrillation	Helpful Standard Gases	Necessary	Unnecessary	Unnecessary	Helpful	Unnecessary
Ventricular tachycardia	Helpful Standard	Helpful	Unnecessary	Unnecessary	Necessary	Helpful Electrophysiologic studies
Premature ventricular contractions	Unnecessary	Unnecessary	Unnecessary	Unnecessary	Helpful	Helpful Electrophysiologic studies
Heart block	Unnecessary	Unnecessary	Unnecessary	Unnecessary	Necessary	Helpful Electrophysiologic studies
Confounders						
Anxiety	Helpful Standard	Unnecessary	Unnecessary	Unnecessary	Helpful	Unnecessary
Vasomotor syncope*	Unnecessary	Unnecessary	Unnecessary	Unnecessary	Helpful	Unnecessary
Rare confounders						
Long QT syndrome	Unnecessary	Unnecessary	Unnecessary	Unnecessary	Helpful	Additive Electrophysiologic studies
Right ventricular dysplasia	Unnecessary	Helpful (MRI bottor)	Unnecessary	Unnecessary	Helpful	Unnecessary

*Tilt table test most helpful for diagnosis of vasomotor syncope.

Table F-17.   Cardiac Causes of Chest Pain Due to Myocardial Ischemia

Diagnosis / Subtypes	Etiology	Precipitating Factors	Location	Timing (Onset, Duration)	Relief	Quality
Angina pectoris	Coronary artery disease emboli or atherosclerosis Aortic stenosis	Exercise Anger	Substernal	Onset during or immediately after exercise 5–15 min	Rest Nitroglycerin	Choking Squeezing "Band across chest" Pressure Dull ache Tightness
Variant angina (Prinzmetal's)	Coronary artery spasm	Plaque rupture	Substernal	Immediate onset 5–15 min Cyclic, morning	Rest Nitroglycerin	Pressure Ache
Acute MI 1. Q wave 2. Non Q wave	Coronary artery disease	Thrombus and/ or rupured plaque	Substernal	Constant for 30–60 min but can last intermittently for days Most common in morning	Morphine Beta-blocker Completion of MI	Heavy pressure Squeezing

Table F-18.   Cardiac Causes of Chest Pain Due to Myocardial Ischemia

Diagnosis / Subtypes	Radiation	Associated Symptoms	Aggravating Factors	Pathophysiology	Comments
Angina pectoris	Left arm Jaw Neck	Dyspnea	Cold weather Smoking Heavy, large meal	Increased myocardial O_2 consumption or decreased O_2 supply	Increased suspicion with claudication, multiple risk factors Possibly due to aortic stenosis if murmur present
Variant angina (Prinzmetal's)	Left arm Jaw Neck	Nausea Dyspnea	Early AM Hormone surge	Coronary artery spasm	More common in women Angina pattern does not correlate with activity

continued

Continued from previous table — Acute MI row:

- **Diagnosis/Subtypes:** Acute MI; 1. Q wave; 2. Non-Q wave
- **Left arm, Neck, Jaw**
- Anterior/lateral: CHF, shock, tachycardia; Inferior/posterior: bradycardia, heart block; Diaphoresis; Nausea/vomiting; Dyspnea
- Increased myocardial oxygen demand
- Decreased O_2 supply due to coronary occlusion
- **Risk factors:** Diabetes, High BP, Claudication, Stroke, Hyperlipidemia

Table F-19. Cardiac Causes of Chest Pain *Not* Due to Coronary Artery Disease

Diagnosis / Subtypes	Etiology	Precipitating Factors	Location	Timing (Onset, Duration)	Relief	Quality
Pericarditis	Viral/bacterial Autoimmune disease External trauma Post MI Postcardiac surgery Uremia Drugs	See Etiology	Precordial Substernal	Gradual onset Hours or days	Sit up Lean forward Shallow respiration Anti-inflammatory drugs	Sharp Pleuritic
Aortic dissection	Connective tissue disorders	Hypertension	Substernal Back Neck	Sudden Hours	Surgery Analgesia	Severe Deep Maximum at onset
Aortic stenosis	Congenital Rheumatic Calcific	Exercise Anger	Precordial Substernal	Minutes	Rest (avoid NTG)	Dull pressure
Aortic aneurysm (without dissection)	Atherosclerosis Marfan's syndrome Hypertension Trauma	See Etiology	Substernal	Gradual onset Hours	Surgery based on size, clinical presentation	Ache

Table F-20.   Cardiac Causes of Chest Pain *Not* Due to Coronary Artery Disease

Diagnosis / Subtypes	Radiation	Associated Symptoms	Aggravating Factors	Pathophysiology	Comments
Pericarditis	Neck Shoulders	Fever Dyspnea	Supine Breathing Turning Swallowing Twisting Coughing	Inflammation of pericardium	Can be chronic or recurring
Aortic dissection	Thoracic or lumbar area of back Abdomen	Transient weakness of legs Syncope Different systolic BP between right/left arms	Hypertension Failure to follow aortic size	Intimal tears due to hypertension and/or cystic medial necrosis	Requires acute treatment Control BP Surgery
Aortic stenosis	Neck Jaw Left arm	Dyspnea Fatigue Syncope	Cold weather Eating Smoking	Obstruction of aortic valve causing decrease in cardiac output	Anginal in character
Aortic aneurysm (without dissection)	Interscapular Abdomen Lumbar	Cough Dysphagia Hoarseness	Dissection	Dilation of thoracic aorta	Abdominal aorta can also develop aneurysm

Table F-21. Gastrointestinal Causes of Chest Pain

Diagnosis	Etiology	Precipitating Factors	Location	Timing (Onset, Duration)	Relief	Quality
Ruptured esophagus	Mallory-Weiss	Severe retching and vomiting Esophageal procedure Esophageal cancer	Site of perforation (cervical, thoracic, abdominal) Epigastric pain	Immediate onset Hours	Surgery	Severe
Esophageal reflux	Hiatal hernia	Recent meal	Substernal between xiphoid and suprasternal notch	Gradual after ingestion 10–60 min	Antacid H_2 blockers	Burning
Esophageal spasm	See Pathophysiology in Table F-22	Recent meal Anxiety Emotional stress	Substernal	Immediate onset 5–60 min	Nitroglycerin Spontaneous	Dull Sharp Squeezing
Peptic ulcer/duodenal ulcer	Gastritis Smoking Alcohol Emotions	ASA NSAIDs	Epigastric	Gradual after ingestion Hours	Food Antacid Bismuth/metronidazole	Burning
Biliary disease	Cholecystolithiasis Cholecystitis	Diet Gallstones	Right upper abdominal quadrant	Episodic onset Hours	Spontaneous Analgesia	Colicky
Pancreatitis	Alcohol Biliary tract disease	Binge drinking	Epigastric	Gradual onset Hours	Lean forward	Steady ache

NSAIDs = nonsteroidal anti-inflammatory drugs.

Table F-22. Gastrointestinal Causes of Chest Pain

Diagnosis	Radiation	Associated Symptoms	Aggravating Factors	Pathophysiology	Comments
Ruptured esophagus	Between scapula	Dyspnea Tachycardia Diaphoresis Mediastinal crepitation Cyanosis Pallor	Lack of immediate treatment	Perforation of esophagus, causing bleeding into mediastinum	"Tearing sensation" after vomiting
Esophageal reflux	Rare	Nausea	Bending over Supine position Valsalva's maneuver	Regurgitation of acid due to weak sphincter	"Heartburn"
Esophageal spasm	Back Arms Jaw	Dysphagia	Cold fluid *Not* exercise	Neuromuscular disorder (achalasia)	Mimics angina Localized to actual level of spasm
Peptic ulcer/duodenal ulcer	Rare	Nausea	Lack of food Spicy food	Increased acid production *Helicobacter* infection	Diagnosed by endoscopy
Biliary disease	Lower back	Dyspepsia Indigestion Fever Nausea Vomiting	Fatty foods Spicy foods	Obstruction of ducts by stone Inflamed gallbladder	Diagnosed by abdominal ultrasound
Pancreatitis	Back	Fever	Alcohol ingestion	Inflammation of pancreas	Rebound tenderness

Table F-23.   Pulmonary Causes of Chest Pain

Diagnosis	Etiology	Precipitating Factors	Location	Timing (Onset, Duration)	Relief	Quality
Pleuritis Sticking	Viral Autoimmune defect Pulmonary embolus	Infection Pneumonia	Lateral thorax	Gradual onset Hours	Rapid, shallow breathing	Sharp
Pneumothorax	Chest trauma Pulmonary disease	See Etiology	Lateral thorax	Sudden onset Hours	Thoracentesis Sit upright	Sharp
Pulmonary embolism Pleuritic	Venous thrombus/emboli	CHF History of embolism Surgery Malignancy Immobility Pregnancy	Lateral thorax	Sudden onset Hours	Analgesia	Sharp
Mediastinal emphysema	Pulmonary disease	Coughing	Upper thorax	Sudden onset Hours	Spontaneous	Sharp
Pulmonary hypertension	CHF Valvular disease Pulmonary embolism COPD Systemic high BP Atrial septal defect	High altitude Hypoxia Increased LV pressure Chronic lung disease	Substernum to neck	Sudden onset Minutes	Relaxing Nitroglycerin	Tight

Table F-24.   Pulmonary Causes of Chest Pain

Diagnosis	Radiation	Associated Symptoms	Aggravating Factors	Pathophysiology	Comments
Pleuritis	Diaphragmatic to shoulders	Fever, Dyspnea	Inspiration	Inflammation of pleural surfaces	
Pneumothorax	Diaphragmatic to shoulders	Sudden dyspnea, Hypotension, Tachycardia	Lack of immediate treatment	Rupture of lining due to weakened surface	Younger adult, Hyperlucency on chest x-ray
Pulmonary embolism large	Diaphragmatic to shoulders	Cyanosis, Dyspnea, Tachypnea, Hemoptysis	Inspiration	Embolus to pulmonary vasculature	Can be life-threatening when acute and
Mediastinal emphysema	Neck	Mediastinal crepitation	Inspiration	Pulmonary alveoli rupture allowing air to dissect	
Pulmonary hypertension	Neck, Throat	Shortness of breath, Fatigue, Dyspnea	Exercise	Elevated pulmonary artery pressure	

Table F-25.   Neuromuscular-Skeletal Causes of Chest Pain

Diagnosis	Etiology	Precipitating Factors	Location	Timing (Onset, Duration)	Relief	Quality
Herpes zoster (shingles)	Viral infection	Chickenpox Immune system deficiency Cancer Radiation	Specific dermatome of thorax	Gradual Hours/days before rash presents	Analgesia Aluminum subacetate (Domboro) soaks	Radicular Gripping Burning Superficial
Musculoskeletal inflammation	Myositis Arthritis	Increased activity Thoracic surgery	Anterior chest	Gradual onset Hours/days	Physical therapy Heat Massage Analgesia NSAIDs	Gripping
Costochondritis (Tietze's syndrome)	Unknown	Thoracic surgery	Costochondral joints	Gradual onset Hours/days	Spontaneous NSAIDs Steroid injection into joint	Superficial
Thoracic outlet syndrome	Rib abnormalities Cervical arthritis Cervical disk disease Peripheral neuropathy and vascular disease	Arm movement over head	Upper extremities Anterior chest wall (rare)	Gradual onset Hours/days	Heat Muscle relaxants Decreased movement of arms Analgesia Surgery	Radicular

NSAIDs = nonsteroidal anti-inflammatory drugs.

Table F-26.   Neuromuscular-Skeletal Causes of Chest Pain

Diagnosis*	Radiation	Associated Symptoms	Aggravating Factors	Pathophysiology	Comments
Herpes zoster	None Pain pattern follows a dermatome	Itching Rash Hyperesthesia	Touch	Viral disease of spinal ganglia and vesicular eruption at dermatome	Common in elderly
Musculoskeletal inflammation	Variable	Recent strenuous activity	Movement Palpation	Dependent on etiology	
Costochondritis (Tietze's syndrome)	Shoulder	Swelling at affected joints	Palpation Movement Coughing	Inflammation of costochondral joints	
Thoracic outlet syndrome	Neck Shoulder Scapula Axilla	Altered sensation Muscle atrophy Vascular insufficiency	Palpation over supraclavicular space	Compression of neural and vascular structures that exit superior rim of thoracic cage	Usually age 30–40 Female > male

*Other possible diagnoses of chest pain to be considered include mediastinal tumor, neuritis, and a broken rib.

Table F-27.   Psychological Causes of Chest Pain

Diagnosis	Etiology	Participating Factors	Location	Timing (Onset, Duration)	Relief	Quality
Anxiety	Panic attacks Neurocirculatory asthenia	Claustrophobia History of psychological problems	Left inframammary region Substernal	Gradual onset Seconds to hours	Tranquilizers Spontaneous	Stabbing Tightness Dull
Hyperventilation	Associated with anxiety	History of psychological problems Claustrophobia Panic attacks	Precordial chest	Gradual onset Seconds to hours	Rebreath CO_2 ("brown bag") Spontaneous	Stabbing Tightness
Depression	Situational Endogenous	History of psychological problems Sedentary Recent stress	Left anterior chest	Gradual onset Minutes to hours	Counseling Medication	Variable

Table F-28. Psychological Causes of Chest Pain

Diagnosis	Radiation	Associated Symptoms	Aggravating Factors	Pathophysiology	Comments
Anxiety	Throat Left arm	Choking sensation Breathlessness Palpitations	*Not* exercise Uncertainty	Syndrome related to sympathetic nervous system fight/flight response	Most common cause Fear of exercise
Hyperventilation	Neck Left arm	Inability to take satisfying deep breath Tingling and numbness of hands, lips Near syncope	Fearful situation	Tachypnea causes repiratory alkalosis	
Depression	Variable	Despair Agitation Insomnia Lack of concentration Decreased libido Decreased appetite	Lack of resolution of stressor	Clinical or situational depression	Flat affect can obscure angina

Table F-29.   Cardiac Causes of Dyspnea

Diagnosis	Onset	Associated Symptoms	Precipitating Factors	Relieving Factors	Aggravating Factors	Clinical Factors	Etiology
Valvular heart disease	Chronic, progressive	Syncope Chest pain	Exercise Arrhythmias	Rest Medications Surgery when indicated	Noncompliance with diet and medications	Degenerative Rheumatic Congenital HLA tissue capability	Stenosis Insufficiency
LV failure	Chronic or acute	PND Fatigue Edema Tachycardia Weight gain Cough Orthopnea	Sodium intake Excess fluids Viral illness Noncompliance	Diuretics Afterload reduction	Beta-blockers Alcohol Other medications that depress LV function (flecainide, verapamil)	Systolic or diastolic dysfunction Right-sided involvement History of cancer treatment	Myocardial damage/ dysfunction Hypertrophy Infiltrative
Coronary artery disease (CAD)	Chronic or acute	Substernal chest pain	Exercise Anger Noncompliance with regimen	Nitroglycerin Rest	Cold weather Smoking Heavy, large meal	Increased suspicion with claudication, risk factors Dyspnea can be angina equivalent	Acute MI or severe ischemia causing myocardial stunning
Arrhythmia	Acute	Syncope Palpitations	Abnormal electrolytes Exercise "Holiday heart"	Medication Pacemaker Correcting electrolytes	Digoxin toxicity Diuretic therapy Ischemia Dilated cardiomyopathy	Associated with CHF	Atrial flutter/ fibrillation Ventricular tachycardia Heart block Pacer malfunction
Pericardial disease	Gradual onset Hours or days of duration	Substernal or precordial Chest pain Fever	See Etiology	Sit up Lean forward NSAIDs	Supine Breathing Turning Swallowing Coughing	Nonanginal description ST elevation PR depression Low T waves	Viral/bacterial infection Autoimmune diseases Rheumatic fever External trauma MI Cardiac surgery Uremia Drugs

PND = paroxysmal nocturnal dyspnea; NSAIDs = nonsteroidal anti-inflammatory drugs.

Table F-30.   Systemic Causes of Dyspnea*

Diagnosis	Onset	Associated Symptoms	Precipitating Factors	Relieving Factors	Aggravating Factors	Clinical Factors	Etiology
Anemia	Chronic Acute	Fatigue Bloody stools Melena Hemoptysis Hematuria	ASA or NSAID use Blood loss anticoagulation	Transfusion Iron supplements Erythropoietin	Alcohol use Poor diet	See Etiology	Peptic ulcer disease Surgery Diet deficiency Chronic illness
Deconditioned	Chronic	Fatigue	Exercise Chronic illness Injury	Rest	Bed rest	Primary due to sedentary lifestyle Secondary due to chronic disease	Acute/chronic illness Surgery No exercise schedule
Obesity	Chronic	Fatigue Sleep apnea LV dysfunction	Exercise Large abdominal girth	Rest Sitting Weight loss	Persistent weight gain	Decreased motivation to exercise	Associated with chronic illness limiting activity (COPD, CHF) Associated with diabetes Eating disorder

NSAID = nonsteroidal anti-inflammatory drug; ASA = aspirin.
*Other systemic causes of dyspnea include metabolic acidosis (diabetic acidosis), pregnancy, hyperthyroidism, and hypothyroidism.

Table F-31. Psychogenic Causes of Dyspnea

Diagnosis	Onset	Associated Symptoms	Precipitating Factors	Relieving Factors	Aggravating Factors	Clinical Factors	Etiology
Hyperventilation	Acute	Tingling of arms and hands	Claustrophobia Fearful situation Emotional instability	Rebreath CO_2 ("brown bag") Tranquilizers Counseling Deep sighing	Loss of control	History of anxiety, psychological problems	Panic attacks Depression Neurocirculatory asthenia

Table F-32. Pulmonary Causes of Dyspnea

Subset Diagnosis	Onset	Associated Symptoms	Precipitating Factors	Relieving Factors	Aggravating Factors	Clinical Factors	Pathophysiology
Asthma	Sudden	Fatigue of accessory muscles Wheezing Cough	Exertion Allergens Inhaling cold air	Inhalers Medications	Smoke Dust Pollens	Onset in childhood history of respiratory infection	Obstruction of upper intrathoracic airways
Bronchitis	Chronic/ sudden	Cough Sputum	Infection	Antibiotics Inhalers Clear secretions	Smoking Allergens	Smoker	Inflammation of bronchial tubes causing obstruction
Chronic obstructive pulmonary disease (COPD)	Chronic	Use of accessory muscles Wheezing Cough Sputum Orthopnea	Long history of smoking Exertion	Clear secretions Inhalers Steroids	Smoking Allergens	Infection common cause for exacerbation	Airway collapse

Parenchymal	Gradual	Cough Fever Hemoptysis Wheezing	See Clinical Factors Inhaled irritants Infection Congenital	Steroids Antibiotics	Lack of serial follow-up	Pneumonia Alveolitis Drug induced Metastatic disease Pneumonitis Pulmonary fibrosis	Variety of factors causing alveolar and interstitial lung disease
Pulmonary edema	Sudden	Diaphoresis Cyanosis Tachypnea Frothy sputum Rales	Minimal exertion Salt overload Excess fluids	Sit upright Supplemental O_2 Diuresis Tourniquet	Lack of treatment	Pulmonary embolus Cardiac cause High altitude ARDS Lymphatic insufficiency Drug induced	Interstitial/alveolar fluid accumulation
Cor pulmonale	Chronic	Hepatomegaly Cough Orthopnea Peripheral edema	See Clinical Factors	Oxygen Decreasing hematocrit	Smoking Pulmonary infection	Sleep apnea COPD Obesity Pulmonary hypertension Fibrosis Pulmonary stenosis Embolus	Increased pulmonary vascular resistance due to vascular damage
Pulmonary hypertension	Gradual	Peripheral edema Abdominal swelling Hepatic congestion Palpitation Syncope	Exercise	Rest	Exercise	Repeated episodes of pulmonary embolism Primary or secondary cause Associated with right-sided heart failure Atrial septal defect	Increased pulmonary vascular resistance

continued

Table F-32. Pulmonary Causes of Dyspnea (Continued)

Subset Diagnosis	Onset	Associated Symptoms	Precipitating Factors	Relieving Factors	Aggravating Factors	Clinical Factors	Pathophysiology
Pulmonary emboli	Sudden	Cyanosis Hemoptysis Palpitation Pleuritic chest pain Shallow, rapid breathing Dizziness/ syncope	Long period of sitting Trauma CHF Thrombo- phlebitis Pregnancy	Heparin Oxygen Warfarin during follow-up	Lack of immediate treatment	Associated with right-sided heart failure Higher risk with history of cardiomyopathy, atrial fibrillation, stroke, heart valve	Vascular occlusion Hypoxemia
Pleural effusion	Gradual	Sharp chest pain	See Clinical Factors	Shallow inspiration Thoracentesis	Deep inspiration	CHF Cirrhosis Pulmonary infection Metastatic disease Nephrotic syndrome	Inflammation of parietal pleura Increased end-diastolic pressure
Pneumothorax	Sudden	Pleuritic chest pain	Chest wall injury Surgery	Oxygen Sit upright Thoracentesis	Lack of immediate treatment	Usually younger adult Associated with COPD	Rupture of pleural lining
Chest wall injury	Sudden	Signs of trauma Point tenderness	Accident or surgery	Medications	Lack of immediate treatment Deep breath	Severe trauma Broken ribs	Related to injury
Restrictive lung disease	Chronic	Fatigue	Asbestos Exposure Infection Tuberculosis	Oxygen therapy	Progression of disease Allergens Infection Environmental pollution	Paralysis of respiratory muscles Kyphosis Obesity Abdominal distention	General alveolar hypoventilation

ARDS = adult respiratory distress syndrome.

Table F-33. Cardiovascular Causes of Syncope

Diagnosis	Etiology	Associated Symptoms	Precipitating Factors	Relieving Factors	Aggravating Factors	Clinical Factors	Pathophysiology
Arrhythmias							
Carotid sinus sensitivity	Hypersensitivity of vagal response from stimulation of carotid sinus baroreceptor	Dizziness Bradycardia Mild hypotension	Tight collar Neck turning Direct manual pressure to carotids Shaving	Remove pressure causing autonomic stimulation	Continued massage or pressure	Atherosclerosis Male Elderly	Increased vagal response causing drop in heart rate and BP
Sudden death, ventricular tachycardia	Valve disease Drugs Myocardial disease Ischemia	Pale Pulseless	*Not* positional	Cardioversion, chemical or electrical	Medication Abnormal electrolytes	Antiarrhythmic drugs Cardiomyopathy Drugs	Isolated areas of myocardium Re-entry
Bradycardia, heart block	Conduction system disease	Hyperemia No premonitory symptoms	*Not* positional Arrhythmia	Normal heart rate	Medication Abnormal electrolytes	CAD Cardiomyopathy Elderly Rapid recovery	Degeneration of conduction system Cerebral ischemia
Other							
Valvular heart disease	Aortic stenosis IHSS Mitral stenosis	Atrial and/or ventricular arrhythmias Chest pain Dyspnea	Exercise	Stop exertion	Overexertion	Murmur	Decreased arterial pressure with CO limited vasodilation Decreased cerebral perfusion

continued

378 F. Differential Diagnosis in the ADVIsE Approach

Table F-33. Cardiovascular Causes of Syncope (Continued)

Diagnosis	Etiology	Associated Symptoms	Precipitating Factors	Relieving Factors	Aggravating Factors	Clinical Factors	Pathophysiology
Other (cont.)							
Vasovagal faint (common faint)	None Cerebrovascular disease Anemia Drugs Bed rest Sight of blood or injury	Blurry vision Pallor Sweating Nausea Bradycardia Hypotension	Heat Hunger Emotions Fatigue Venipuncture	Supine position Raise legs	Recent blood loss Quick return to upright position	Young individuals Most common cause of syncope Lingering weakness	Vagal inhibition Autonomic overactivity Decreased peripheral vascular resistance
Orthostatic hypotension	Autonomic deficiency Neuropathy CNS disease	No sweating No nausea Dizziness	Erect posture	Gradually increase periods of activity Elastic stockings	Long periods of bed rest Excess medications	No increased heart rate Decreased BP with standing Elderly	Limited hemodynamic compensation due to autonomic factors

Hypovolemia due to dehydration or blood loss usually is easily recognized by clinical history and laboratory tests. IHSS = idiopathic hypertrophic subaortic stenosis; CAD = coronary artery disease; CO = cardiac output.

Table F-34. Pulmonary Causes of Syncope

Diagnosis	Etiology	Associated Symptoms	Precipitating Factors	Relieving Factors	Aggravating Factors	Clinical Factors	Pathophysiology
Pulmonary stenosis	Congenital legion	Chest pain Palpitations Fluid retention Dyspnea	Usually congenital	Surgery depending on gradient	Exertion	Associated with RV hypertrophy	Reduced lung perfusion due to stenosis
Primary pulmonary hypertension	Chronic embolization COPD	Tachypnea Dyspnea Fatigue Chest pain	Exercise	Nitrates Anticoagulants	Exercise	Associated with RV hypertrophy or dilation	Reduced cardiac output
Severe coughing (posttussive) syncope	Increased intrathoracic pressure decreases venous return	Dizziness	Vigorous coughing Bronchial irritation Atmospheric conditions Postnasal drip	Treatment of cough Smoking cessation	Smoke Allergens Irritants	Middle-aged male COPD Smoker Alcohol use	Decreased cerebral perfusion Decreased venous return
Hyperventilation	Neurogenic	Smothering Tight chest Suffocation Panic attack Numbness of extremities	Anxiety	Rebreathe CO_2 ("brown bag") Anxiety relieved	Helplessness	Can last 30 min	Decreased cerebral blood flow and alkalosis due to hypocapnia
Hypoxia	Anemia Lowered atmospheric pressure	Visual disturbances Headache Breathlessness Cyanosis Tachycardia	High altitude (<10,000 ft)	Go to lower altitude	Remaining at high altitude Exertion	Earlier symptoms if anemic, or if pulmonary and cerebrovascular disease present	Decreased oxygen saturation and pressure

RV = right ventricle.

Table F-35.   Neurologic Causes of Syncope

Diagnosis	Etiology	Associated Symptoms	Precipitating Factors	Relieving Factors	Aggravating Factors	Clinical Factors	Pathophysiology
Seizures	Infection Head injury Alcohol use Hepatic failure Uremia Congenital	Postictal drowsiness Tonic-clonic movement Incontinence Preceded by aura No decreased BP	Metabolic Meningitis Encephalitis Head trauma Sleep deprivation Drugs Noncompliance Alcohol withdrawal Tumor	Self-resolved Antiseizure medications	Alcohol Noncompliance with regimen Electrolyte disorders	History of epilepsy Alcohol use General vs focal type	Cerebral arrhythmia Neuroleptic discharge
Transient ischemic attack	Atherosclerosis Cerebral or carotid Vascular disease Inflammatory disorder	Hemiparesis Dysarthria Visual disturbance Paresthesias	Emboli Thrombus	Anticoagulation Carotid artery surgery	Carotid stenosis	Carotid bruit Lasts 5–10 min.	Cerebral ischemia Carotid stenosis vs vertebral basilar insufficiency
Cerebrovascular accident	Cerebral infarction or hemorrhage	Hemiparesis Dysarthria Weakness Aphasia	Thrombus Hemorrhage Emboli High BP	Anticoagulation Carotid artery surgery	Elevated INR Congenital vascular abnormalities	Increased risk with high BP, atrial fibrillation and hyper-coagulation states	Cerebral ischemia or infarction
Vertigo	Viral infection Inner ear tumor or disorder Meniere's disease CNS disease	Sensation of movement Loss of balance Normal heart rate and BP Tinnitus	Infection Systemic illness	Self-limited Antihistamines Anticholinergic agent Phenothiazines	Sudden rapid head movement	Associated with nystagmus	Vestibular disease

Index

Note: Page numbers followed by *f* indicate figures; those followed by *t* indicate tables.